THE AYURVEDIC GUIDE
TO
DIET & WEIGHT LOSS

THE SATTVA PROGRAM

SCOTT GERSON, M.D.

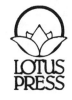

LOTUS PRESS

Twin Lakes, WI

DISCLAIMER
This book is not intended to treat, diagnose or prescribe. The information contained herein is in no way to be considered a substitute for your own good common sense, or as a substitute for a consultation with a duly licensed health care professional.

First Edition, 2002
Printed in the United States of America

LIBRARY OF CONGRESS CATALOGING-IN-PUBLICATION DATA
Gerson, Scott
The Ayurvedic Guide to Diet & Weight Loss, The Sattva Program
ISBN: 0-910261-29-6
1. Subject   I. Title
Library of Congress Control Number: 2001135593

Cover, page design and layout: Kerry P. Hopper, KPComm

Published By:
Lotus Press
P.O. Box 325
Twin Lakes, Wisconsin 53181
Web: www.lotuspress.com
E-mail: lotuspress@lotuspress.com
(800) 824-6396

TABLE OF CONTENTS

PART I

    The Five Basic Elements: The Pancha Mahabhutas

    Energies Which Create Your Ayurvedic Constitutional Type
    The Body Energies: The Three Doshas
    The Mental Energies: The Three Gunas

        The Seven Body Tissues: The Sapta Dhatus
        The Three Waste Products: Malas
        The Digestive Fire: Agni

PART II

        Homeostasis
        Digestion and Toxicity: Jathagni and Ama
        Pathogenesis of Obesity: The Six Stages of
          Any Disease
        The Three Doshas and Their Gunas
        Diets Don't Work

Overview

The Ayurvedic Approach to Weight Loss: The *Sattva Program*

The Intelligent Holistic Program To Lose Weight Effortlessly in Just Weeks

O h my God! Is this yet *another* book on weight loss? Could there possibly be anything new left to say?

Not only new, but also louder. I have always regarded myself as a type of "step-up transformer" whose simple role is to amplify the wisdom of a still robust ancient Eastern tradition which here in the West has been reduced to an almost inaudible whisper. This book succinctly integrates an authentic Indian medical tradition, Ayurveda, with current modern research on nutrition and weight loss to create a message that will undoubtedly deliver true benefit to all that read it. I know this to be true because I have applied it to hundreds of my own patients over the past fifteen years and have seen its efficacy. This program of weight control has been proven effective by literally hundreds of thousands (without exaggeration) of individuals who have followed these uncomplicated principles for several thousand years. More recently, over the years I have documented that in addition to weight loss, the other benefits of this lifestyle program include lower LDL-cholesterol, improved LDL-cholesterol/HDL-cholesterol ratio, lower serum triglycerides, more efficient glucose metabolism, more vitality, greater stamina, normal libido and improved general health.

The main feature of *The Sattva Program*® is that not all individuals require the same regimen in order to lose and maintain their weight. Each of us has a unique combination of biological, physiological and emotional components that makes our path to balance and health equally singular. To help us identify the specific characteristics of our own physiology, Ayurvedic Medicine, the holistic health system practiced in India, provides us with remarkably precise descriptions of the *three body types* and their variations. This knowledge gives us the understanding of the specific qualities and needs of our own bodies.

As the only physician in North America who has also been fully and formally trained in Ayurvedic medicine, I find myself in a unique position in this country. First and foremost, I am an internist and someone who keeps abreast of the most recent clinical research relating to diet and health. For example, how many physicians out there are aware of a study published in December, 1998 in *The Journal Of Applied Nutrition* which documented the benefits of whole grain cereal breakfasts in reducing heart disease? For me this kind of information is not only interesting and relevant to my busy medical practice—it's my passion. Perhaps that is why I devote a significant amount of time to my own clinical and basic science research, conducted primarily at the National Institute Of Ayurvedic Medicine in Brewster, New York. Over the past fifteen years I have undertaken more than thirty clinical and laboratory studies which have certainly added—albeit modestly— to the solid bedrock foundation of knowledge which is slowly accruing to support alternative medicine therapies. I am interested in leaving behind for our children at least a few bits of information that is true, that is scientifically supported, and that can be used in a safe and effective manner.

The program described in this book succeeds where others fail. Whether it's the "low-fat, high carbohydrate" or the "high-protein, low carbohydrate" or some other strategy of the moment, they all fail to recognize one thing: the uniqueness of each individual's metabolism and rhythms. Ayurveda recognizes three distinct types of individuals each with different requirements. *The Sattva Program*® teaches us to live in accord with our own unique biological patterns instead of trying to apply one system of weight loss to every-one. Given the obvious differences in our physical appearances, genetic backgrounds, and our physiological set-ups, it is not even logical that one single program of weight maintenance could apply to everybody. The fact is, the strategy that suits *me* would possibly have you fighting against *your* distinct rhythms. The only possible outcome is emotional stress, physical discomfort, and eventual failure that comes from all of these "this-will-work-for-everyone" cookie-cutter weight-loss programs.

This book starts out by explaining, with the help of clear and simple tables and charts, the basic concepts upon which this important medical system is based. Reading these ideas makes so much sense even to the uninitiated. Why? Because Ayurvedic Medicine is rooted in observational truth. This is not some novel and imaginative system based on "blood types" or some other nonsense; it is a medical system with over three thousand years of verification and elimination of what is ineffective or unsafe.

After learning the basic principles of Ayurvedic medicine, you are provided with a comprehensive but fun and simple questionnaire to fill out. This will give you accurate information about your *constitutional type*—an important component of using the program. The program, which is called The Sattva Program, alludes to *sattva*, a Sanskrit word meaning balance or harmony. The main idea is to promote balance in the physiology of every individual through measures that take into account his/her unique physical characteristics, mental tendencies, or in other words, his/her Ayurvedic constitutional type.

Armed with the knowledge of your constitutional type, the book takes you on an exploration of the concept of obesity in Ayurveda and a discussion of human energy metabolism. We will describe the six stages of obesity—a concept unique to Ayurveda and uncannily accurate. This leads to a section on homeostasis—another of the central ideas in this program. This is the notion of your body achieving balance and optimum function from a regimen of foods, herbs, activities, etc. which are unique for you. We will also discuss the concepts of Agni—the digestive fire and how to promote and maintain it, and Ama—digestive toxins and how to eliminate them.

The next section of the book gets to more practical information. This includes specific dietary information and herbal information for each constitutional type, as well as additional valuable lifestyle information. I have also provided some clear, honest, and succinct information on subjects covered in confusing ways in other books: insulin and glucagon, complex vs. simple carbohydrates, low-fat vs. high-fat, high protein vs. high carbohydrate, etc.

Having reviewed what is clearly the wrong approach to weight loss, I then proceed to outline *The Sattva Program*®. I list specific foods in a very complete Food List. I then go on to what most will consider the core of the book—the dietary recommendations for each specific constitutional type. Here you will find not only food recommendations, but also specific herbal preparations, exercises, and mind-body approaches for each type.

After a discussion on the benefits of a whole foods vegetarian diet I have provided an extensive chapter of recipes. I have personally collected most of these delicious recipes from the wives of many of my professors of Ayurveda and colleagues in India. I have modified them to meet dietary needs in this country. They are truly delicious and effective in rapidly reducing weight.

I conclude with a chapter on Panchakarma therapies, which are the famous and luxurious spa therapies of Ayurveda including deep oil massage with warm herbalized oils, mud treatments, steam baths, enemas, laxative therapies, nasal oil therapies, and many other procedures designed to promote detoxification, weight loss, and rejuvenation. I conclude with an Appendix reviewing recent medical research on obesity to balance the Ayurvedic presentation with a dose of modern science. That represents, after all, who I am.

I urge you to utilize the information and practical approaches of *The Sattva Program*® without reservation because in the fifteen years of treating patients with it I have never had a patient who has not lost weight and improved their well being. Almost all patients reach their ideal weights. This program is especially for individuals who have tried other systems of weight loss and have been disappointed with the results. By focusing on achieving balance in life, a balance that is unique for *you*, you will not only see striking weight loss results, but also experience life-changing benefits throughout all aspects of your mind and body.

CHAPTER 1.

INSPIRATION FOR THIS BOOK

*T*he inspiration for writing *The Ayurvedic Guide to Diet & Weight Loss: The Sattva Program* arose from my work and study as a physician for the past twenty years in the field of Ayurvedic Medicine. During the time in the 1970's when I was engaged full-time in the study of Ayurveda in some of India's most prestigious institutions, I became intensely interested in the subject of nutritional healing—the use of specific foods to heal various diseases. At that time this was a subject that was completely unrecognized in the western medical establishment. Today it still is in its infancy and receives far less attention than it merits.

In Ayurvedic Medicine as practiced in India, it is common to prescribe food regimens as medicine. In fact, in colleges of Ayurveda this is given the name Kitchen Pharmacy and is a very important facet of both ancient and modern Ayurveda. I initially was fascinated by how certain simple dietary modifications could often stimulate the detoxification and revitalization of an individual without specialized medicines or therapies.

In fact, for just about every disease condition of the human body or mind, Ayurveda has established effective means of treatment with foods. Sometimes conditions can be addressed with diet as the chief treatment; sometimes it is one of several components of the treatment.

I have witnessed hundreds of examples. One such example is a condition known in ancient India as "Amlapitta", or gastritis. This is a condition caused by the excessive formation of acid in the stomach, which creates a burning sensation in the upper abdominal, chest, and throat regions. Among the many effective Ayurvedic recommendations for the cure of this condition are the following dietary measures:

Food articles to favor: Basmati rice, barley, wheat, red phaseolus bean, mung dal (a common legume), milk, bitter gourd, ripe banana, pomegranate, patola (a variety of small cucumber), vetasasuga (root of the cane plant commonly used as a vegetable), cabbage, garlic, and licorice root.

Food articles to reduce: Heavy and sour foods, newly harvested cereals, sesame seeds, black beans, excessive oil, goat's milk, wine, and tea.

Ayurvedic physicians have always observed profound improvements in health when their patients were able to make appropriate dietary changes. In 1988, for the first time in our history, the Surgeon General of the United States acknowledged the deficiencies in the typical American diet and called for change. He stated that two-thirds of all deaths in the nation are directly influenced by poor diet and that poor eating habits play a large role in our nation's largest killers: coronary heart disease, stroke, atherosclerosis, diabetes, and cancer. In western industrialized nations, and increasingly throughout the world, it is becoming easier and easier to become overweight and to stay that way! In contrast to the effort required to obtain sufficient amounts of food to sustain us before the industrial revolution, today people in many parts of the world can find an abundance of food within a few blocks walking distance. Much of these foods are highly processed and high in fat and the media is there to constantly remind you to go out and get them. To compound the problem, more of us than ever before have sedentary jobs and work longer and longer hours. We must often make the distressing choice in our shrinking leisure time whether to engage in physical activity or to just recuperate from the demands of the work week. It is no surprise, therefore, that recent estimates suggest that 1 in 2 adults, or about 80 million people, in the United States are overweight or obese.

In my years as a primary care physician integrating the wisdom of Ayurveda with that of conventional medicine, I have evolved an understanding of how to select wholesome foods to promote weight loss and maintenance. The selection of which foods to eat is not arbitrary. Foods act according to their various energetic attributes. The effects of foods on the human biology are the same categories of effects of herbs and medicines, however foods are generally less potent, less specific, and require a longer time to act. Thus we know of foods which are hypolipidemic (fat reducing), antacid, tranquilizing, anticarcinogenic, laxative, antidepressant, etc.

As I have used these principles first on myself and my family and then on hundreds of patients, I have witnessed positive results which not only include weight loss, but also improvement and often cure of other health conditions including high cholesterol, osteoarthritis, high blood pressure, diabetes, hypoglycemia, chronic fatigue syndrome, fibromyalgia, depression, asthma, constipation, irritable bowel syndrome, allergies and many other co-existing problems. In addition, the results are generally quick, unambiguous and long-lasting. Over the years, I have continued to refine and modernize the program, especially by expanding the original food choices. By and large, the original wisdom of the ancient Indian physicians has been left intact and unmodified.

CHAPTER 2.

THE FUNDAMENTAL PRINCIPLES OF AYURVEDA

*A*yurvedic Medicine has its origins shrouded in the mists of time and is one of the most ancient organized systems of medicine in the world. Its written knowledge dates back to approximately 1500 BC to an Indian historical period known as the Vedic Period, at which time fragments of medical information were recorded in ancient scriptures known as the *Rigveda* and the *Atharvaveda*. Over the next millennium, up to the dawning of Christianity, Ayurvedic Medicine flourished in what has become known as its classical age. It was during this time that Ayurveda evolved into a highly organized medical science with specialized methods of diagnosis and treatment. There is also archeological evidence that Ayurvedic principles may have spread beyond the borders of India during this classical age where it influenced the medical traditions of eastern Asia, Persia, and Greece. Ayurveda continued to flourish in India until well into the Medieval Period, when due to several centuries of political and military upheaval, it experienced a dramatic decline. Today, Ayurvedic medical thought is preserved primarily in two sets of original authentic textbooks, known as the Major and Minor, respectively. Each set consists of three books:

The Major Set:
The Charaka Saṁhitā (600 B.C.)
The Suśruta Saṁhitā (500 B.C.)
The Aṣṭāṅga Hṛdaya and Saṁgraha of Vagbhata (500 A.D.)

The Minor Set:
Madhava Nidānā (900 A.D.)
Sarngadhara Saṁhitā (1300 A.D.)
Bhavaprakasha (1600 AD)

All of these original texts were written in the Sanskrit language and provide us with great detail regarding the Ayurvedic approach to maintaining health and treating disease.

9

Over the last century, Ayurvedic Medicine has experienced a rebirth and has continued to evolve its holistic approach to health in accordance with the scientific advances of the day. Classically, Ayurvedic Medicine was conceptualized and practiced as eight major clinical subspecialties of medicine in addition to numerous adjunctive specialties. The eight major subspecialties continue to be taught today and they include:

1. Internal Medicine
2. General Surgery
3. Otorhinolaryngology
4. Pediatrics and Obstetric/Gynecology
5. Psychiatry
6. Toxicology
7. Nutrition, Detoxification and Rejuvenation
8. Fertility and Virility

Another feature of Ayurvedic writing that deserves mention is the way in which the authors of these ancient texts described diseases. For every condition there is information regarding: definition, etiology (causes), prodrome (earliest signs), clinical symptoms, pathophysiology (disease process), prognosis (forecast), principles of management, medicines, diet, lifestyle recommendations, and even etymology (name derivation). This approach is strikingly similar to that of modern medicine.

Today, there are approximately 100 Ayurvedic medical colleges in India, which is the only place to obtain an authentic and complete education in this discipline. The majority of the colleges are sponsored by the Central Government of India; the remainder are private institutions. All of the programs are four to five years in duration and require passing a standardized examination in order to receive the Bachelor in Ayurvedic Medicine and Surgery (B.A.M.S.) degree. Other respected degrees, which indicate accredited training in Ayurvedic Medicine, are the Fellowship degrees, Masters of Philosophy in Ayurveda (M.Phil., Ay.), and the Doctor of Philosophy in Ayurveda (Ph.D., Ay.). There are currently several institutions of Ayurvedic medical training *outside* of India, which are in various stages of assessment for accreditation by the Central Government of India including those in the United Kingdom,

Italy, Australia, and the United States. Further information on accreditation and regulatory matters can be obtained from the National Institute of Ayurvedic Medicine (Brewster, New York 845-278-8700).

Current Perspective of Ayurveda in Modern Medicine

Today Ayurveda does not enjoy the same status as it did in the pre-Christian era. Part of the reason for this was the emergence of a great philosophical and scientific renaissance in the early part of the nineteenth century. At that time, Cartesian scientific materialism began to permeate all facets of human thought and activity. Thus physicians and scientists of the day developed methods for reducing complex observations into their component parts and began analyzing each in isolation. Thus began the search, which continues today, for *single* causes of diseases and *single* molecules to combat them. Modern medicine had become a reductionist science and lost the art of understanding the patient as a whole. Observations, as astute as they might be, and intuitions, born of years of experience, became meaningless unless validated by scientific method and statistical analysis. This led to losing sight of the forest while studying the individual trees.

Despite this need in the medical community for experimental analysis, the last three decades have witnessed a strong revival in awareness about traditional systems of medicine throughout the world. There are diverse reasons for this trend but prominent among them is the dissatisfaction on the part of both the modern physician and patient with the conventional allopathic approach. Undeniably, synthetic chemical drugs have given mankind the arsenal to combat many more diseases than in the past: chemotherapy's, antibiotics, corticosteroids, anti-arrhythmic, and anti-depressants to name a few. However the high incidence of side effects associated with these drugs and the subsequent prescription of additional drugs to manage those effects, have added tremendously to the risk and cost of the modern approach to treating disease. In addition, people are becoming skeptical about the reductionist approach of treating the symptom of a disease or treating a "laboratory result" discovered by an automated and expensive computerized analytical machine. More and more people are turning to Ayurveda as a system of health care which emphasizes self-healing, safe and natural methods, and a view of each individual as a unique whole. However, the Ayurvedic physician is aware of the limitations of this approach. While often effective for chronic, recurrent conditions, metabolic disorders, and degenerative diseases where modern medicine has little to offer except symptomatic treatment, Ayurveda is not as effective for acute infections, injuries, or other life-threatening conditions.

Some efforts have been made to scientifically validate Ayurvedic therapies. These pioneering research efforts, however, have centered around isolating the active components in various Ayurvedic herbal medicines. Table 1 summarizes some of the fruits of that research.

TABLE 1.
AYURVEDIC AND OTHER PLANT-DERIVED MODERN MEDICINES

Modern Drug	Plant Source
Atropine	*Hyoscamus niger*
Codeine	*Paperver somniferum*
Colchicine	*Colchinum actmnale*
Cromyln	*Amni visnaga*
Digitoxin	*Digitalis purpurea*
Digoxin	*Digitalis lanata*
Emetine	*Cephaelis spp.*
Hyoscamine	*Hyoscamus niger*
Pilocarpine	*Pilocarpus jaborandi*
Quinidine	*Chinchona spp.*
Reserpine	*Rauwolfia serpentina*
Vinblastine	*Vinca rosea*
Vincristine	*Vinca rosea*
Taxol	*Taxus brevifolia*

Considerable research work is currently underway on different aspects of Ayurvedic medicinal plants. Phytochemists are reporting novel organic structures in plants and physiologists are exploring their proposed mechanisms of action. Guggulipid, a hypocholesterolemic (cholesterol-reducing) agent, is an important example of the work of Indian scientists at the Central Drug Research Institute (CDRI) which began systematically screening Ayurvedic plants for biological activity in 1964.

Unfortunately, due to the current resurgence of scientific research into the clinical efficacy of Ayurvedic medicinal plants, the public perception of what the Ayurvedic medicine system is has become distorted. Herbal medicines, although important, are not the heart and soul of this medical system. Instead it emphasizes a wholesome style of life which encompasses adherence to immutable laws of nature. To be effective, besides taking the prescribed herbal remedies, one must understand and apply the Ayurvedic principles of living in its totality.

BASIC PRINCIPLES OF AYURVEDA

Ayurveda is a holistic medical science that provides a unique conceptual framework for understanding the nature of disease and offers a variety of treatment modalities to promote recuperation. The concepts of health and disease are based on several fundamental concepts relating to the structure of human beings.

As Above, So Below

Ayurveda is a system of human health care that is derived from observations about the immutable universal laws of nature. One of its most defining concepts is that of *loka-puruṣa-samya* or the connection between the individual and the universe (literally: *loka* = universe, *puruṣa* = individual, *samya* = balance). According to Ayurveda, the individual is a microcosm of nature and falls under the same laws. Both man and the universe are composed of five basic elements, or *pancha* (5) *mahabhutas*:

The Five Basic Elements (Pancha Mahabhutas)

Space	(Akāśa)
Air	(Vayu)
Fire	(Teja)
Water	(Jala)
Earth	(Pṛithivi)

These five elements comprise a dynamic *continuum of energy* which ranges from the most solid, dense form (earth element) to the subtlest vibration (space element). *Earth element* is the grossest form of energy, which is compact and has smell, taste, form, sensation, and sound. When transformed into a higher vibration, earth element becomes *water element*. It loses its compactness and solidity and becomes liquid; it loses the quality of taste but still retains the qualities of form (adapting to that of its container), sensation, and sound. As the energy level increases further along this continuum, movement and friction within the substance produces heat and light; liquidity disappears as does taste, leaving only form, sensation and sound. This is *fire element*. Increasing movement and friction dissolve the quality of form, leaving only sensation and sound as we reach the realm of the *air element*. Ultimately, as energy vibrates at its highest and most subtle level, we reach the *space element*, beyond the scope of sensation and form, where only sound exists. At this level of energy, individual particles of substance have reached a vibration that is beyond cohesive forms of matter.

There is a constant interrelationship between the individual and the universe and a constant co-exchange of elements in order to maintain a normal and balanced state (homeostasis). Furthermore, this exchange of materials reflects the principle of *sāmānya-viśeṣa* or "similar-dissimilar". This principle reflects the observation that matter of a specific nature increases when acted upon by a substance of a similar composition and will decrease with addition of substances of dissimilar compositions. This exchange between individual and nature proceeds in an appropriate and mutually beneficial manner as we eat, drink, breath, eliminate wastes, and perform our activities of life. Health is maintained provided this interaction is harmonious; when the harmony is disrupted disease can arise. The primary object of treatment is to re-establish homeostasis of the five elements within the individual and between the individual and the environment.

Ancient Indian physicians have always maintained that there is a fundamental connection between the individual, the planetary, and the universal realms. Examples of these connections are obvious to us all: the wind and the breath; the earth and the body; the moon and the oceans, the sun and the phenomenon of vision. They felt we could discover universal patterns that would also reveal the nature of the universe by exploring and decoding the energies and forces of our own bodies.

Ayurveda understands life to require four requisite dimensions that occur together in space and time: physical body, mind, five senses, and consciousness. Thus every human being is conceived of as a complete psycho-physiological-spiritual aggregate that is in a dynamic and constant interrelationship with the universe. The five elements of Ayurvedic doctrine represent nothing less than a primitive, yet complete, energetic theory of physics, which incorporates the five essential attributes of matter (Table 2):

TABLE 2.
THE FIVE ELEMENTS AND MODERN PHYSICS

Space	represents the Unified Field
Air	represents Motion and Acceleration
Fire	represents Radiant Energy and Heat
Water	represents Cohesive Forces and Gravity
Earth	represents Mass

The Three Doṣas

In living systems, the five elements become organized into three fundamental biological energies known as the *three doṣas* (pronounced "doshas") or *tridoṣa*. Their names are **Vata, Pitta, and Kapha.**

The elemental composition of the three doshas is depicted in Table 3. Vata dosha comes from space and air, Pitta dosha from fire and water; and Kapha dosha from water and earth. Vata, Pitta, and Kapha result from the combination of the five elements. All living cells, tissues, organs, and organisms consist of all three of the doshas. In fact, life itself has the minimum requirement of at least one unit each of Vata, Pitta, and Kapha.

TABLE 3.
Elemental Composition of the Three Doṣas

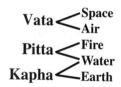

Vata—which governs motion and activity—is said to be at the basis of all movement in the physiology. It controls functions such as blood circulation and the expansion and contraction of the lungs and heart; intestinal peristalsis and elimination; activities of the nervous system; the contractile process in muscle; ionic transport across membranes (such as the sodium pump); cell division; and unwinding and pairing of DNA during the processes of transcription and replication. Vata energy is of prime importance in all movements at all levels of structure.

Pitta governs bodily functions concerned with heat and metabolism, and directs all biochemical reactions and the processes of energy exchange. For example, it regulates digestion, the secretions of the exocrine glands and the endocrine hormones, and intracellular metabolic pathways such as glycolysis (glucose metabolism), the tricarboxylic acid cycle (conversion of citric acid to energy), ATP metabolism (the body's principle source of energy), and the respiratory chain.

Kapha governs the structure and cohesion of the organism. It is responsible for physical and biological strength, natural tissue resistance, and proper body structure. Microscopically, it is related to anatomic connections in the cell, such as the intracellular matrix, cell membrane, cellular receptors, and synapses. It is the energetic principle that holds things together, gives us substance, and connects us to the intelligence of Nature.

In the Ayurvedic view, the human being consists of a physical body with mass and density (*Kapha*) serving as the substratum for a milieu of intricate chemical processes (*Pitta*), connected by a subtle energetic force of movement and motion (*Vata*). The three doshas dynamically co-exist in a genetically determined proportion for each individual and function in a harmonious manner for the ultimate benefit of the whole organism. The qualities of the three doshas can be perceived at the gross level of the physical body as a whole (e.g. nervousness or dryness = *Vata;* febrile or inflammatory conditions = *Pitta;* congestion or lethargy = *Kapha*) as well as at the cellular, molecule and atomic levels.

Thus, a neuron in the Central Nervous System (CNS) might have a higher proportion of Vata energy than the other two doshas, while a hydrochloric acid-producing gland in the stomach would be predominantly Pitta, and a skeletal muscle cell relatively more Kapha. Similarly, the mass-possessing protons and neutrons of an atom represent Kapha energy, the electrons whipping around in shells represent Vata energy, and the potentially explosive forces within the atom is the Pitta energy.

We Are All Unique

As an Ayurvedic physician, I have always been aware of the heterogeneity (varied), complexity, and idiosyncrasy of individual health habits. All of us are so unique in the patterns we've formed in consuming foods, imbibing liquids, exercising our bodies, using herbs, prescription medications, and vitamins, getting rest and relaxation, and just about every other facet of human existence. We subtly but inexorably develop our own personal preferences and aversions. Recognizing these differences among people is vitally important to treating their illnesses and correcting their imbalances. In fact one of the most outstanding differences I've found between modern Western medicine and Ayurvedic medicine is Western medicine's exclusive preoccupation with categorizing differences among the myriad of human diseases, while almost completely failing to recognize the importance of unique differences and similarities among individual human beings. Most physicians can tell you about the six different types of Herpes virus infections or the four different categories of kidney stones. But the person in whom these stones are forming is a complex miniature universe of unique emotional energies, mental energies, memories, hormonal shifts, nervous impulses, and metabolic processes occurring at individually determined rates and according to unique rhythms. How successful the prescribed therapy for those kidney stones will be could be profoundly affected by how that individual will respond to the weather that week, a brand new love relationship, being criticized by the boss, attending a symphony performance or even a funeral. All of these events will generate an energetic backdrop that arises from within. This book focuses on creating necessary changes in these inner energetic patterns. As with all elements of life, people respond differently to food both physiologically and psychologically. The extraordinary approach of Ayurveda is that it requires that every aspect of a successful weight control program must be tailored to the constitution of each unique individual.

How do preferences and aversions develop? How do preferences evolve into needs and aversions magnify into repugnance. When do needs become addictions? Why do some people become addicted to certain behaviors while other people are capable of stopping at will?

We now know that our early environment, personality development, upbringing, and education influence our preferences and aversions to some extent. However, in exploring these observations of individual tendencies over the course of the past twenty years, I have witnessed another factor far more powerful than acquired circumstances, social environment, or parental models that create our deeply unique psychophysiological patterns. That factor is what is known as each individual's unique *constitutional type*.

What Is "Constitution?"

Our constitutional type is determined by the combination and proportion of three fundamental biological energies that regulate our physiological functions and three fundamental psychospiritual energies that determine our mental and emotional nature. Although Western conventional medicine has no terminology to describe these energies in a cogent manner, they are nevertheless quite familiar and real to us all. Most of us have noticed that on a slightly cool and breezy day some people are already dressed in heavier jackets, hats, scarves, and even gloves while others are comfortably wearing tee-shirts. Similarly while a cup of coffee may make some people nervous and shaky, others are just pleasantly more alert, and still others are completely unaffected. And have you ever experienced a situation where both you and a friend hear a joke that you find witty and hysterically funny while your friend finds it infantile and dumb? What is the cause of all this diversity? Can it be measured with sophisticated blood tests, seen under the electron microscope or revealed with a CAT scan? The answer is of course, no. But these differences among people are nonetheless undeniable and observable. In Ayurvedic Medicine, an elegant and coherent terminology exists to describe the energies that constitute an individual's physiology and psychology. We will first discuss in more detail the set of energies that operate within the physiology—the physical aspect of human beings. As we have already mentioned, these are called the three *doshas*. Then we will describe another important set of energies that operate in the psychology—our mental aspect. They are known as the three *gunas*.

CHAPTER 2. THE FUNDAMENTAL PRINCIPALS OF AYURVEDA

Energies Which Create Your Ayurvedic Constitutional Type

A. The Three Doshas: Energies of the Body

The physiological energies are called the *Doshas,* which are three in number. As a reminder, the names and general meanings of the three doshas are:

1) **Vata**—the energy of all movements in the physiology
2) **Pitta**—the energy of digestion, heat, and transformation in the physiology
3) **Kapha**—the energy of strength, cohesion, and stability in the physiology

All human beings have all three of these vital energies, but it is the *proportion* in which they occur that determines one's constitutional type. This is important information because anything that you do with the intention of losing weight must be undertaken with a clear understanding of your specific constitutional type in mind and all the specific nuances and requirements that arise from it. This gives us an immediate understanding of which foods are best for us, what types of exercise we should do and for how long, which herbs will help promote weight loss, and how to maintain a balanced mind and body throughout our entire lives.

The proportion of the three doshas that determines your constitutional type also determines your biochemical idiosyncrasies, metabolic patterns, disease disposition, and every innate physiological tendency that has been coded into your specific mind/body complex. Knowing your Ayurvedic Constitutional Type will guide you towards practical, simple measures that will reduce and maintain your body weight as well as your general health. Every time you eat a specific food—say an apple—a specific impulse of communication is created in your physiology. This communication is partially determined by the qualities of the specific food (one apple contains 80 kcal of energy, 0.3 g protein, 21 g carbohydrates, 2.0 g fiber, 4.5 mg calcium, 12 mcg folic acid, 135 IU Vitamin A, etc.) and partially by the unique characteristics of your own mind and body. In my physiology that apple, with its Vitamin A content, could stimulate the retinal epithelium into repair of a minor lesion; in you the same apple could stimulate red blood cell synthesis in the bone marrow (folic acid) or a gentle laxative effect (fiber). It all depends on how your mind/body *interprets* that apple in terms of its specific needs.

In simple language, we can accurately say that the common language between an apple and the human physiology that permits information to flow is the *doshas*. The individual has a specific doshic make-up and the apple also has a specific doshic make-up. This is what determines what effect the apple will have when it interacts with a specific person. Besides regulating the limitless rhythms and processes that occur continuously in your mind and body, doshas are found throughout the entire scope of nature as well. The doshas are literally everywhere—in plants, pets, mountains, lakes, the climate, the seasons, and of course in foods. These three energetic principles connect you as an individual to the entire natural world. As we say in Ayurveda, "As above, so below" implying the connection between the microcosm and the macrocosm. Individual human beings and Nature are in perpetual contact with each other and exchange materials and energies in order to maintain stability and balance. This exchange of substances happens in a natural way as we breathe in and out, consume food and water, and excrete wastes. In essence, at the most fundamental level, what is being exchanged and balanced throughout our lives are the three doshas.

The three doshas have well-established functions and features in the human organism:

Function		Qualities
Regulates functions concerned with movement	**VATA**	Moving, quick, light, cold, dry, rough, minute
Regulates functions concerned with digestion, heat, metabolism	**PITTA**	Hot, sharp, acidic, light, unctuous
Regulates functions concerned with strength, structure, fluids	**KAPHA**	Heavy, solid, oily, slow, dull, cold, steady, soft

Vata Dosha

The term *vata* stems from a Sanskrit word vyu (vayu) which means "that which moves things;" it is sometimes translated as wind. It is composed of the elements space and air—the lightest and subtlest of the five elements. It is considered in some ways to be the most influential of the three doshas because it is the moving force behind the other two doshas, which are incapable of movement without it. Vata dosha is responsible for all the somatic activities and sensations. It is the intelligence that channels perceptions (temperature, pressure, sweetness, lightening, violin music, etc.) through the appropriate sensory organs, converts them into internal psychological events, and then orchestrates the appropriate response via the organs of action. It is responsible for all movements in the mind and body: the movement of air in and out of the lungs, the flow of blood through the circulatory system, nutrients through the alimentary tract, and thoughts through the mind. Vata promotes a healthy balance between thought and emotion and gives rise to creativity, activity and clear comprehension.

Because, among other functions, Vata regulates the nervous processes involved with movement, thoughts, emotions, eating, drinking, elimination, and our general functioning, its disturbance can often have far-reaching consequences.

Here is a table that summarizes the manifestations of a balanced or unbalanced (excessive) Vata dosha:

Effects of Vata Dosha

Effect of Balanced Vata	*Effect of Unbalanced (Excess) Vata*
Proper coordination of all body functions	Body functions impaired or disorganized.
Normal movements associated with eating	Movements for eating, digestion, and elimination, digestion, and elimination disturbed (bloating, constipation, gas)
Mental activity controlled and precise	Mental agitation, confusion; impaired memory

Effects of Vata Dosha *(Cont'd)*

Effect of Balanced Vata	*Effect of Unbalanced (Excess) Vata*
Control of the organs of perception and organs of action	Perception and action are inappropriate; senses that are dulled; responses untimely
Stimulation of digestive juices	Deficiency of the digestive juices
Desire to lead an active life; vitality, curiosity and natural interest	Loss of energy and joy for life
Normal drying of occasional mucous discharges	Persistent bodily discharges
Normal respiratory function	Shortness of breath, dry cough, disturbance in respiratory movements, hiccup
Normal sleep pattern	Insomnia, light or interrupted sleep
Excellent energy level	Non-specific fatigue, anxiety, worry, cold intolerance, depletion of Life Force

Pitta Dosha

The term *pitta* comes from the Sanskrit word pinj (pinj) meaning "to shine" (according to Sir Monier-Williams its exact entomology is a mystery). It carries the meaning of "that which digests" and is associated with the idea of being yellow-tinged or bilious. In its widest sense, Paittika digestive function includes all chemical and metabolic transformations in the body as well as processes that promote heat production (i.e. conversion of iodine to triiodotyrosine in the thyroid gland). Pitta also governs our ability to digest ideas and impressions and to therefore perceive the true nature of reality. It stimulates the intellect and creates enthusiasm and determination. Pitta is often regarded as the "fire" within the body. Think of it as the energy stored in the chemical bonds of all the organic substances that make us up: it is encoded in our hormones, enzymes, organic acids and neurotransmitters. *Charaka Samhita*, an ancient Ayurvedic text, teaches that pitta functions in digestion, heat production, providing color to the blood, vision, and skin luster.

Here is a table that summarizes the manifestations of a balanced or unbalanced (excessive) Pitta dosha:

Effects of Pitta Dosha

Effect of Balanced Pitta	*Effect of Unbalanced (Excessive) Pitta*
Strong and complete digestion	Incomplete digestion; poor differentiation between nutrients and wastes
Normal heat and thirst mechanisms	Irregular body temperature, disturbed perspiration, unregulated fluid intake
Excellent vision	Impaired vision
Good complexion; healthy facial tone	Variable, blotchy skin color, coloration inflamed; unhealthy appearance
Hair lustrous and usually slightly wavy	Hair dry; premature graying or baldness
Courageous, cheerful, focused	Irritable, anxious, driven, obsessed
Stimulated, open intellect	Dullness of reasoning faculty
Steadfast concentration on the truth; disciplined, responsible	Spiritually impoverished
Efficient assimilation of foods	Heartburn, peptic ulcer, irritable bowels,hemorrhoids, diarrhea, alcoholism

Kapha Dosha

The term kapha derives from the Sanskrit word "shlish" which means "that which holds things together; to embrace; coherent." In fact, one of the other designations for kapha appearing in some of the older literature is *shleshma*. It is the force that provides structure to everything from an individual atom or cell to the sturdy musculoskeletal frame. It gives strength, stability, and endurance—both physical and psychological—and promotes human emotions and capacities such as love, compassion, empathy, understanding, forgiveness, loyalty and patience. One very important function of Kapha dosha in the human body is that it governs immunity and resistance against disease; it's energy promotes self-healing and the ongoing processes of self-repairs of which we are largely unaware. Where Vata and Pitta effects become active in the body, Kapha acts to limit and control these two forces and prevent their excessive activity. The two elements that compose Kapha are water and earth. Together, these two prototypical elements form the fundamental protoplasm of life. Kapha imparts mind-body-spirit stability and resilience. It is the anabolic force in the body that governs the formation of neuropeptides, stomach linings, and all new cells and tissues of the body that are constantly being destroyed and re-created. Its excess is the principal cause of overweight and obesity.

Here is a table that summarizes the manifestations of balanced and unbalanced (excessive) kapha dosha:

Effects of Kapha Dosha

Effect of Balanced Kapha	Effect of Unbalanced (Excessive) Kapha
Excellent nutritional status; firm musculature, strong bones	Poor nutritional status, flabby, fatigued, "feeling old"
Adequate moisture and lubrication throughout the body	Dry; decreased mucous and saliva
Well-knit joints	Loose joints, prone to sprains
Stable, compact, and strong physique	Soft and weakened physique; obese

Effects of Kapha Dosha *(Cont'd)*

Effect of Balanced Kapha	*Effect of Unbalanced (Excessive) Kapha*
Sexual potency, strong immunity	Sexual impotency, sedentary, diminished immunity
Calm, forgiving, understanding, patient	Intolerant, insecure, jealous, rude
Strong digestion, regular appetite	Slow digestion, appetite unregulated
Physiological amounts of respiratory moisture	Excess mucous production

Each of us are constituted from all three of the doshas; they are all essential to support life. What makes us all unique is the proportion in which the doshas occur. Sometimes one dosha clearly dominates; more often two doshas combine to dominate; infrequently all three doshas can be found in equal proportion.

Here are some brief descriptions of the features and behaviors that define the three doshas in their purest manifestations. See if you can begin to recognize which type (or types) best describes you. Later in this chapter you will determine this more precisely.

VATA
Vata Characteristics

- Thin, light physique
- Walks and performs activities quickly
- Meal times and quantities tend to be irregular
- Sleep is light, interrupted; insomnia
- Memory is erratic
- Unable to sit still for very long, restless, fidgety, bites nails
- Makes rapid, choppy hand gestures when speaking
- Leaves sentences unfinished, as new thoughts fill the mind
- Tendency towards hasty decisions
- Often dissatisfied with or unable to sustain friendships
- Excitable, changeable moods

- Tires easily, tendency to do too much
- Understands new information quickly but can easily forget it

Vata Behaviors

- Has different bedtimes and mealtimes
- Digests food well at times and incompletely at others
- Experiences intense emotional states for short times, then quickly forgets
- Seeks out new experiences and loves frequent change
- Can become hungry at any time of the day or night
- Joins new organizations or careers often and with great enthusiasm but for short times
- Can be cruel at times and destructive to property

PITTA
Pitta Characteristics

- Medium physique and height tending towards slender
- Moderate endurance and strength
- Sharp onset of hunger and thirst; very strong digestion; cannot miss meals
- Tendency to perspire freely
- Tendency towards anger, frustration, and impatience
- Hair is light brown, blond, or reddish and tends to fall out prematurely
- Aversion for extremely hot weather
- Highly intelligent, good speakers, leaders in their fields
- Reddish or yellowish complexion, often with freckles or moles

Pitta Behaviors

- Stops all other activities when it is time for meals
- Punctual and strongly dislikes wasting time
- Finds oneself in positions of responsibility and group leadership
- Earns a living through his/her own personal device and effort
- Can be feared at times by others
- Can lose interest in sexual pleasure
- Usually are very learned, brave, and respectful individuals
- Can be judgmental, sarcastic, jealous, and egocentric
- Display determination and discipline with regards to spiritual practices

KAPHA

Kapha Characteristics

- Strong, muscular, and well proportioned physique with thick bones and muscles
- Tendency towards overweight
- Face tends to be round and attractive
- Appetite regular and food intake relatively small due to efficient digestion
- Calm and steady demeanor; does not become easily frustrated or anxious
- Large, dark, tranquil eyes
- Thick, dark, wavy hair
- Strong sexual drive and attraction for sensual pleasures
- Reaches slow, well-considered decisions over time
- Speech is clear and melodic

Kapha Behaviors

- Will sleep long and deeply if given the opportunity
- Can seek emotional comfort from eating
- Is slow to change habits, jobs, relationships
- Will procrastinate and take a long time to complete projects
- Holds a grudge forever and may finally find cunning ways to get revenge
- Displays affection freely; has long-standing friendships; loyal
- Does not use foul or harsh language
- Does not get sick often and heals quickly
- Movements are slow, coordinated, and graceful

B. The Three Gunas: Energies of the Mind

Ayurveda acknowledges universal forces of Nature that operate both within us and outside of us. These forces or energies of Nature can be observed to be a dynamically shifting equilibrium by anyone who takes the time to notice. Whereas the three *doshas* can be understood to create the physical constitution, the *gunas*, which are also three in number, create the qualities of the mind. These energies constitute the deepest and most subtle nature of all sentient beings. Accustomed as we all are in the West to acknowledge only those external phenomena that are perceivable by the five senses (seeing, hearing, smelling, tasting, or touching), we are less familiar with these subtle energies that exist within and around us. However, the ancient Indian sages regarded an understanding of these energies to be tantamount to knowing about healing disease of any kind. Once again Ayurveda finds in its original language, Sanskrit, a vocabulary to beautifully describe these primary energies. As a group they are known as the *gunas*, which translates to "quality, attribute, peculiarity, or property; a chief property of all existing things". Their individual names and general meanings are:

1) **Sattva** — Intelligence, Light (not Dark), Harmony
2) **Rajas** — Activity, Movement, Action
3) **Tamas** — Materiality, Substance, Inertia, Darkness

The gunas are very real forces that are inherent in the very nature of Universal Energy, which operate not only on the mental but also on the spiritual levels of existence. By this it is meant that these qualities determine the nature and emotional texture of one's thoughts, the subconscious drives that ultimately create our lives. The *gunas* are said to be the way in which our past deeds (karmas) encode themselves in our lives and generate our desires and aversions in each succeeding incarnation. Whereas the three doshas are the agents of determining physical and biological attributes of living beings, the three *gunas* have their effects at a deeper and more fundamental level and allow us to comprehend the qualities of energies at the spiritual and mental dimensions. In fact, the gunas are anterior to and create the doshas.

Just as all individuals consist of diverse and unique proportions of the three doshas, all known objects in the entire universe are composed of combinations of the three gunas.

Rajas is what creates activity, change, movement, and excitement in Nature. It is the force that stirs things up and creates a disharmony within an existing state of harmony. Rajas is an unstoppable force which seeks to move outward towards disintegration and division. It is the force of impulse and passion and though it leads one powerfully in a single-minded pursuit of pleasure and stimulation, it eventually culminates in disharmony and discomfort if it is unopposed. It is what leads one away from one's comfort zone, away from one's truth and true nature.

Tamas is what creates resistance to movement and causes inertia in nature; it is obstructing and slow in quality. It is also what veils the true nature of things from one's intellect, what causes darkness, ignorance, dullness, stagnation and attachment to material things. Tamas manifests as the force of gravity and prevents thoughts and objects from evolving and moving; it is the force that stabilizes the world and prevents changes in form and structure. Tamas unopposed will create a downward spiral of destruction and dissolution wherever it dominates; it brings about disorder, ignorance, and blasphemy of the intellect. It promotes separation, selfishness, spiritual sleep and lower levels of consciousness. It pulls awareness down from the heights of subtle energies and perceptions to the gross and material aspects of existence.

Sattva is what creates harmony, intelligence, balance, light, virtue, truth, and lasting joy in Nature. It can be known when one is pure and clean in mind, heart, and body. It is an uplifting force that enlightens the mind and enlivens the individual soul. Sattva is the song of the birds, the rays of sunlight, the pristine perfection of a snow-covered mountain; it is the principle that brings scope, clarity, and openness to the mind, the force that creates peace and love in the heart.

Let's elaborate a little further on these three subtle universal energies. Rajas and Tamas are energies that cause agitation and delusion, respectively. Sattva, in contrast, provides the mind with the clarity to see things as they really are and the steadfastness and resolution to act in harmony with Nature. Rajas drives us to constantly seek happiness *outside* of ourselves and discourages awareness of the inner needs. Rajas, when it dominates, leads to emotional turmoil, irresistible desires, and excessive activity. We know Rajas is ascendant when all our energies seem to be directed towards the pursuit of outer and sensory goals.

Tamas weakens our creative urges and ability to understand the events and patterns of our lives. It veils us from our own inner intuitive wisdom and disconnects us from the wisdom of Nature at large. Tamas throws us into a perception of life as a purely physical experience. Life is understood only in terms of the physical body and the laws that govern that domain; there is no appreciation for subtler things that can be known by means other than the five senses; the "sixth sense" in life becomes vestigial. Tamas creates identification almost exclusively with the material aspects of existence and restricts us to darkness and limitation.

Sattva is the equilibrium point between the activating energy of Rajas and the stabilizing energy of Tamas. Sattva is the state of balance in the physical, mental, emotional, and spiritual realms of life. By creating and increasing Sattva in one's life, one promotes harmony and efficiency in the biological processes of the body and mind. When Sattva prevails in our energetic profile, there is an opportunity to comprehend our true Nature and our unique make-up.

CHAPTER 3.

DETERMINING YOUR AYURVEDIC CONSTITUTIONAL TYPE

*F*rom the viewpoint of Ayurveda, the first step in the treatment of any diet-related condition is to determine your individual constitutional type. This is determined by the proportion of each dosha and guna that occurs in each individual. The dosha/guna that is predominant will reflect the energies and metabolic tendencies within. Knowing what your Ayurvedic Constitutional Type is will allow you to understand your mind and physiology and will allow you to interpret with great specificity your metabolic signals.

The questionnaire below is provided to help you determine your Ayurvedic Constitutional Type. It is divided into three parts: Vata, Pitta, and Kapha (V, P and K). Some answers will be obvious such as those asking about objective physical characteristics (i.e. hair color, height, dry skin, etc.). For emotional and behavioral characteristics which can be more subjective and variable, try to answer according to how you have felt and behaved over the course of your lifetime, or at least for many years, and not based on the past few months.

Select one choice (V, P, or K) for each numbered item. At the end of the questionnaire record the number of V's, P's, and K's. The proportion of the three is your Ayurvedic Constitutional Type.

AYURVEDIC CONSTITUTIONAL TYPE QUESTIONNAIRE

1. Physique   **V**   I am taller (or shorter) than average and thin with a rather under-developed physique.

   P   I am average in height with a moderately developed physique.

   K   I am thick, large, and broad, with a well-developed physique.

2. Weight	*V*	I am thin; my bones tend to be prominent (knuckles, elbows, knees, facial bones, etc.)
.	*P*	I am of moderate weight with a slight tendency toward overweight.
	K	I am heavy and easily tend towards overweight or obesity.

3. Hair	*V*	My hair is two or more of these: dry, kinky, curly, coarse, black, dark brown.
	P	My hair is two or more of these: Red, light brown, blond, soft, fine, prone to premature gray or balding.
	K	My hair is two or more of these: Thick, oily, wavy, medium to dark brown.

4. Teeth	*V*	My teeth are two or more of these: crooked, large, protruding,with large spaces, with receding gums.
	P	My teeth are two or more of these: medium-sized, yellowish, gums bleed easily.
	K	My teeth are large, straight, and white.

5. Eyes	*V*	Small, dry, brown and I tend to blink a lot.
	P	Sharp, penetrating, green, blue, or gray, with reddish or yellowish sclerae.
	K	Large, attractive, charming, with white sclerae, brown or deep blue.

6. Eyebrows	*V*	Thin, not bushy, dry, and firm to touch.
	P	Medium in all respects.
	K	Thick, bushy, oily, soft.

7. Nose	*V*	Thin, small, bumpy, and slightly crooked.
	P	Medium-sized, reddish, large pores.
	K	Large but proportionate, oily, thick.

8. Lips	*V*	Thin, can be dry or chapped, darkish, and somewhat unsteady.
	P	Medium, soft, pink.
	K	Thick, moist, large, smooth, firm.

9. Shoulders   **V**   Not very broad or thick and down-sloping.
          P   Medium.
          K   Thick, broad, firm.

10. Chest   **V**   Thin and not muscular. Breasts are small (women).
          P   Medium in all respects.
          K   Muscular, thick, over-developed, breasts are large.

11. Arms   **V**   Thin, long, and the bones are prominent.
          P   Medium, strong and wiry.
          K   Large, thick, and well-developed.

12. Hands   **V**   Cool, dry, and well-lined, sometimes tremulous, knuckles prominent.
          P   Medium, warm, pink, moist, soft.
          K   Large, thick, long, well developed, knuckles smooth.

13. Calves   **V**   Small and firm.
          P   Moderately firm and long.
          K   Long, firm, shapely, rounded.

14. Feet   **V**   Small, dry, cool, and rough.
          P   Medium-sized, soft, warm, pink.
          K   Large, thick, solid, moist.

15. Nails   **V**   Dry, small, tend to chip or crack, darkish, surface rough.
          P   Pinkish, medium-sized, soft.
          K   Large, thick, smooth, white, hard.

16. Joints   **V**   Thin, prominent, dry, and make cracking sounds, prone to fracture.
          P   Medium, soft, loose, prone to sprains.
          K   Large, thick well-knit, strong.

17. Bowel Movements   **V**   Hard, dry, accompanied by gas, tendency towards constipation.
          P   Regular, tends towards loose and soft or diarrhea, abundant.
          K   Regular, large, oily.

18. Urine	V	Small amounts very frequently throughout the day.
	P	Abundant, deep yellow, occasionally slightly burning.
	K	Moderate, concentrated.

19. Perspiration	V	Scanty, no strong odor.
	P	Profuse, strong odor.
	K	Moderate, sweet odor.

20. Appetite	V	Unpredictable and erratic; I sometimes am not hungry at mealtimes and very hungry between meals.
	P	Sharp, acutely aware of mealtimes, dislikes delaying meals, enjoys and can digest large quantities of food.
	K	Constant, can miss a meal comfortably, feels best with smaller quantities of food.

21. Activity Pattern	V	I perform activities very quickly, I can become distracted easily or may not always complete things I begin.
	P	I perform activities intensely and efficiently. I am a perfectionist. I am likely to become aggravated if interrupted or encounter difficulties.
	K	I do things slowly, deliberately, and calmly.

22. Learning Pattern	V	I seem to learn new things very quickly; I can forget things if I don't use them for a while.
	P	I learn moderately quickly after hearing new material two or three times.
	K	It takes me a little longer to really learn things, but once learned I never forget.

23. Immunity	V	Low, I get minor illnesses fairly often.
	P	Moderate, I usually do not get sick.
	K	High, I seem resistant to disease.

24. Disease Pattern	V	Fatigue, nervous system, insomnia, weakness, dryness.
	P	Fevers, inflammations, ulcers, skin conditions.
	K	Congestion, respiratory conditions, benign growths, obesity.

25. Speech   V   I tend to talk a lot and show enthusiasm in my speech by nature.

P   Argumentative, precise, convincing, sharp, direct speech.

K   Slow, sometimes monotonous, low-pitched, rhythmic speech.

26. Social   V   More often than not I am insecure and nervous in new social situations.

P   I am outgoing and usually assertive and accessible around people.

K   I usually do more listening than speaking in new situations, but people are attracted to me nonetheless.

27. Gait   V   I usually walk quicker than most people with short light steps.

P   Stable, purposeful pace at moderate speed.

K   Slow, unhurried, and graceful strides.

28. Voice   V   Low volume, hoarse, vibrato, cracking, not really deep or resonant.

P   Sharp, loud, captures attention.

K   Pleasant, deep, harmonious, resonant.

29. Temperament   V   Nervous, changeable, never seems to be content.

P   Always seems to be struggling, achieving; highly self-motivated.

K   Usually happy, slow to desire or see the need for change.

30. Sleep   V   Often light or interrupted, insomnia, 5-7 hours per night.

P   Sound, 6-8 hours per night.

K   Deep, uninterrupted, difficulty waking.

31. Memory   V   Short, forgets relatively easily.

P   Average, clear on details.

K   Long.

32. Concentration   V   Easily distracted.

P   Rarely distracted, intensely engaged.

K   Moderate levels of concentration.

33. Truthful-ness	V	Will often harmlessly lie to avoid uncomfortable situations.
	P	Usually tells the truth.
	K	Never lies, there is no reason to ever do this.
34. Will Power	V	Weak, I often start out very determined but later give in.
	P	Moderate, I am very self-critical when I fail to follow through.
	K	Strong, if I make a decision I stay with it.
35. Spiritual Reading/ Study	V	I go through periods of interest and periods when I lose interest.
	P	I have surprising discipline and constancy in spiritual matters.
	K	I have never really pursued any spiritual avenues.
36. Emotional Reaction to Stress	V	Fearful, anxious and worried.
	P	Anger, aggressiveness, irritability, demanding, uncompromising.
	K	Complacent, steady, calmly seeks solutions, may become depressed.
37. Mental Tendency	V	Questions everything, theorizes as to the cause of events, creative.
	P	Discriminating, judging, suspicious.
	K	Logical, stable, reasonable, slow to evaluate.
38. Forgive-ness	V	I forgive and forget easily and often.
	P	It takes me a very long time to forgive; I tend to hold grudges.
	K	I understand that people make mistakes; it rarely upsets me.
39. Love	V	I fall in and out of love easily.
	P	I have had relatively few but intensely passionate love affairs.
	K	I feel I am hungry for love and affection; long-term relationships.

40. Dreams	V	Flying, running, fear, searching, traveling.
	P	Passion, violence, light, anger, jealousy, the sun, colors.
	K	Romance, water, ocean, sadness, empathy.

41. Sex Drive	V	Frequent desire, low stamina.
	P	Moderate desire, dominating, passionate.
	K	Cyclical, sometimes insatiable, excellent stamina.

42. Hygiene	V	Very clean and neat, intolerant of sloppiness, uncleanness.
	P	Moderately clean, but secondary to other concerns.
	K	Can be dirty and sloppy for periods of time.

43. Work Habits	V	Selfless, often volunteers to help out.
	P	Works intensely, especially to achieve personal goals.
	K	Procrastinates, sometimes lazy, takes time to complete projects.

44. Recreation	V	Exercise, travel, movies, dancing, parties, skating, visiting friends.
	P	Attending sporting events, competitive athletics, reading, building or repairing, woodworking, playing musical instruments.
	K	Attending concerts, dining out, television, sleep, sex, food, literature.

45. Financial Behavior	V	Spends impulsively, spends on trifles, feels poor.
	P	Spends moderately, enjoys luxuries, gourmet meals.
	K	Frugal, saves money, spends freely on food, entertainment.

46. Weather Intolerance	V	Cold, windy, dry.
	P	Hot, humid.
	K	Cold, damp, rain.

47. Disease Tendency	V	Nervous system, pain, mental instability, arthritis, fatigue, weakness, hearing loss.
	P	Febrile illness, inflammations, infections, skin disorders, heart disease, ulcer disease, hemorrhoids, alcoholism.
	K	Respiratory diseases (bronchitis, asthma), obesity, high cholesterol, sinusitis.

48. Pulse   **V**   Rapid, thready, light.

                P   Bounding, strong, superficial.

                K   Slow, broad, strong.

49. Tongue   **V**   Thin, surface with several or more furrows, dark pink, blue-tinged (especially on undersurface).

                P   Moderately thick, reddish especially near the tip, moist.

                K   Thick, whitish coating, pink.

Record the total numbers of each response below:

Number of V's (Vata)   _____

Number of P's (Pitta)   _____

Number of K's (Kapha) _____

Using Your Questionnaire Score to Determine Your Ayurvedic Constitutional Type

By adding the scores for Vata, Pitta, and Kapha you have determined your Ayurvedic Constitutional type. Although there are only three doshas, they can combine in ten possible ways to give ten possible Constitutional Types. These are enumerated below.

If one score is much higher than the other two, you are a single dosha type.

Single Dosha Type (3)
Vata
Pitta
Kapha

Examples: If you scored Vata <u>38</u>, Pitta <u>8</u>, Kapha <u>4</u> you would be considered a Vata Type.

                     If you scored Vata <u>10</u>, Pitta <u>35</u>, Kapha <u>5</u> you would be considered a Pitta Type.

                     If you scored Vata <u>9</u>, Pitta, <u>8</u>, Kapha <u>33</u> you would be considered a Kapha Type.

Generally, the single dominant dosha must be at least 2.5 times as much as the other doshas for an individual to be considered a single dosha type. There are rare exceptions to this rule but you may feel confident by applying it.

If no single dosha is dominant, you are a bi-doshic type.

Bi-doshic Types (6)

Vata-Pitta	Pitta-Vata
Pitta-Kapha	Kapha-Pitta
Kapha-Vata	Vata-Kapha

Examples: If you scored Vata 20, Pitta 24, Kapha 8 you would be considered a Pitta -Vata Type.
If you scored Vata 6, Pitta 18, Kapha 26 you would be considered a Kapha-Pitta Type.

In practice, the majority of individuals are bi-doshic types. The dosha with the relatively highest score is your primary dosha, but its manifestation in your mind and body is significantly colored by the secondary dosha. There can also be a few traits that are attributable to the third dosha (i.e. thick bushy eyebrows in a Vata-Pitta individual) but these will be few, if any.

If all three scores are nearly equal, you are a tri-doshic type.

Tri-doshic Types (1)

Vata-Pitta-Kapha

This doshic type is truly rare and requires all three dosha to score within 10% of each other. Remember also that the questionnaire should be supported by the descriptions given above for each type. If the questionnaire says you are a Pitta type yet you feel from the descriptions that you are definitely a Vata type, re-take the test the next day, or have a close friend or family member take it with you. The odds are you will be a bi-doshic type.

| VATA | PITTA | KAPHA |

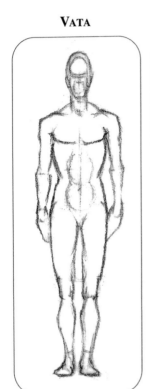
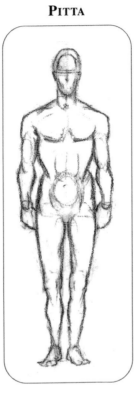
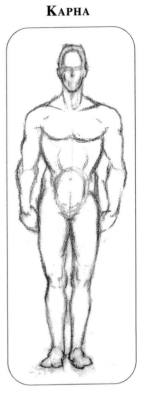

CHAPTER 4.

ADDITIONAL IMPORTANT AYURVEDIC CONCEPTS

*T*o further our understanding of Ayurvedic Medicine, which is the basis of the Sattva Program for Weight Loss and Maintenance, let us examine just a few more important concepts of this system.

The Seven Bodily Tissues—Sapta Dhatus

The dhatus are the basic varieties of tissues that compose the human body. The word *dhatu* comes from a Sanskrit word which means "that which enters into the formation of the body"; the root *Dha* means "support, that which bears".

The primary Dhatus are seven in number. They are:

1. Śukra dhātu   (reproductive tissues)
2. Majjā dhātu   (bone marrow and nervous tissues)
3. Asthi dhātu   (bone)
4. Meda dhātu   (fatty tissues)
5. Māṁsa dhātu   (muscle tissues)
6. Rakta dhātu   (formed blood cells)
7. Rasa dhātu   (plasma)

The most unique feature of Ayurvedic histology (concept of tissue formation) is that each human tissue is formed from the previous tissue in ascending order of complexity. Thus when food is ingested it is digested until, in the small intestines, it becomes a liquidy, chyme-like material known in Ayurveda as *āhāra rasa*, or food essence. With the help of ahara rasagni (each dhatu has its own agni, or digestive enzymes), this ahara rasa is converted into Rasa dhātu (blood plasma)—the first and most simple tissue.

Now, Rasa dhātu—catalyzed by Rasagni—is transformed into Rakta dhatu (formed blood cells), the second fundamental bodily tissue. Rakta dhatu in turn, with the help of raktagni, becomes mamsa

41

dhatu (muscle), and so on. Table 5 illustrates the sequence of tissue formation.

TABLE 5.
THE SEVEN TISSUES

Śukra dhātu (reproductive tissues)

∧

∧∧

Majjā dhātu (bone marrow and nervous tissues)

∧∧∧

∧∧∧∧

Asthi dhātu (bone)

∧∧∧∧∧

∧∧∧∧∧∧

Meda dhātu (fatty tissues)

∧∧∧∧∧∧∧

∧∧∧∧∧∧∧∧

Māṁsa dhātu (muscle tissues)

∧∧∧∧∧∧∧∧∧

∧∧∧∧∧∧∧∧∧∧

Rakta dhātu (formed blood cells)

∧∧∧∧∧∧∧∧∧∧∧

∧∧∧∧∧∧∧∧∧∧∧∧

Rasa dhātu (plasma)

Together, the dhātus and *upadhātus* make up the physical bulk of the body. Upadhatus are secondary tissues that add support and function structurally but usually are not implicated in metabolic disease conditions of the body. The upadhatus include hair, nails, ligaments, cartilage, etc.

Each dhātu consists of countless infinitesimal paramanus (cells) that are units of structure and function. Each paramanu contains innumerable suksma srotas (channels, pores) through which it receives nutrients and subtle energies and eliminates waste materials. Because dhatus are saturated with pores, the human body can also be said to be filled with pores (srotomaya). The srotas of each dhatu are unique in their structure and function and in the materials that move through them. The state of health of each dhatu as well as its relative vriddhi/kshaya (excess/deficiency; increase/decrease) is assessed by the physician.

Waste Materials—Malas

As a consequence of foods that we take into our bodies from the external world and the normal biological processes that take place internally, we generate different kinds of waste materials, or malas, which must be excreted. Ayurveda generally recognizes two kinds of malas:

1. *ahara mala* or wastes from food
2. *dhatu mala* or wastes from the tissues

The *ahara malas* include feces, urine and sweat. These are the three main malas. The *dhatu malas* include the various secretions of the nose, eyes, ears; lactic acid, carbon dioxide, and other metabolites of cellular respiration; exfoliated hair, skin, and nails. Although these are all waste products, they serve a role in maintaining health as long as they are normal in their quantity, qualities and function. However, if the malas become abnormal in some regard (i.e. increased or decreased) they become a factor in creating disease. When the dhatus and malas become unbalanced they are called dushyas (soiled tissues). The malas are composed predominantly of different elements. Feces is composed mainly of earth element; urine, mainly water and fire; sweat, primarily water. Of course, all five elements are contained in every mala.

The Channels—Srotas

Srotas, meaning channels or pores, are present throughout the visible body as well as at the "invisible" or subtle level of the cells, molecules, atoms, and subatomic strata. It is through these channels that nutrients and other substances are transported in and out of our physiologies. It is also through these channels that information and intelligence spontaneously flow. When the flow of appropriate nutrients and energies through these channels is unimpeded, there is health; when there is excess, deficiency, or blockage in these channels disease can take root. Some srotas have obvious correlates with western concepts (e.g. both Ayurveda and allopathy recognize the anna vaha srota, or gastrointestinal channel and the prana vaha srota, or respiratory passageways.) Other srotas have no western correlate: artava vaha srota or udaka vaha srota, carrying the monthly menstrum and the pure water in the body, respectively.

Together with knowledge of the doshic imbalances, the dhatus (tissues) involved, the state of the agni (digestive fire), and other diagnostic means, assessment of the srotas is one of the means in Ayurveda by which diseases can be distinguished. By knowing which srotas are affected and the nature and extent of their disturbance, one can understand a great deal about the disease process.

The *Charaka Samhitā* describes thirteen srotas. *Three* srotas connect the individual to the external environment, by bringing air, food, and water into and out of the body. *Seven* srotas are associated with the seven bodily tissues (sapta dhatus). Another *three* srotas direct wastes out of the body. That makes thirteen. However, other ancient authorities recognize *three* additional srota relating to lactation, menstruation, and the flow of thoughts through the mind. This brings the total number of srotas to sixteen, which is the accepted description.

Following is a list of the *sixteen srotas* of the human being:

Three srotas connect the individual to the external world:

Prana vaha srota	the channels carrying prana, the breath.
Anna vaha srota	the channels transporting solid and liquid foods.
Udaka vaha srotas	the channels transporting water (no Western equivalent).

Seven srotas represent channels to and from the tissues (dhatus):

Rasa vaha srotas	the channels carrying plasma and lymph.
Rakta vaha srotas	the channels carrying blood cells and specifically hemoglobin.
Mamsa vaha srotas	the channels carrying muscle nutrients and wastes.

Meda vaha srotas	the channels supplying the various adipose tissues of the body.
Asthi vaha srotas	the channels bring nutrients to the bones and transporting wastes.
Majja vaha srotas	the channels supplying the bone marrow and nerves including the brain.
Sukra vaha srota	the channels carrying the sperm and ova and supplying their nutrients.

Three srotas regulate the elimination of metabolic waste products:

Purisha vaha srotas	the channels which carry the feces.
Mutra vaha srotas	the channels which carry the urine.
Sveda vaha srotas	the channels which carry perspiration.

Two srotas are specific for women:

Artava vaha srotas	the channels which carry the menstrum.
Stanya vaha srotas	the channels carrying the breast milk during lactation.

One srota is associated with the mind (manas):

Mano vaha srota	the channels which carry thoughts, ideas, emotions, and impressions.

The Digestive Fire—Agni

Agni is the fire constantly burning within our minds and bodies, which kindles all the biological processes of life; it is the fire that powers the transformation of one substance into another. The most obvious function of agni is to promote digestion. But for living beings, everything depends on it—our appearance, body temperature, auto-immunity, awareness, understanding, intelligence; our health, our energy, our lives. Many diseases are connected directly or indirectly to an abnormality of agni. Not only is agni responsible for the breakdown of food substances, but also for neutralizing toxins, bacteria, and viruses that can disrupt our immune system.

When agni is healthy there is excellent digestion, normal elimination, proper tissue formation, good circulation, high energy, strong immunity, good complexion, pleasant body odor and breath, intelligence, enthusiasm, and perception.

When agni is unhealthy however, digestion is inefficient and incomplete and all the functions mentioned above are disturbed. Most importantly, when agni is disturbed, incompletely digested food forms an internal toxin known as *ama*. This substance can further putrefy and ferment within the intestinal tract and can spread throughout the body to cause disease. Thus, without exaggeration, the care of agni is central to maintaining health and treating diseases.

There are thirteen forms of agni, the most important of which is *jatharagni*, which regulates and contributes a part of itself to the other agnis. Sometimes jatharagni is referred to as kosthagni (*kostha* = digestive tract) or pachakagni (*pachana* = cooking). A principal function of jatharagni is to cook the ingested food and separate the *sara* (nutrients) from the *kitta* (waste). The sara is also known as *ahara rasa,* which is the substrate for the first bodily tissue, rasadhatu.

The other twelve agnis are the dhatagnis (7) and the bhutagnis (5), which are related to the tissues and the five subtle elements, respectively. The dhatagnis regulate the physiological processes in each of the seven tissues, while the bhutagnis regulate the further digestion and assimilation of the pancha mahabhuta contained in the ingested foods.

The Ayurvedic texts mention factors that disrupt agni. These include eating at inappropriate times, overeating, undereating, eating devitalized foods, eating before the previous meal has been digested, excessive sleep, anger, grief, immoral behavior, consumption of excess fluids, or frequent changes in dietary habits.

Agnis are classified into four categories according to how they manifest in the human being: sharp, mild, irregular and regular.

Tiksnagni (sharp) implies strong digestion, circulation, and immunity. Impurities, if they accumulate, tend to do so in rasa and rakta dhatus (plasma and formed blood cells). These people have a tendency toward inflammations and acidity. This condition is usually seen in pitta constitutions.

SAMAGNI (NORMAL)

MANDAGNI (LOW)

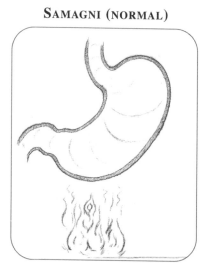

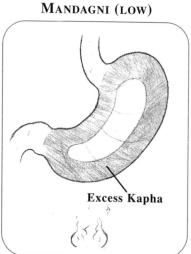

Excess Kapha

Mandagni (mild) usually manifests as slower digestion, low appetite, cravings for heavy or sweet foods, and a tendency to carry excess body weight. Circulation may be slow and excess secretions often form. Usually seen in Kapha constitutions.

Visamagni (irregular) can promote irregular appetite, with intense periods of hunger alternating with lack of interest in food. There is often intestinal bloating, gas, constipation, or abdominal discomfort. Immunity is often diminished, especially with regard to the nervous system, bones, and upper respiratory tract. Not surprisingly, this type of agni is common in vata constitutions.

Samagni (regular, balanced) occurs in individuals who are well-balanced, eat proper amounts and kinds of foods, exercise and rest appropriately. One sees normal appetite, satisfaction surrounding meals, normal bowel movements, endurance, (mental) clarity, and (emotional) stability.

This completes our survey of the most important principles of Ayurvedic Medicine. For further information and more complete discussions of any of the concepts in this chapter you can read any of the references listed in the Appendix.

CHAPTER 5.

THE CONCEPT OF OBESITY (STHAULYA) IN AYURVEDA AND WESTERN MEDICINE

A. GENERAL CONSIDERATIONS

*O*besity, or *sthaulya*, is a multifactorial complex of imbalances affecting both an individual's physiology and psychology, which results in an increase of body weight to more than 30 per cent above "normal". This increase is due to the systemic accumulation of fat throughout the body. I hesitate to use the term "normal" because this is difficult to determine. Who is a "normal" person and what does he or she look like? The standard tables used in modern medicine which take into account age, height, and weight are certainly not applicable to everyone. According to Ayurveda, three 48 year old women, each of them an identical 5'4" in height, should have somewhat different ideal body weights if indeed they happen to be of different constitutional types. It would be "normal", for example, for the vata-type woman to weigh 110-118 while the kapha-type woman would be more comfortable and happy at 123-130; the pitta-individual would most likely find her "normal" weight somewhere between these two ranges.

Body Mass Index (BMI)

Today, obesity is usually defined in terms of the *body mass index* (BMI), which is the weight (in kilograms) divided by the height (in meters). The normal range of BMI is 18.5 to 24.9. Overweight is defined as a BMI of 25.0 to 29.9. Obesity is currently defined as a BMI of >29.9. BMI is very closely correlated with the amount of body fat. Although this sounds very precise and scientific, there is no solid medical or physiological evidence for these criteria and many feel these numbers are arbitrary.

The BMI can also be determined using pounds and inches with the following formula:

$$BMI = \frac{\text{Weight in Pounds} \times 703}{(\text{Height in Inches})^2}$$

or

$$\frac{\text{lbs}}{\text{in}^2} (\times 703)$$

TABLE 3.
OBESITY CLASSIFICATION BY BMI

	BMI
Underweight	<18.5
Normal Weight	18.5–24.9
Overweight	25–29.9
Mild Obesity	30–34.9
Moderate Obesity	35–39.9
Severe Obesity	>40

Waist Circumference

Measurement of your waist circumference is yet another independent method of determining if your weight is creating a higher risk for certain health conditions. Large waist circumference (for men: >40 inches; for women: >35 inches) indicates that you have a greater than normal proportion of your body fat in the central and upper part of your body. This central obesity is associated with several health risks collectively termed "metabolic syndrome," which include: hypertension, blood clotting abnormalities, glucose intolerance, insulin resistance, high levels of insulin, increased serum triglycerides and LDL cholesterol, and decreased HDL cholesterol.

To determine your waist circumference use a tape measure to take a measurement at the level of your navel (the bottom of the ribs in the back).

CHAPTER 5. THE CONCEPT OF OBESITY (STHAULYA) IN AYURVEDA AND WESTERN MEDICINE

Health Consequences of Obesity

More than ever before, there is a growing awareness of the role of obesity and overweight in causing disease and shortening our lifespan. In fact a recent study (1999) published in the *New England Journal Of Medicine* which included over 1 million Americans revealed that the risk of death from all causes increases with moderate and severe overweight for both men and women in all age groups. (Calle EE, Thun MJ, Petrelli JM, et al. Body-mass index and mortality in a prospective cohort of U.S. adults. *NEJM* 341:1097, 1999). Clearly, it is no longer acceptable for us to sit back and deal with the secondary consequences of obesity or to place "losing weight" midway down our list of personal goals and priorities.

Overweight and obesity are associated with virtually all of the most common diseases that have been on the rise over the past 50 years: type-2 diabetes, high blood pressure, hyperlipidemia, coronary heart disease, polycystic ovary disease, hyperandrogenism, gallstones, osteoarthritis, infertility, fatigue, low back pain, shortness of breath, esophageal reflux, depression, colon cancer, postmenopausal breast cancer, and endometrial cancer. One recent survey showed that approximately 55% of Americans are overweight and, even more distressing, 22% suffer from obesity. (Kuzmarski RJ, Flegal KM, Campbell SM, Johnson CL. Increasing prevalence of overweight among U.S. adults. The National Health and Nutrition Examination Surveys, 1960 to 1991. *JAMA* 272:205, 1994.). Contrast this to what science is discovering about restricting calories and losing weight. When caloric intake is restricted to about 65% of their usual intake, mice and rats lose significant amounts of fat tissue and the animals *live as much as 50% longer* than animals fed *ad libitum*. (Barzilai, N, Gupta, G. Revisiting the role of fat mass in the life extension induced by caloric restriction. *J Gerontol A Biol Sci Med Sci*, 54(3):B89-96, 1999).

From a biological point of view, all obesity has a common metabolic cause: the intake of more calories than are needed to provide energy for all the metabolic processes. Like modern medicine, Ayurveda understands that if you consume more than the required amount of calories, those unutilized calories are simply transformed into fat in the body. But that is where the simplicity ends. The interesting observation that has gone unexplained by modern medicine is that different individuals burn calories more easily than others. The intricacies of the human metabolism, when approached from the modern reductionist viewpoint, remain incompletely understood. Modern science does not understand why some people who eat a relatively high-calorie diet maintain a constant weight even if they are physically inactive, while others gain significant amounts of weight on a calorie-controlled diet and regular exercise. You may be reading this and recognizing this to be your situation.

Ayurveda understands this phenomenon to be related to the constitutional type of each person. While the vata-type individual will often consume large amounts of calories and burn them quickly, the kapha-type person will sometimes eat very little yet consistently gain weight little-by-little. In fact, studies show that obese groups and normal weight groups have approximately the same daily caloric intake per kilogram, after adjusting for body weight. I have witnessed this many, many times over the course of my medical career. The reason is simply that these kapha-types utilize calories more efficiently; it is due to their inherent metabolic make-up. These individuals, if left to their own ways, will naturally have a greater tendency towards increased fluid retention and fat storage and decreased fat mobilization. The reasons for this are not understood in the paradigm of allopathic medicine.

How many calories of energy are appropriate also varies over time for the same individual, being partially determined by a complex interrelation of a person's age, hormones, psychological situation, stress level, activity level, and other metabolic changes. Research also seems to indicate that part of the problem may be genetic as well. For example, a mutation in the chromosome that controls the beta-3 adrenergic receptor has been associated with a syndrome including diabetes, obesity, and insulin resistance. (Clement, K, Vaisse, C, et al. Genetic variation in the beta-3 adrenergic receptor and an increased capacity to gain weight in patients with morbid obesity. *NEJM* 333:352, 1995). This receptor is involved with promoting heat production and energy expenditure in the body. We now understand that generally speaking there are two major sub-types of obesity that take into account both the *number* and *size* of the fat cells in the body.

The first sub-type is known as *hypertrophic* or adult-onset obesity. This condition features a normal and fixed number of fat cells; individuals gain weight exclusively through the hypertrophy (increase in size) of these cells. Hypertrophy occurs as a consequence of fat deposition inside these cells. People with this type of obesity are almost always amenable to weight reduction. Over 85% of obese individuals fall into this category.

The second sub-type of obesity, which is relatively uncommon, is known as *hyperplastic-hypertrophic* and is characterized by increases in both the *absolute number* and size of the fat cells. These changes usually occur during childhood or early adolescence and are typically difficult to reverse. In persons with this type of obesity a high level of failure is anticipated and our efforts are directed towards minimizing the potential metabolic consequences (coronary artery disease, hypertension, respiratory problems, gall stones, diabetes, musculo-skeletal problems, depression, and some forms of cancer.)

B. Balance vs. Imbalance: The Real Solution

Energy Storage vs. Release

One of the most important and completely overlooked features of the human physiology is our capacity to actually store excess energy that we obtain from our food for later use and then release it in an organized manner. Think about how different our days would be if that were *not* the case. By analogy, you would then be identical to a lamp that must be plugged in at all times in order to work. In other words, if we couldn't store food energy, we'd have to be eating all the time— even during activities. Imagine needing to be eating while you were mowing the lawn or riding your bicycle. And if you tried to eat a large meal just prior to that bicycle ride, that strategy would fail. It would be like plugging in the lamp for an hour before using it and then unplugging it, and trying to turn it on. If the lamp can't *store* energy, then it must always be connected to an energy source. To take the analogy a step further, what if we ate too *much* food at one time? It might be like plugging our 115-volt lamp into a 230-volt outlet and could burn out our circuits.

Fortunately, human beings evolved in such a way that we do indeed have the capacity to store energy from our food intake. As you know, we humans have the extraordinary physiological machinery to use the energy from our foods to meet our immediate requirements and store the remainder for later. We can do this by virtue of an internal rechargeable battery that we all are created with: our body fat. We recharge and replenish this stored energy depot every time we eat more than we need and we drain it every time we need additional biological energy. On the average, most of us store enough energy in our fat tissues for us to jog from New York City to Chicago without consuming a thing.

The Other Functions Of Fat

Adipose tissue, for many decades considered an inactive, quiet storehouse of energy, is now understood to be a truly complex and metabolically active component of the neuro-immuno-endocrine axis. Fat cells secrete cytokines and peptides, which are biologically active and are definitely related to specific disease conditions. One of these cytokines is tissue necrosis factor alpha (TNF-alpha). Studies have revealed that TNF-alpha may contribute to insulin resistance, which leads to an increased risk of diabetes mellitus as well as atherosclerosis. Leptin is another cytokine secreted by fat cells which plays an important, if incompletely understood, role in body composition, immune response, and metabolism. One function of leptin is its ability to redistribute fat from the visceral depots to subcutaneous areas. In addition, fat tissues secrete peptides, which act as messengers between fat cells and other body tissues. Thus it appears probable that the excess or deficiency of fat cells and their biologically active products plays a vital role in the disease and healing processes.

What gives us the ability to store and release food energy as required? The answer lies in the complex and counter-regulatory hormones, enzymes, and neurochemicals that have evolved to create the human neurohormonal system. We now know that insulin and glucagon are the chief hormones involved in these processes. When we eat a meal, insulin promotes the storage of any excess food energy as fat for later use. When energy is required, glucagon stimulates the release and breakdown of the stored carbohydrate and fat (and if the need is sufficiently great, protein) to provide energy. But there are many other pairs of opposites with equally important effects on our fat stores, and hence our weight.

Because of their importance to a complete understanding of the issues of weight loss, we will describe them here in some detail: sympathetic vs. parasympathetic nervous predominance, lipase vs. l-carnatine, cortisol vs. adrenocorticotropic hormone (ACTH), NADPH vs. NADH, acetyl coenzyme A vs. acetyl coenzyme A carboxylase, adenosine diphosphate vs. adenine triphosphate, and many other unpublicized yet vitally important enzyme systems.

Being overweight means you have developed an imbalance in one or more of these physiological enzyme/hormone pairs in the direction that favors energy storage. Simply losing weight will not correct this imbalance and the amount of weight loss will always be limited because the underlying problem has not been corrected. However, creating balance in these energetic processes will result in an easy and permanent maintenance of a weight that is natural for you. And the beauty is that to accomplish this balancing act is simple.

Homeostasis

If you go out for a thirty minute walk your pulse rate is likely to increase by 20 to 50 percent depending on how fast you walk and what kind of shape you're in. After you stop walking, however, your pulse rate automatically returns to its initial resting rate. In fact, every process in your body has a "set point" which is normal for you. Physiologists refer to this ability to maintain a precisely constant level of function as *homeostasis*. Other common examples of homeostasis in operation abound. It's the reason your body maintains its internal temperature of 98.6°. despite being in the cold or heat. It is also why, if you are healthy, your blood sugar, calcium, and potassium levels stay so perfectly constant. Everything in the human body operates according to many complex natural laws that have been perfected over millions of years of human evolution.

One important example of homeostasis at work in your body is the function of your pancreas. The pancreas is made up of thousands of individual round islands of cells called *Islets of Langerhans*. The outer cells in each little islet produce glucagon while the inner cells make insulin. It is these tiny structures buried deep within your pancreas that perfectly balance a large number of critically vital processes in your body including blood glucose levels, providing nutrition for the entire brain, carbohydrate and fat metabolism, cholesterol production, arterial smooth muscle proliferation, and the ratio of storage and burning of energy.

Another example of homeostasis in the physiology is actually something very pertinent to this book: *body weight*. Believe it or not, your weight is really regulated with almost perfect precision. Consider that during the average lifetime, the average individual consumes approximately 60 million kcal. A gain or loss of 25 pounds (equivalent to 86,000 kcal) represents a deviation of *approximately 0.001%*. This lifetime regulation of body weight occurs not only in non-obese people but in obese people as well. In obesity, the "set point" is elevated and the obese individual's weight is in relation to that.

When you stop and think about it, its quite inexplicable how hundreds and thousands of these biological processes are maintained day after day, year after year in such precise sequences and measures. And then consider that they do not occur in isolation but must be perfectly coordinated in order to sustain health, and you begin to understand the utter miracle of homeostasis.

The approach in Western science that has been attempted for the past three centuries is to reduce each individual process down to its minute details and to try to determine what chemicals and processes account for homeostasis in each one. It would be a monumental task to do so, even if it were possible. It is not. This reductionist approach can only lead to an infinite chain of unexplainable observations, which will require more and more research and never produce full understanding. The reality is that we are more than just an admixture of biological processes and set points. There is within each of us an innate intelligence that regulates and coordinates all of these processes in a way that is uniquely perfect for us. That intelligence is your Ayurvedic Constitutional Type, determined by the proportion of the three doshas and gunas you were born with. Just as the unique proportion of the three doshas and gunas determines your physical characteristics and your mental tendencies, they also determine the individual "set points" for all of these vital physiological and biochemical processes. In other words, your constitutional type is your master setting—it is your balance point, your homeostasis.

Just as the conversion of glucose to fat is maintained in homeostasis by the pancreas, all of the thousands of physiological processes throughout your body are determined by the original setting of your doshas. Unfortunately, we have no direct way of communicating with our pancreas to shift it into fat-burning mode of operation. Studies of biofeedback techniques, hypnosis, acupuncture, herbal medicines, and many other modalities have failed to prove effective. Nor is it possible to take oral glucagon or insulin pills because they are quickly degraded by digestive enzymes.

However, you can directly and profoundly communicate with and modify your doshic balance. We are not talking about modifying your Ayurvedic Constitutional Type—that is permanent throughout your entire lifetime and cannot be altered. It is your original setting. It is when you begin to aggravate one or more doshas and acquire an excess or deficiency of those doshas that you develop imbalances and diseases, such as obesity. It is this doshic imbalance that can be influenced and modified. Through The Sattva Program you will learn how to adjust your doshas so that they can be the agents of homeostasis for every process in the body, including maintaining your ideal weight.

C. DIGESTION AND TOXICITY: JATHAGNI AND AMA

One of the most important realities about our bodies that we must understand is that we are not frozen and unchanging masses of flesh and bones but rather we are constantly changing. This idea is acknowledged by both modern science and ancient wisdom. Today we know that we break down and build up our body tissues every moment of each day; in medical parlance these processes are known as catabolism (breaking down) and anabolism (building up). Even nervous tissue, which until recently was regarded as a tissue that did not undergo these processes, is now known to be able to regenerate under optimum conditions.

How this regeneration of tissues takes place is of great interest to researchers investigating obesity because the processes that build up tissues can do so either in a fat-increasing manner or fat-reducing manner. What determines which pathway these processes will take is the state of the *cellular digestion*. Every time we eat we send our food through a complex and intricate cascade of biochemical transformations which incorporate the "foreign" food substance into our own "self". Digestion and assimilation of our food is an amazing and precise activity that has not been adequately understood by modern western medicine. What *is* known is that digestion is an energy-dependent process that begins even before we put anything in our mouths. Digestion begins in the *mind* with what is termed the cerebral phase of digestion. This means that in anticipation of the meal the brain sends signals to begin the manufacture and release of digestive juices and enzymes. The quantity of these juices may be determined by how strong one's appetite is. Appetite, according to Ayurveda, originates from a set of digestive fires known as *agnis*. Agni is a Sanskrit word that means "fire". Actually, the modern understanding of digestion and the Ayurvedic understanding are remarkably similar up to a point. Ayurveda describes the process of digestion as requiring a precise amount of fire (agni), neither too little or too much. When your appetite is strong it means your fire is burning high; conversely, when the body requires nourishment it signals agni to burn higher, which creates a heightened appetite. When agni is burning high, then the digestive organs and the individual cells of all bodily tissues can best digest and assimilate food substances and convert them into tissues and energy and not fat and toxins.

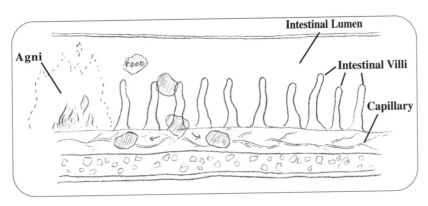

FOOD ABSORPTION

In the Ayurvedic teaching, digestion refers not only to the (gross) absorption of foods through the lining of the small intestine and into the blood stream, but also includes the assimilation of that food at the (subtle) cellular and sub-cellular—i.e. mitochondrial—level. Individuals who have weight problems always have disturbances in their gross and subtle digestion. Improper and inefficient digestion creates a toxic endogenous byproduct known as *ama*. Ama has attributes of both an energy and a substance. It is a white, sticky material that adheres to and obstructs the various channels through which bodily nutrient and wastes flow throughout the body. Cholesterol plaques in the arterial walls would be an accurate way of visualizing one example of ama. Another common example of ama is the white, sticky coating you may see on your tongue—especially in the morning—which comes from the blood. However, besides blood and lymph ama also blocks the circulation of *energies* throughout the body. Due to its widespread capacity to disrupt normal flows and communications in the physiology, ama is the common cause of a wide variety of diseases and conditions. In overweight individuals it creates so many of the symptoms we see including fatigue, resistance to exercise, dullness, lack of resolve, compulsive eating patterns, irregular eating patterns, bloating, food cravings, and obesity.

This chapter will explore why we must address the problem of *ama* and improve and balance the *agni* before we can significantly and permanently create weight loss.

D. PATHOGENESIS OF OBESITY: THE SIX STAGES OF ANY DISEASE

Obesity is caused by an excess of Kapha dosha. Individuals with a Kapha constitution are born with an inherent attraction to food, especially sweet, heavy, oily, and cooling foods. The same is true for people who *acquire* a Kapha imbalance. Some foods that cause an accumulation of Kapha dosha include: milk, curd, butter, sugar, flesh of animals from wet regions, dates, avocados, coconuts and most oils. Similarly, Kapha types also tend to somehow circumvent adequate physical exercise, enjoy sleep, may abstain from sexual intercourse for extended periods of time, and will surround themselves with comforts and luxuries when given the opportunity. However, individuals of any Ayurvedic constitutional type can accumulate excess Kapha dosha and thus become obese. It is important for all of us to identify (and correct) the unique factors which have created the tendency to accumulate excess Kapha dosha. These factors can be exacerbated by genetic predispositions to obesity, emotional imbalances, and concurrent diseases such as hypothyroidism, Cushing's syndrome (hypersecretion of cortisol), or lesions within the hypothalamus. Simultaneous with measures to eliminate excess Kapha we must also incorporate measures to address our other specific and unique constitutional imbalances.

The Sattva Program derives from Ayurvedic Medicine—a comprehensive system of health care that originated approximately 3500 years ago and is still practiced in India and worldwide. As a complete system of medicine, Ayurveda has an elaborate and detailed philosophy of disease and treatment. It is not necessary to describe all of these philosophies at length here. The interested reader should refer to the appendix for a list of excellent reviews of the principles of Ayurvedic medicine.

It is relevant, however, to discuss the Ayurvedic understanding of the pathogenesis of disease—how disease arises in the human physiology. You will get a good idea from this one small example of Ayurvedic philosophy how profound the understanding was of these ancient physicians of the nature of disease.

The Six Stages Of Disease (*Sat Kriyakala*)

Ayurveda precisely identifies six stages of any disease process which describe the disturbance and movement of the aggravated doshas in the physiology. They are named:

1. Accumulation
2. Aggravation
3a. Spread
3b. Remission
4. Localization
5. Manifestation
6. Permanent Change

This procession of six stages gives us an understanding of how the doshas undergo an increase as a result of aggravating factors (diet, lifestyle, climate, emotional stress, seasons, etc.). Each dosha initially accumulates in areas of the body that are their respective normal sites (i.e. Vata = colon, mind, heart; Pitta = small intestines, blood, liver, skin; Kapha = stomach, lungs, joints.) If the body cannot eliminate the increasing dosha(s) and maintain homeostasis, it will begin to accumulate (Stage 1) slowly and in small quantity. If no measures are taken to correct the situation, the process continues into the next stage in which the accumulated doshas provoke and irritate the local tissues (Stage 2). If the process is allowed to proceed, the doshas will fill to capacity in the region of accumulation and finally begin to overflow and spread (Stage 3a) throughout the body. This is a critical stage in the disease process. If simple remedial measures are taken at this time, the aggravated dosha can easily recede (Stage 3b). If not, depending on the dosha and the constitution of the person, the spread can be relatively localized or, if the doshas reach the bloodstream, nervous system and other channels, quite widespread. While spreading, the doshas can mix with various tissues (e.g. muscle, tendons, nerve, pancreas, etc.) and waste products. Eventually, the disseminating dosha(s) relocate in one or more different sites where they begin to manifest symptoms of disease (Stage 4). Usually the site of relocation is determined by the existence of some previous weakness or insult at that site which may have compromised the defense mechanisms. So, for example, we know that cigarette smokers are more prone to bronchitis than non-smokers. At this stage the relocated doshas rapidly become more concentrated at the cellular and organ levels than in earlier stages. When the now established dosha(s) re-accumulate and alter the structure and/or function at the site, clinical manifestations of the disease appear (Stage 5). This is normally the point at which people realize something is wrong and seek medical attention. At this stage we can often recognize and name the disease: asthma, arthritis, overweight, etc.. If no intervention takes place, the disease fully matures and accelerates and can permanently and irreversibly alter the function of the tissues affected (Stage 6). Complications that are unique features of the particular disease process can now manifest. For example, untreated diabetes mellitus evolves into kidney, nerve, and retinal degeneration.

According to the Ayurvedic concept, it is always easier to treat the excess doshas while they are still in their original sites (Stages 1 and 2). The stage of spread (Stage3) is the transitional stage. As the doshas first relocate (Stage 4), there is still strong defensive energy available, so treatment is still very effective. In the final two stages, where the disease manifests and matures (stages 5 and 6), treatment becomes more difficult but still possible. If progression is permitted to the latter stages of Stage 6, the disease is incurable.

The Six Stages of Obesity

The specific evolution of obesity according to Ayurveda is as follows:

The excessive use of foods with sweet, heavy, oily, moist, bulky, slimy, soft, and cooling qualities, in addition to the factors enumerated above, causes an increase in Kapha dosha. This Kapha excess is the initiating factor.

One of the sites in the human body where Kapha dosha will accumulate is the stomach. When this accumulation reaches a critical point, the entire digestive process is impaired.

The impairment of digestion is due to a deficiency in *jathagni*, the main digestive fire, which results from the excess Kapha in the stomach "extinguishing" the fire. (see p. 47)

The deficiency of Jathagni results in incomplete digestion of ingested foods that result in a digestive residue being left behind. This residue is known as *Ama*.

The Ama initially combines with the blood plasma just as it is created from the ingested foods being absorbed in the small intestines; this Ama-Plasma complex circulates throughout the body and settles in the fat tissues.

This accumulation of Ama in the fat tissues (Meda dhatu) causes a disturbance in the way in which fat metabolism occurs. It creates disturbances in important enzymes (dhatwagnis) and other factors involved with fat utilization.

Consequently, fat tissue increases throughout the body and the pro-
dromal symptoms of obesity begin to manifest followed by the actual
symptoms (rupas).

E. The Twenty Gunas: The Qualities of Matter

Ayurveda teaches us that all organic and inorganic matter, as well as
all thoughts, feelings, and actions have distinctive qualities, or *gunas*,
which characterize them. There are ten pairs of gunas, each pair consisting of a specific quality and its opposite. For example dry and oily,
hard and soft, etc. Throughout the whole of nature, we can see the play
of so many of these pairs of opposites occurring together in balance:
man and woman, day and night, sympathetic and parasympathetic
nerves, land and sea, and so forth. In each pair, the two elements are
indispensable to each other and one cannot exist without the other. In
fact, the entire universe has been described as the interplay of two great
antagonistic forces which eternally creates, sustains, and destroys all
that exists. The ancient Chinese called these two forces Yin and Yang;
the ancient Hindus called them Rajas and Tamas and also perceived a
third balancing force, Sattva. All great traditions describe these two
complementary forces in their own way. As these two Universal Forces
manifest down at the level of the material world, they differentiate into
the ten pairs of qualities (gunas) listed below. Note that half of these
qualities promote an increase in total tissue mass and hence body
weight and the other half promote a decrease in total tissue mass and
body weight.

The Ten Pairs Of Gunas

NOURISHING	LIGHTENING
1. Cold	Hot
2. Soft	Hard
3. Oily	Dry
4. Heavy	Light
5. Dull	Sharp
6. Gross	Subtle
7. Smooth	Rough
8. Stable	Moving
9. Turbid	Transparent
10. Solid	Liquid

The next piece of information to know is that the three doshas (Vata, Pitta, and Kapha) also have these qualities as shown in the table below. Foods, herbs, substances, or actions that consist of the same qualities as a particular dosha, will increase that dosha and even aggravate it.

The Three Doshas and Their Gunas (Qualities)

VATA	PITTA	KAPHA
Cold	Hot	Heavy
Dry	Sharp	Solid
Moving	Liquid	Stable
Light	Moving	Oily
Rough	Subtle	Cold
Hard	Light	Dull
Transparent	Soft	Smooth
Subtle		Soft
		Gross
		Turbid

If you associate with substances and activities that have qualities that are the same as the qualities composing a particular dosha, that quality will increase; if you associate with things that have qualities opposite to those which make up a dosha, that dosha will not accumulate excessively and will eventually decrease. This is known as the principle of *samanya-vishesa.*

It is important to appreciate what is being said here. It is possible to easily understand the qualities of substances if you simply become aware of the mind and senses, for they are the keys to any form of understanding and knowledge. Observe, for example, what information the senses and mind offer if you consume a large piece of cheesecake with a generous scoop of vanilla ice cream. If attention is rested on the body as a whole, one will instantly sense fullness, coolness, solidity, and perhaps lethargy and a resistance to move from the couch! These sensations are referable to the gunas of heavy, soft, cold, dull, stable, gross, solid, and so forth which are contained in those particular foods. Compare this to the sensations you might experience after having a generous amount of broccoli, bok choy, or other green vegetable. Soon after eating these vegetables you are likely to be light, warm, content, clear-minded, and energetic. Several hours after such a meal, depending on your digestive capacity you (and those around you) might experience an additional sensation: intestinal gas! These sensations are all referable to the gunas of lightness, warmth, clear, etc. contained in those foods.

Through an understanding of the twenty gunas and their relationships with the doshas, you can easily predict which qualities will promote weight loss and gain. You will also gain great insight into which foods and substances will balance your constitution and thereby promote health in general.

Why It Is Important To Understand Doshas and Gunas

The principal theme of this book is the relationship of the diet to the vitality of the body and mind. The foundational concepts of Ayurveda summarized above have been used for over 3000 years to effortlessly guide individuals towards proper food selections, preparation, and weight control as well as health in general. As we enter the twenty-first century people from many parts of the planet are searching for a lifestyle plan and dietary program that promotes optimal physical health and emotional/spiritual growth as well. *The Sattva Program* derives from the wisdom of Ayurvedic Medicine and provides an effective method for weight loss and maintenance that is precisely adaptable and sensitive to individual requirements. The program is a comprehensive guide to lifestyle recommendations and nutrition that takes into account specific constitutional needs while effectively addressing weight loss issues. Although *sattva* is a uniquely Hindu concept, its principles can be recognized in the core ideas of almost every ancient health system from the Chinese to the Native Americans. The common features in such traditions have been access to higher states of consciousness, peaceful societies, and long, healthy lifespans.

Diets Don't Work

There is now no dispute within the medical community that restrictive diets are rarely, if ever, successful over the long run in helping people lose and maintain their weight at a healthy level. From the simplest forms (self-supervised calorie-counting or over-the-counter appetite suppressants) to the more intricate forms (proprietary weight loss programs, physician- or dietitian-supervised programs, or one of the new fad high-protein diets), research shows a similar pattern. Most individuals will lose a small amount of weight initially with *any* of these unnatural regimens. However, within 1-2 years most people gain all of the weight back, and many gain even more. Despite these statistics, dietary products and weight loss programs have grown into a *50 billion-dollar* industry in the United States alone. We continue to be bombarded with infomercials, books, articles, and testimonials about novel diets that don't work in the long run.

The general consensus that now exists regarding the ineffectiveness of dieting in producing long-term weight loss for the majority of people gave rise to the conclusion reached at the recent National Institutes of Health Consensus Conference (1992) that the treatment of obesity should emphasize "strategies that can produce health benefits independently of weight loss". Although most of the pundits at this conference probably never heard of Ayurveda, their search could realistically end there if they only knew.

In 1991, it was estimated that at any given time 65 million Americans are dieting. Some achieve modest short-term weight reduction. Yet, according to the National Institutes of Health (1992), one-third to two-thirds of this weight is regained within one year and almost all is regained after five years. At the same time that we have all these millions of people dieting, the prevalence of obesity in this country has increased alarmingly from 12.0% in 1991 to 22.5% in 1994, and this is considered a conservative estimate (Third National Health and Nutrition Examination Survey).

It seems obvious that the explanation for the failure of the current dietary approaches to weight loss and maintenance lies in the fundamental defect in the general conventional paradigm that defines health in the modern world. Modern medicine has convinced most of us that health is a uniquely physical state. Ayurveda, in its wisdom, teaches that health requires the integration of the mental, emotional, spiritual, environmental, as well as the physical aspects of life. We must always keep the proper perspective. Weight is only one element of physical well-being, and physical well-being is only one element of complete well-being. Rather than a limited focus on pounds and body fat percentage, a successful approach must be more holistic in nature focusing on eating in a natural, calm manner, participating in fun physical activities, and treasuring your life to the fullest extent. That holistic approach has been followed for many centuries by those aware of Ayurveda—it is called *The Sattva Program*®.

CHAPTER 6.

HOW TO GET STARTED: TEN EASY STEPS

Writing this book has been a magical and rejuvenating experience for me. This is chiefly because I made a resolution one year ago to personally follow *The Sattva Program*® for the duration of the writing process. I actually did this for two very pragmatic reasons.

The first was that I myself had a need to lose a little excess weight (10 kg or about 22 pounds) which had accumulated over the past several years. I honestly have followed an Ayurvedic lifestyle for more than twenty years and am in excellent general health. However, I come from a family that has been prone to overweight (and in some cases obesity) and due to this my tendency toward this condition is apparently particularly strong. Reflecting upon my life prior to this writing, I realized that certain aspects of my daily routine had slipped and could be improved and reoriented to specifically promote weight loss and maintenance. So I have taken this opportunity to re-establish balance and correct this situation through *The Sattva Program*®.

The second reason was that I knew that as the weeks and months went on, it would give me continuous insight into the practicality and potential obstacles to the many Ayurvedic recommendations that comprise the program. Ayurveda provides wisdom and guidance for becoming skillful in creating balance and healing through diet, lifestyle modification, and mind-body awareness. However, as you have probably realized if you have read through this book, the synthesis of *all* of the facets of this program can initially seem a little daunting for busy Westerners. To fully implement this program, it requires most people to learn a substantial amount of new material regarding food, diet, exercise, fasting, herbal medicine, and other areas. It also imposes, in its complete form, a variety of behavioral changes that might be difficult to accomplish all at once. Therefore, I realized that an essential section of this book would be a short chapter representing a distillation of *only the most important recommendations* for actually beginning the program. Having myself followed the program for more than a year now, I feel qualified to finally write this short but important chapter. I can tell you that had I not actually applied the recommendations to myself, this section would certainly have been different. I hope the personal insights I have gained prove to be helpful to you as you begin this program for weight loss. That is what follows below. By the way, I did indeed lose the 22 pounds—in fact, over the last twelve months I actually lost *30 pounds* (13 kg)! I want nothing more than for you, the reader, to share in this experience as well. For like all of Ayurveda, *The Sattva Program*® can certainly lead you to health, balance and harmony at a level far beyond your expectations.

More and more people around the world are seeking a nutritional and lifestyle plan that promotes both a high level of physical vitality and integrity as well as emotional, mental and spiritual evolution. A major unifying theme of this book, in fact, is the direct relationship and influence of not only our diet but of many diverse aspects of our lives to our weight, and ultimately our health. *The Sattva Program*® for weight loss is an excellent, time-tested model of life-affirming holistic principles that are highly adaptable to individual needs for weight management.

The Program in its entirety should be thought of as a goal towards which we all can aspire. *The Sattva Program*®, as you know, presents comprehensive behavioral and spiritual practices developed over many millennia in addition to its dietary and lifestyle guidelines. As we begin the program, however, we may prefer to start with a comfortable and natural combination of recommendations that we can easily incorporate with little or no effort—without compromising on effectiveness or results.

Here are the ten most important recommendations for an easy start to *The Sattva Program*®. Where appropriate an item will contain information about the place in the text where you can read about it in more detail. Some are simply self-explanatory. If you do nothing more from this program than follow these ten recommendations, you will unquestionably see results within two weeks. So I exhort you to disregard your past failures, rid yourself of any poisonous doubts, and begin this exciting and simple program of healing and weight loss today.

1. After determining your Ayurvedic Constitutional Type using the questionnaire found in Chapter 3, begin to follow the specific diet for your constitution (Vata, Pitta, or Kapha).
These three diets are all found in Chapter 12.

2. Use the *Sattvic Satiety Scale* and do not exceed a level of "7.5" at any meal.
Please, please familiarize yourself with this scale; it will change your life. The most important number on the scale is "7.5". This corresponds precisely to the sensation of being satisfied with the amount of food you have taken in without being either too full or still hungry.

THE SATTVIC SATIETY SCALE

	Begin Eating						Optimal Satiety (Stop Eating)		
0	1	2	3	4	5	6	7	8	9	10

Very Hungry   **Very Full**

The other important level to remember is "2.0," which is the level at which one should be when beginning a meal. It corresponds to the feeling of noticeable hunger and the desire for food. It normally occurs 5-6 hours following the previous meal. See p. 83 for complete description.

3. If you currently are a non-vegetarian, begin the transition towards a more plant-based diet.
Limit the intake of any type of flesh foods (e.g. meats, poultry and fish) to 4-5 ounces per meal. This is approximately equivalent to a portion equal in size to the palm of your hand. Eventually try to limit the consumption of flesh foods to only once a day.

4. Consciously limit processed sugar and other sweeteners as much as possible (sucrose, corn syrup, dextrose, maple syrup, etc.)

5. Do not eat after dinner.

6. Begin the Walking Program as described in Chapter 10.
Your initial goal should be 20 minutes of walking five days per

week (100 minutes per week). Walking is becoming recognized by a growing number of medical professionals as an important first step in restoring harmony and regaining control over one's weight. It is not a minor feature of this program but a specific therapy which is multi-dimensional and which brings benefit to many different areas of human function. For example, we now know that a simple walking program, such as the one outlined here, promotes and maintains weight loss, improves insulin resistance, improves circulation, protects and strengthens the heart, increases the respiratory capacity, increases HDL-cholesterol, increases muscle coordination and flexibility, and may even up-regulate the immune system. Besides these effects, we all know the tremendous amount of self-esteem we feel when we exercise regularly!

7. Sip warm water (Pitta types) or hot water (Vata, Kapha types) frequently throughout the day.

Keeping the body free from toxic accumulations in the various tissues is an important aspect of optimal health. One of the main benefits of sipping hot or warm water throughout the day as opposed to cold water is the dilating effect this will tend to have on the tissues and channels of the body. Dilation, in turn, makes it easier for toxins to be removed through natural physiological processes. Common experience teaches us that trying to clean any surface with hot water is far more efficient than when using cold water.

8. Consciously see to it that your total water intake each day is 6 to 8 12-ounce glasses (approximately 3 liters).

As I will point out in the last part of Chapter 7, the sensations of thirst and hunger are felt together to indicate the brains needs for additional immediate energy. Drinking adequate water throughout the day before and after meals will reduce the intensity of the thirst and hunger and therefore help prevent overeating. When water intake is insufficient, you are likely to feel more "hungry" and eat larger portions of food at more frequent intervals in an effort to supply necessary sugar to the brain. On the other hand, if the brain senses an adequate volume of water in the body, the risk of over-eating weight gain is greatly reduced.

9. Herbal supplementation.
As a minimum, everyone should begin taking the *Sattvic Basic Formulation* described on p. 180 for the initial three months.
It is extremely well-tolerated, effective, safe, and appropriate for all constitutional types. It can be obtained from The National Institute of Ayurvedic Medicine by calling toll free (888) 246-NIAM or by visiting their website at http://www.niam.com.

As I have already stated, Ayurveda contains a reliable and increasingly evidence-based databank on herbal medicines that promote and maintain detoxification, general balance and weight reduction. Herbs are generally best used in combination to support lipid metabolism, blood cleansing, tissue cleansing, thermogenesis, or to strengthen the function of the immune system. In addition to herbal materials, Ayurveda also uses common medicinal spices to help direct and intensify the effects of the treatment. Ayurveda does not abandon the achievements of medical science but rather integrates it with knowledge gained over the millennia and shapes a rational and intuitive synthesis of ancient and modern knowledge. The Sattvic Basic Formulation is an example of this integration and is an easy way to begin. At any time you feel comfortable, add the other more specific herbs for your constitution to your regimen. (See Chapter 12 for the Vata, Pitta, and Kapha specific herbal formulations.)

10. Cultivate the habit of performing The Attention Exercise described on p. 91 at least once each day.
Ayurveda certainly recognizes that there is no limit to the potential power of the mind. The only limitations are one's that we self-impose. Along with thoughts, our emotions are an aspect of our mind which carry tremendous force. This force can be directed by the human will to achieve positive (or negative) aims. We must all begin to realize that thoughts and feelings are not some vague, impotent aspect of human life, but rather are what creates our reality. Thoughts become things. Positive thoughts become positive things; negative thoughts become negative things. That is why it is very important to be aware of what we think and feel. Ayurveda ultimately promotes yoga and meditation practices as a method for understanding how we may be using our deepest thoughts and emotions against ourselves. However, it may take a while for many people to develop a strong interest in these very dis-

ciplined practices. In the meantime, The Attention Exercise represents an excellent and powerful way to develop a higher level of awareness of the inner workings of our mind. Learning to shift our attention from a narrow focus where, often out of habit, it remains "captured" by some sensation or stimulus to a wider focus where our attention is "free" to observe our immediate situation can provide a view into the deeper layers of the mind. By simply opening up our attention, we experience a calm awareness—a heightened level of consciousness that can sometimes give us a simple insight into thoughts and emotions that are controlling our behavior.

Chapter 7.

The Sattva Program® for Permanent Weight Loss

The Sattva Program®

S attva is a Sanskrit word meaning harmony and balance; it also connotes purity and goodness. Ayurveda has for centuries described practices that increase the sattva in one's life and thereby bring about a state of balance and health. Sattvic practices nourish the mental, emotional and spiritual base of an individual regardless of religious orientation. Because no therapy can ever be effective over the long run without improving these deep aspects of life, *The Sattva Program®* is the key to all weight maintenance programs. Because a chief consequence of sattvic practices is to strengthen, discipline, and delight the mind it is clear that this approach must be at the foundation of every successful weight management plan.

The Sattva Program® is a program that combines general principles of sattvic living with specific individualized constitutional guidelines. Overweight conditions are effectively addressed by understanding these conditions for what they truly are—an accumulated toxin with both physical and mental roots that are unique for each person. The molecular structure of human fat which deposits in different individuals may be identical, but the unhealthy habits, attitudes, misconceptions, and stored emotional experiences which promulgate obesity are unique and singular.

The first step in using *The Sattva Program®* is to determine your Ayurvedic Constitutional Type. You have been shown how to do this in Chapter 3. In this Chapter, we will describe the tenets of the Sattvic lifestyle which are common to individuals of all constitutional types who desire long-term weight loss.

Finally, in Chapter 12 we will describe what specific measures are recommended for each specific constitutional type. In addition to the general program described here, these measures will include specific recommendations for diet, exercise, Ayurvedic herbal supplements, breathing exercises, and many other simple yet powerful weight-management techniques based on your constitutional type. Once you make a firm resolution to lose your excess weight by following this program based on sound nutrition and healthy living, weight loss will result in every case—I have not yet seen it fail.

The General Sattva Program For All Constitutional Types

The original Ayurvedic text outline clear instructions for daily living. These recommendations are called the Ayurvedic daily regimen. There is also information given which suggest ways that we should adapt to each season of the year; this group of suggestions are called the Ayurvedic seasonal regimen, and are described later in Chapter 13. The concept being put forth is that by adhering to the cycles of nature and acting appropriately throughout the day and the year, our doshas will achieve and maintain balance and excellent health will arise naturally.

The Sattva Program integrates the time-tested wisdom of Ayurveda with the most scientifically up-to-date knowledge of weight-loss and weight maintenance techniques.

Individuals of all Types should follow the daily regimen given here. It is the core of the Sattvic Program to lose weight and maintain it. You will modify some of these practices according to your Ayurvedic Constitutional Type when indicated below.

Morning

Establish the habit of waking up between 5:30 and 6:30 AM.

Upon arising drink an 8 oz. glass of filtered water into which you have squeezed the juice from half a lemon.

Evacuate the bladder and bowels, wash the hands and face, the eyes, brush the teeth, scrape the tongue.

Perform a five-minute Garshana Self-Massage every day before bathing. (see pg. 93)

Perform a fifteen-minute Abhyanga Self-Massage following Garshana Massage. (see pg. 95)

Exercise for twenty minutes: outdoor walking, treadmill, calisthenics, aerobics, or yoga according to the recommendations for your Ayurvedic Constitutional Type. (see Chapter 3)

Bathe or shower. Shave if necessary. Wash the entire body two separate times.

Dress in clean fresh clothes; use perfumes, jewelry, and ornaments according to the recommendations for your Ayurvedic Constitutional Type.

Rest in meditation for 20-30 minutes preceded by pranayama (breathing exercises; see sections on specific Constitutional types).

Take morning dosage of any appropriate herbal supplements. (see Chapter 12)

Breakfast: whole grain cereals (preferably hot, but cold is acceptable), fresh fruits and fruit juices are the healthiest choices. Specifically millet, brown rice, amaranth, quinoa, or buckwheat are the best cooked whole grains for breakfast. (see "Recipes" Chapter 15 for delicious and simple ways to prepare these items.)

Sip hot water frequently (about every 30-60 minutes) throughout the morning. Herbal teas that are recommended for your Type are also acceptable.

Afternoon

Determine your Ayurvedic Caloric Needs based on your Ayurvedic Constitutional Type, sex, frame size, and activity level. (see Chapter 9)

Eat a plant-based, primarily vegetarian diet based on your Ayurvedic caloric needs.

Observe the principles of Ayurvedic Food Combining described in the next chapter. The one most important Ayurvedic principle is *never to eat protein and starch at the same meal.* Another way of stating this point: never eat two heavy foods (i.e. concentrated foods) at the same meal. A heavy food is anything other than a fruit or a vegetable. It is really simple once you get the hang of it.

Reduce the intake of fat, especially saturated fat (red meat, butter, cheese, egg yolks, whole milk, coconut, peanuts).

It is, however, essential to have 1-2 tsp. per day of unrefined, cold pressed flaxseed oil or alternatively 1-2 tablespoons of flaxmeal (ground flax seeds). Either can be sprinkled on grains or vegetables. Flax seeds contain omega-3-fatty acid which increases the metabolism of fat. Keep the oil and/or ground seeds refrigerated.

Always clean the hands, feet, and mouth before eating.

The dining table and dining room must be clean and the atmosphere cheerful, light, and well-ventilated. Always ensure that the dining room is warm and have candles on the table whenever possible.

Before or at the beginning of lunch and dinner have a small amount (approximately 1/8 tsp.) of fresh grated ginger root with a few drops of fresh lemon juice. Follow with a few sips of water to wash it down.

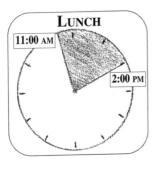

Make lunch the largest and main meal of the day and always eat it between 11:00 AM and 2:00 PM.

For lunch, strongly consider proper combinations of: soups of all kinds (especially bean soups), fresh salads, steamed or stir-fried vegetables, whole grain bread (i.e. pita, chapati), beans and other legumes.

There is a sequence in which foods of different tastes should be eaten. Foods having either a sweet taste (whole grains) or having a high protein content (legumes, soy) should be consumed first, then foods with sour and salty tastes, followed by pungent tastes and finally by foods with the bitter and astringent (most vegetables) tastes. A *small* amount of the sweet taste is acceptable at the conclusion of the meal.

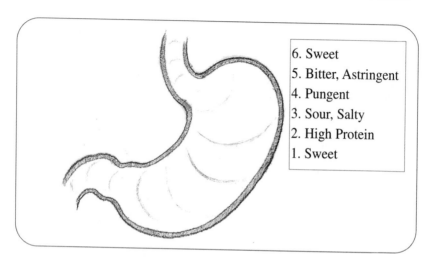

6. Sweet
5. Bitter, Astringent
4. Pungent
3. Sour, Salty
2. High Protein
1. Sweet

Limit your intake of animal foods to 4-6 oz. per day if you choose to have any at all. Regard animal foods as condiments used to supplement your meal in small amounts. Favor fish and skinless poultry. Omit red meat altogether.

There should be an interval of approximately 4 to 5 hours between breakfast and lunch and 5 to 6 hours between lunch and dinner.

Sip hot water frequently throughout the afternoon. This is an important part of the program. We recommend obtaining a stainless steel thermos to keep the hot water very accessible.

Drink between 6 and 8 glasses of filtered water or herbal teas each day. If you can make all of the water *hot*, this is optimal; if not, make up the difference with room temperature water.

Avoid daytime sleep.

Evening

If it suits your schedule, exercise in the late afternoon. Up to thirty minutes prior to dinner is an excellent idea since it naturally modulates appetite and increases the daily energy expenditure. This practice is not mandatory but certainly worth trying very hard to establish either as your main exercise time or as an additional period.

Evening meditation for 20-30 minutes before dinner.

Dinner should be lighter and less rich than lunch and not later than 7:30 PM.

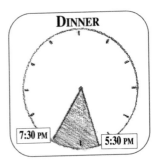

Dinner: fresh vegetable salads, cooked vegetables, soups, whole grains, legumes. (See Chapter 15)

Never retire to bed sooner than 2 hours after the evening meal; the ideal interval to wait is 3 hours or more.

After dinner consume no further food. Only herbal teas and water are permitted.

Try to avoid stressful or strenuous activities in the evening.

Try to establish a bedtime of 10:00 to 10:30 PM.

Additional Points of The Sattva Program

Sattvic Eating Behavior At Home

1. Establish specific times and places for eating and eat *only* according to these conditions. For example, when at home eating should be restricted to *the dining room* at 7:30 AM and 6:30 PM. If you normally are also at home for lunch, eat at a set time.

2. Never eat while in the kitchen.

3. Never eat in response to guests coming to visit unexpectedly; learn to serve guests food without compromising your own discipline.

4. Establish the good habit to *always* say some form of grace before any meal *or snack*. This will emphasize to the mind the importance and true significance of each meal, which is to provide nourishment for our mind and body through the generosity of Nature.

If you do not know any appropriate sayings, one very nice Ayurvedic grace before meals is: "Om Paramatmane Namah" which simply means "We acknowledge the Divine Spirit in ourselves and in all things".

5. Always wash the hands and face before meals and snacks.

6. During meals concentrate on eating. Establish the etiquette of not discussing intense subjects or personal problems during meals.

7. Put all the courses on the table at the start of the meal. This will permit everyone to see the entire meal and avoid overeating items that are served early in the meal because they weren't aware of items to follow.

8. After you (and others at the table) have filled your plate with portions of the various foods being served, remove the bowls and platters of food from the dining table. This may seem like an awkward inconvenience at first, but it is a very important habit to establish.

Athletic and hard laboring members of the family should go into the kitchen and serve themselves extra food if necessary.

9. *Thoroughly* chew each bite of food and swallow completely before taking another bite.

10. Make a conscious effort to *eat slowly* and never bolt food down. The average time to eat a meal is 30 minutes.

It takes the brain approximately twenty minutes to register the degree of fullness in the stomach. If you eat too fast, your stomach will be full but your brain won't yet know it and you will overeat—only to realize a few minutes later that you are *stuffed!*

11. Always provide ample time for all meals and never eat in a hurry.

12. After the meal, remove leftovers from the table immediately and store or discard them appropriately. Never provide opportunities for nibbling to continue after the meal.

13. According to Ayurveda, the proper amount of food to be consumed at any meal is that amount which would fit comfortably into both hands when placed together and held outstretched. This amount of food would fill the stomach 50%. Each individual's hands are uniquely proportional to his or her own stomach.

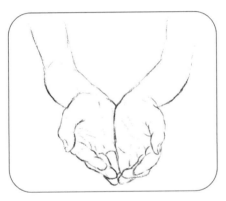

Another way of saying the same thing is that at every meal, the stomach should be filled 50% with solid or semi-solid foods, 25% with liquid beverages sipped throughout the meal, and 25% left empty—or more precisely left with air, which is necessary for any process of combustion.

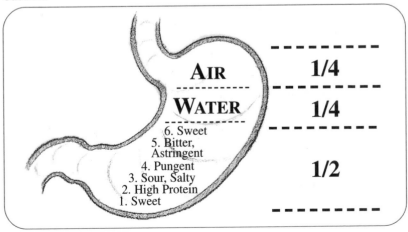

AIR — 1/4

WATER — 1/4

6. Sweet
5. Bitter, Astringent
4. Pungent
3. Sour, Salty
2. High Protein
1. Sweet

1/2

CHAPTER 7. THE SATTVA PROGRAM FOR PERMANENT WEIGHT LOSS

There is yet a third method of monitoring the quantity of food we take in at any meal, which may be the most useful of the three. This is a mind-body method that I learned long ago from the then assistant dean at the College of Ayurveda in Thiruvanathapuram, Professor Mrs. P.G. Cherdolhar. I have continued to employ this technique over the last twenty years with consistent success.

The technique utilizes the satiety scale illustrated below which is pictured in the mind.

THE SATTVIC SATIETY SCALE

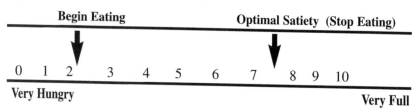

The Sattvic Satiety Scale is a measure of how hungry you are feeling at any time.

Level 0 represents the most hungry that you can be. There is no food in the stomach and you are feeling *very* hungry. In theory, you should eat before this point and never reach this level.

Level 10, on the other hand, represents the point at which you could not eat another morsel of food. You are experiencing abdominal distention and heaviness. People commonly experience Level 10 when having Thanksgiving Dinner at their mother's home.

Level 7.5 is the optimal point in any meal when you should stop eating. It represents the point at which you are satisfied but not stuffed. You feel light, alert and happy and ready for your next activity. ***Important: The difference between Level 7.5 and 8 or 9 can be as little as one or two forks of food.*** That is why it is important to pay attention to the eating process throughout the meal.

Level 2 represents the level at which the food from the previous meal has been completely digested and assimilated and now the stomach has emptied and the body is requiring more energy as food. You feel hungry. This is the point when you should begin to eat. According to Ayurveda, one should not eat unless the Satiety Scale has come down to Level 2.

Levels 3, 4, 5 are increasing levels of "fullness" and satiety as you eat a meal. These are also levels which are experienced "on the way down" the scale after you've eaten and the meal is being digested over the next several hours.

Level 6, 7 represent degrees of satiety; 7.5 is optimal.

Levels 8, 9 are the levels at which you have definitely over-eaten. There is fullness, heaviness, abdominal distention, resistance to movement and mental lethargy. This is the average point at which most people are conditioned to stop eating. Learn *not* to reach these levels by cultivating attention during meals.

Hunger is a subjective feeling by which the body signals the mind that energy to sustain its life processes is required. Hunger also occurs when the digestive system, which is of course responsible for the digestion and initial metabolism of food, is in a state of readiness. Ayurveda teaches that we should eat only when we are hungry. Just as arising and starting the day early in the morning near sunrise is an example of becoming more in tune with natural cycles and rhythms, so is eating only when one is hungry.

The Sattva Satiety Scale will help you harmonize your eating patterns with your hunger level. After just a few days of working with this scale, you will be able to accurately determine your satiety level (i.e. hunger) at any moment. This mental exercise is simply one example of how we can use our attention to access knowledge about our world. Whenever we are able to rest our *full attention* on any person, object, or situation, *knowledge* arises spontaneously and guides us to take whatever action is appropriate.

I recommend that everybody who is interested in losing weight conduct the following exercise.

Chapter 7. The Sattva Program for Permanent Weight Loss

For one entire week, using the Sattva Satiety Scale, *eat whenever your hunger level reaches 2 or below—as many or as few times a day as this occurs.* This means that instead of paying attention to the usual external cues which signal us to eat (assigned lunch hours, dinner dates with friends, family schedules, etc.), for this one week you should only pay attention to your actual hunger levels. You will eat when your hunger level dips below 2, and stop eating at 7.5.

This exercise may possibly cause you to eat at unusual times during the day, to eat very small quantities, and even to skip meals altogether. But it is very important to try to complete an entire week of this exercise because it will help reconnect your eating behavior to your actual bodily needs. To assist you, I have included on the next page a copy of the chart I provide to my patients to track their eating patterns for the week. Use this chart to record your hunger level and emotional state before and after each meal or snack and the time you ate. As much as possible, simply record the information without blame, praise, guilt, or judgment of any kind. Just observe and record. Naturally, our eating behavior has strong effects on our emotions and recording this data may bring up feelings. It is certainly advisable to acknowledge your feelings but try not to get too caught up in them during the week.

After the week ends, it is time to re-adjust your eating schedule to the normal breakfast, lunch, and dinner times. If you wake up and begin your day at a reasonable early time and have only a light breakfast, you will indeed find that your satiety scale quite naturally reaches 2 and you become hungry right around lunchtime and dinnertime. Eating only until you have reached 7.5 soon becomes an indelible good habit. Patients with whom I've lost contact for years often tell me how this method has remained with them and has become instinctive even when other good habits have long since fallen by the wayside.

Weekly Record of Hunger Levels and Emotional States

Instructions: Record the time, hunger levels, and emotional states each time you eat whether it's a full meal or a small snack. Start with any day of the week that is convenient.

	Sat.	Sun.	Mon.	Tues.	Wed.	Thur.	Fri.
Time of eating							
Hunger level before eating							
Emotional state before eating							
Hunger level after eating							
Emotional state after eating							
Time of eating							
Hunger level before eating							
Emotional state before eating							
Hunger level after eating							
Emotional state after eating							
Time of eating							
Hunger level before eating							

	Sat.	Sun.	Mon.	Tues.	Wed.	Thur.	Fri.
Emotional state before eating							
Hunger level after eating							
Emotional state after eating							
Time of eating							
Hunger level before eating							
Emotional state before eating							
Hunger level after eating							
Emotional state after eating							
Time of eating							
Hunger level before eating							
Emotional state before eating							
Hunger level after eating							
Emotional state after eating							

	Sat.	Sun.	Mon.	Tues.	Wed.	Thur.	Fri.
Time of eating							
Hunger level before eating							
Emotional state before eating							
Hunger level after eating							
Emotional state after eating							
Time of eating							
Hunger level before eating							
Emotional state before eating							
Hunger level after eating							
Emotional state after eating							

To determine Hunger Levels refer to the Sattvic Satiety Scale

To determine Emotional State, use one or more simple descriptors such as happy, sad, nervous, calm, angry, fearful, content, tense, anxious, frustrated, worried, etc.

HERE'S AN EXAMPLE OF HOW TO USE THIS CHART:

	Sat.	Sun.	Mon.	Tues.	Wed.	Thur.	Fri.
Time of eating	12:15 pm						
Hunger level before eating	2.5						
Emotional state before eating	slightly anxious, restless						
Hunger level after eating	7.5						
Emotional state after eating	calm, alert						
Time of eating	6:30 pm						
Hunger level before eating	2.0						
Emotional state before eating	happy, enthusiastic						
Hunger level after eating	8.0						
Emotional state after eating	slightly lethargic, content but heavy						

Sattvic Eating Behavior When Not At Home

1. *Never* discuss business during meals. Gently and diplomatically request of your business acquaintance that business be discussed directly *after* the meal. Very few people cannot easily complete a meal in 30 minutes or less. Using this small portion of time for just eating

and light small talk might actually prove to be a good and practical investment as well as healthy. Friendly non-business oriented conversation can only help your business relationships.

2. Develop discipline when coaxed by dining companions to have additional food, drink, or dessert. It is more gracious to thank someone for his or her hospitality than to continue to eat everything offered to you with false enjoyment. Always be firm with yourself in these situations.

3. When traveling, plan in advance for your meals. For instance, decide if you will eat before leaving for the airport, at the airport (in that case, leave sufficient time), or on the plane. Do not eat both before *and* during the flight.

4. When ordering in a restaurant, ask for changes in the meal that are consistent with proper food combining principles.

Remember, you are eating the food and in most cases you are paying for it. You can eat whatever you want. For example, if you order eggplant parmigiana, you might ask for it without the cheese and ask the waiter what it comes with. When (s)he says "spaghetti", you could ask "What vegetables do you have today?" The answer will be some variation of "Fresh snap peas, broccoli, and asparagus." You say: "Great! Instead of the spaghetti, bring me the snap peas and asparagus with the eggplant".

Neither the waiter nor your dining companions will think this is strange—in fact most people would be impressed with your care and attention to what you put in your body.

Miscellaneous But IMPORTANT Sattvic Points

Quick stir-frying, light steaming, and baking are the best ways to cook vegetables.

The best oils to use for stir-frying are small amounts (approximately 1 tsp.) of the monounsaturated and to a lesser extent the polyunsaturated oils: olive, canola, sesame, safflower, sunflower, and soybean.

The following foods can be taken as often as desired cooked or raw: alfalfa sprouts, bell peppers, bok choy, cabbage, celery, chicory, carrots, endive, escarole, lettuce, parsley, radish, spinach, turnips, watercress.

Regarding the amount of food to be consumed at any one meal: the stomach should be filled 50% with solid and semi-solid food, 25% with water or other beverage sipped throughout the meal, and 25% should remain empty for air to ensure proper mixing and combustion.

Do a vegetable juice fast once a week for 18-24 hours. (Carrot, beet, celery, parsley, spinach, watercress, green peppers, cabbage, comfrey, artichoke, radish, potato).

Consciously omit processed sugar as well as other "sweeteners" from the diet (sucrose, corn syrup, dextrose, maple syrup, and honey).

Also omit alcohol, egg yolks, soft drinks, carbonated water, artificial flavorings, colorings, preservatives, whole milk, high fat foods, deep-fried foods, and excessive salt.

Exercise. Begin by walking a minimum of 100 minutes a week (twenty minutes five times a week). Increase to 150 minutes a week plus 100 minutes a week of weight/machine training. Read Chapter 10 entitled "Sattvic Exercise" and also see the chapter on your Ayurvedic Constitutional Type for more specific recommendations.

The Attention Exercise

Ayurveda understands the enormous power of mind-body techniques. The one key to all physical, emotional, or spiritual work is *attention*. Learning to adopt new behaviors is fundamentally about learning to shift our attention from our usual limited, obsessive focus to a much more all-inclusive appreciation of the whole. Learning to shift our attention from a narrow focus where, often out of habit, it remains "captured" by some sensation or stimulus to a wider focus where our attention is "free" to observe our immediate situation is an important lesson in life. By simply opening up our attention, we automatically become filled with a calm awareness—a heightened level of consciousness that can be easily known.

Try this simple mind-body *attention exercise* to access this consciousness. For those readers who have not yet been formally trained in a meditation technique, this exercise is a very worthy substitute for both the morning and evening meditations that are recommended.

Sit comfortably in a chair with your back straight but not rigid or tense. Rest your hands on your lap in a natural position; have your feet flat on the floor. Be comfortable.

Keep your eyes open and resting on any object that happens to be 10-12 feet in front of you. Although looking there, without moving your eyes or scanning the room, be aware of everything in your entire field of *vision*.

Become aware of any *smells* in the room that you might not have noticed previously. Also consciously note any *tastes* in your mouth (i.e. sweet, sour, bitter, metallic, etc.)

Now simply become aware of any physical sensations that are known through your sense of *touch*. Feel the hands resting on the lap... the clothing against the skin... the pressure of the back of the legs and buttocks against the chair... the breeze flowing over the face and exposed areas of your skin.

Finally, rest the attention in the *listening*. Hear *all* the various sounds in the room where you are sitting. Do not have any particular interest in any one sound; do not even bother to name the sounds—just be aware of each one as it arises and leaves. Let the listening also expand out of the room to include your entire home. Just sit quietly and listen—again with no judgment or particular focus. And now let your attention run out even farther—include your whole street...then your town...your state...the whole country...the entire planet beneath you. Don't let the mind wonder about how to do this; just let the mind follow these suggestions and it will happen perfectly. Now let your listening expand even farther to the realm of all the planets..the stars...and finally let your listening rest at a place that is beyond even the furthest sound.

Sit in this state of awareness for one or two minutes and enjoy the peace and calm.

What you have just experienced is a state of heightened consciousness which, according to how well you managed to free your attention, brought you a lot of information about yourself and your world. True and real information. Not imagined or as we say nowadays, "virtual", information. By freeing up your attention through this excercise, you can know among other things: if there are aches and pains in the body, if there are subtle odors in your environment, if there are residues in the mouth, what colors are around you and what effect, if any, are they having, and are you being exposed to disturbing noises?

This exercise, if it is done regularly, will refine your attention beyond the physical and can cultivate the higher realms of human intuitive knowledge. However, in this book we are concerned with using attention as a tool for forging a deep connection to our bodies. For everyone the physical body is our most intimate and compassionate, if not inescapable, teacher. It is also the doorway to our spiritual evolution. If we can become aware of the awesome intelligence of our bodies, we soon realize our inseparable connection to the whole earth—in fact, the entire universe.

Unfortunately, many of us who are overweight or obese have become almost entirely desensitized to our bodies and have lost the connection to its messages and intelligence. Instead, we find ourselves exiled into the world of our circling thoughts, consumed by our emotions, and subjugated by our conditioned responses. This simple mind-body technique will help you to reconnect with your body; by learning to listen to and trust in its messages we can discover our true needs.

How to Perform Garshana Self-Massage

Garshana self-massage is a dry massage done with raw silk gloves, mittens, or a loofa. (see Appendix for suppliers) All of these items are slightly rough in texture and that is exactly the point. The rough and dry qualities reduce Kapha, promote circulation in the lymph and skin capillaries, help reduce cellulite, and promote the removal of fat from the tissues. This massage aids in the loosening of toxins and impurities from the tissues. Remember to use vigorous strokes as much as possible except where indicated not to.

The massage requires only three to five minutes and is best done just before doing your daily oil massage and morning shower or bath.

1. Put on the silk gloves or pick up the loofa. Sit on a chair or on the floor.

2. Start with the feet and legs. Use moderately vigorous, moderately quick up and down strokes over the long bones of the body (i.e. tibia, fibula, femur, etc.). Start with approximately fifteen to twenty strokes over each area and gradually increase over a week to forty to fifty. Use circular strokes over the joints—half in the clockwise direction and half in the counter-clockwise direction.

3. Now stand up and massage the hips, waist, and buttocks using a combination of circular and up-and-down strokes. Massage longer in areas of cellulite, fat accumulation, or where you sense a stagnation of energy.

4. Next, massage the lower and middle back areas as far as you can reach using up-and-down strokes.

5. The abdomen should be massaged vigorously first in a clockwise direction, then diagonally from the flanks towards the groin.

6. Move up to the chest area where you should massage very lightly over the heart. The upper chest can be massaged vigorously from side-to-side.
7. Massage the shoulders, arms, elbows, forearms and wrists in one continuous, flowing motion alternating up-and-down and circular strokes over the long bones and joints, respectively.

8. Finally, massage the neck and throat areas (up-and-down), face (gently circular), ears, and head (free-style).

How to Perform Abhyanga Self-Massage

Abhyanga Self-Massage is a type of Ayurvedic oil massage that balances all three doshas, helps regulate the appetite, strengthens the entire body, nourishes the musculature, improves flexibility, brings luster to the skin, stimulates circulation, and truly promotes well-being.

1. Use one of the oils suggested for your Ayurvedic Constitutional Type. Pour some of this oil into a four- or six-ounce plastic bottle with a flip top. Warm the oil by placing the plastic bottle in a pot or other vessel containing hot water, for three or four minutes.

2. Remove your clothes and sit on a small stool or on a towel placed on the floor. Apply oil to the entire body (this is not the massage—only the application of the oil). Apply these initial approximate amounts of oil to each of the following areas:

        head, scalp, and neck ------------ two tsp.
        hands, arms, shoulders----------- one tsp. each for left and right
        front torso ----------------------- one tsp.
        buttocks and back --------------- one tsp.
        legs and feet---------------------- two tsp. each for left and right

Additional warm oil should be applied as needed as the massage proceeds.

3. The massage is performed with the ball and palm of the hand and not with the fingers. Wherever possible, use circular strokes over joints and up-and-down strokes over long bones. Use a moderate amount of pressure so that heat is generated from the strokes except over the heart and abdomen where gentler strokes are used. Start with the head and work systematically down the body (in contrast to Garshana massage, which ascends from the toes to the head).

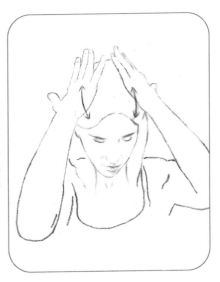

4. Start by massaging the head, using vigorous and rapid front-to-back and up-and-down strokes, as appropriate. Spend between 30 to 60 seconds on the head.

5. Next massage the face and ears, which are massaged by kneading between the thumb and forefinger. Remember to add small amounts of warm oil as needed as you massage each area.

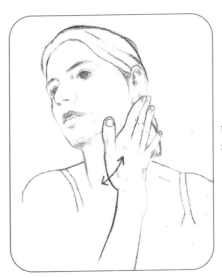

6. Massage the neck and throat areas using up-and down strokes.

7. In a rhythmic, coordinated manner using alternating circular (joints) and straight (long bones) strokes, massage the shoulders, arms and hands on both sides of the body. Create your own rhythm. For example, try massaging with up-and-down strokes for 10 strokes and with circular strokes for 5 strokes. Or make both 7 strokes. See what rhythm feels right and stay with it throughout the massage of the arms and legs. Remember to massage both the front and back aspects of each arm and include the fingertips and fingernails (important!)

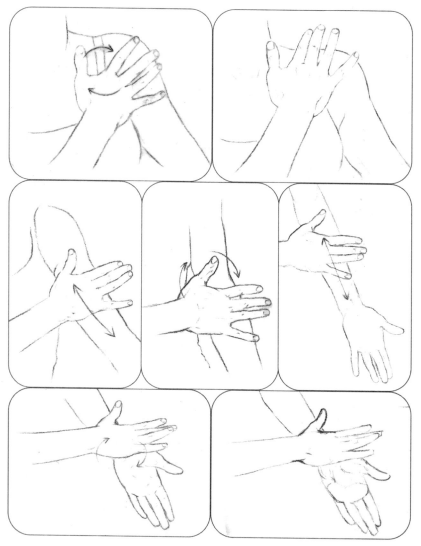

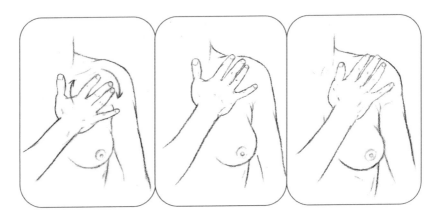

8. Next, massage the chest in a gentle, circular clockwise direction; use about 15-20 strokes.

The abdomen is done in about the same manner, using gentle, circular clockwise strokes. Some people like to massage the abdomen with only one hand, others place one hand on top of the other and use two hands—see which techniques you prefer and stay with it.

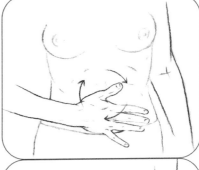

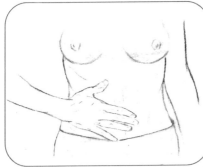

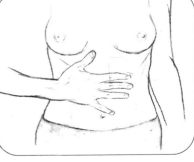

9. Massage as much of the spine, back and ribs as you can reach.

10. The buttocks can be massaged using a combination of circular and straight strokes.

11. The legs are massaged in a similar manner to the arms, using a set pattern of circular (knees, ankles) and up-and-down (long bones) strokes. Use both hands to massage each leg and remember to do both the front and back. Add more oil if needed and massage vigorously.

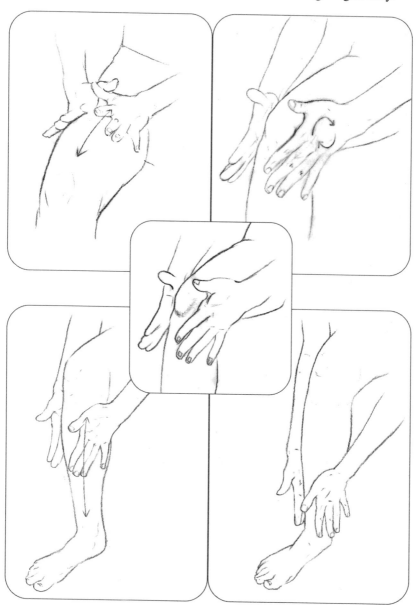

12. Finally, massage the feet. The feet are one of the most important areas to massage and should be given a little more time than the rest of the body. Using the ball of your hand, massage the bottom of the foot vigorously for 30 to 60 seconds. Then do the same for the top of the foot. Massage the toes, web spaces, *and* toenails.

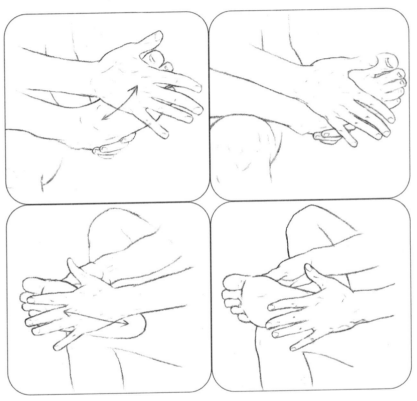

13. The oil should remain on the body for a minimum of 16 minutes. This is almost exactly how long it takes to do the entire massage, so by applying the oil to the entire body before starting the actual massage, you will easily satisfy this time requirement.

14. Following the massage, take a shower or bath using a mild soap. You may wish to purchase a supply of fragrant herbal "utane powder" which efficiently removes the oil, leaves the skin glowing, and has no detergent content. It is used either in place of or along with your favorite soap. (see Appendix for suppliers).

The Importance of Water In Weight Loss

Almost everyone knows that drinking adequate water is good for health. But most people do not understand why this is so and what exactly happens when the body does not get adequate water. Most people believe that we feel thirsty whenever our body needs more water. While this is true, recent research studies have indicated that there are several other indicators of inadequate water in some or all parts of the body.

Up to sixty-five percent of the total body weight is due to water. Although it is present in all parts of the body, it is more abundant in organs such as lungs and brain and fluids such as blood, lymph, saliva and secretions by the organs of the digestive system.

There are three stages of water regulation of the body at different stages of life. These include (a) before birth, (b) between birth and adolescence and (c) in adulthood. Before birth, the unborn baby sends signals to the mother if more water is required for its growth and development. Thus, although the unborn baby sends the signal, the mother experiences the effect. It is believed that morning sickness in a pregnant woman may be the first indicator that the unborn baby needs more water. Water regulation efficiency of the body reaches the peak by the age of twenty years. Subsequently, it gradually declines through life. Thus, the thirst sensation gradually decreases as age advances. This is perhaps why chronic diseases such as obesity, arthritis, high blood pressure, constipation, etc. that are also associated with inadequate intake of water are more common in older age groups. The amount of tea, coffee, alcohol, and carbonated drinks that you consume regularly may also adversely affect the water regulation in later life. The ratio of the water content inside and outside the cells of the various organs is very important. As we get older, water content decreases. Since the water in each cell plays a vital role in its normal function, inadequate water can lead to loss of some cellular functions. Loss of function, in turn, results in demonstrable signs and symptoms.

Normal Volumes of Body Fluids

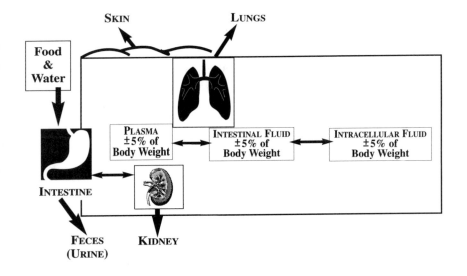

How is the body water regulated?

If you were ever to experience a water shortage in your house, you would prioritize the use of water for essential purposes. For example, you would use the available water for drinking and cooking but reduce the amount of water used for bathing, washing, etc. Similarly, when the body receives insufficient water, *histamine,* a chemical compound present in many cells, initiates a system of water regulation. This physiological system prioritizes the distribution of water to more important organs of the body such as brain, heart, lungs, etc. Histamine influences a system of chemicals called *neurotransmitters.* These chemicals either modify or transmit impulses in the nerves. Histamine directs some neurotransmitters to operate sub-systems to regulate water intake.

These sub-systems use chemical substances that include *vasopressin* and *renin-angiotensin* to regulate water intake and distribution. Vasopressin is a hormone that increases re-absorption of water by the kidneys and therefore decreases the production of urine. Renin is an enzyme produced and stored in kidneys. Whenever the volume of blood decreases, renin initiates a series of chemical reactions that produce a chemical compound, *angiotensin.* Angiotensin causes contraction of the blood vessels of the kidneys and therefore reduces the rate of filtration of blood by the kidneys. Reduced filtration helps the body to retain more water.

Why is water important for maintaining normal health?

As we have said, the water content in various parts of the body regulates their functions. It also helps regulate the functions of the solids such as enzymes, minerals, vitamins, and all substances dissolved in the water. In other words, every function of the body is influenced by the flow of water within and between the various organs. Water serves as a universal vehicle to connect all parts of the body. Adequate distribution of water in all parts of the body ensures that water chemical substances (such as hormones, nutrients, etc.) first reach the more important organs such as the brain, heart, kidneys and lungs.

In addition, modern Ayurveda describes the following roles of water in our body:

1. Water helps maintain the moisture of the lining of the internal organs of the body.

2. It maintains normal volume and consistency of fluids such as blood and lymph.

3. It regulates body temperature.

4. It removes "poisons" or "toxins" from the body through urine, sweat and breathing.

5. Water is essential for regulating the normal structure and functions of the skin.

What is dehydration?

The body loses about three liters of water every day. It is therefore necessary to replenish this volume by drinking at least the equivalent amount of water every day. Inadequate intake of water can lead to dehydration.

Dehydration is excessive loss of water from the body. It results in imbalance in sodium, potassium and chlorides levels. Normally, dehydration is the term used when there is inadequate water in all parts of the body. This is often the result of rapid loss of water due to conditions such as fever, diarrhea, vomiting, etc.

The common symptoms of dehydration of the entire body include increased thirst, increased appetite, loss of skin elasticity, dry skin, decreased urine production, and mental instability and confusion. This is the stage in which the body's natural compensatory mechanisms of water regulation are not able to meet the minimum requirement for the vital organs. As mentioned earlier, dehydration may be present in some specific cells or organs of the body without resulting in these acute symptoms. What are the indications of dehydration? Thirst is an early indicator of inadequate water in the entire body. However, there can be inadequate water supply to some parts of the body without resulting in thirst. Inadequate water in the body cells can adversely affect their functioning. Depending upon the organ affected by inadequate water supply, there are specific signs and symptoms. Chronic pains, fatigue, depression, irritability, heartburn, and allergies are the most common symptoms indicating abnormal function due to chronic dehydration.

Why is adequate water important in weight loss?

The brain is very sensitive to low energy levels available for its functions. Low energy levels cause both thirst and hunger sensations. Normally, hormones are necessary to mobilize energy from stored fat. Since this process takes some time and the brain requires energy quickly and continually, it depends initially on the blood sugar for the energy. It is important to note that only twenty percent of the energy from food reaches the brain; the remaining eighty percent is distributed to the other vital organs and physiological processes. The energy from food that is not used by the brain or by any other part of the body is stored as glycogen and fat. The brain also uses water to produce neuroelectrical signals and transmit its messages to various parts of the body. Thus, the sensations of thirst and hunger are felt together to indicate the brain's needs for more immediate energy. Drinking adequate water throughout the day before and after meals will reduce the intensity of the thirst and hunger and therefore help prevent overeating. When water intake is inadequate, you are likely to feel more "hungry" and eat larger portions of food at more frequent intervals in order to supply necessary sugar to the brain. On the other hand, if the brain senses an adequate volume of water in the body, the risk of weight gain from overeating is greatly reduced.

What is the normal daily requirement of water?

It is very difficult to quantify the exact amount of water each person requires to maintain normal functioning of all the organs of the body. This is because the quantity of water required for the body functions depends on several factors such as age, climate, season, physical activity, type of food consumed, amount of condiments and spices used for cooking, the water content in the food, salt intake, etc.

Normally, our daily diet provides about two-thirds of the body's requirement of water. The remaining one-third of our daily water requirement must come from fluids we consume. Ayurveda suggests that we drink about eight to ten glasses of water everyday to meet this remaining one-third of the body's requirement. You also need to drink additional water when you are tired and/or are sweating profusely.

It is also important to learn when *not* to drink water. It is desirable that you avoid drinking *large quantities* of water while eating food, as it will adversely affect proper churning of the food and the secretion of the saliva. A small amount of liquid consumed during the meal is perfectly fine. The water leaves the stomach within five to ten minutes of drinking it, and therefore if large quantities of water are consumed, the food is also likely to leave the stomach along with the water. Thus, digestion of the food is likely to be adversely affected. Excessive water also may dilute the digestive juices in the stomach to some degree, thus possibly creating incomplete digestion. It is most desirable that you drink most of your water throughout the day and between meals.

Most people tend to drink water in large gulps. Ayurveda recommends that you need to "eat liquids and drink solids". This means that you need to take water sip by sip, and "chew" it in the mouth in order to mix it with the saliva. Avoid regular use of straws for drinking water and/or other fluids.

Other general benefits of water are as follows:

• Regulates body temperature

• Dilutes the blood to an optimum specific gravity and reduces its viscosity to prevent abnormal clotting

• Promotes excretion of toxins via the skin in the form of perspiration

• Stimulates the normal functions of the kidneys and therefore increases the rate of removal of toxins from the body through the urine

• Increases movements of the intestines, thus facilitating formation and passing of soft stools.

• One of the ways to ensure that you are drinking adequate water is to observe the color of your urine. If it is almost white, it means that all parts of your body are well hydrated. A dark yellowish tint to the urine indicates that the kidneys are working harder to conserve water and remove bodily waste products because of inadequate water in the blood. High vitamin B levels can also give a dark yellow color to the urine despite sufficient daily water intake.

• One of the first behavioral modifications for weight loss and control that a patient will learn about upon visiting an Ayurvedic physician will be to optimize all the features of water consumption. It is not an exaggeration to say this is one of the most important things we can do for ourselves to promote a healthy, slim, and vigorous body and mind.

CHAPTER 8.

THE SATTVIC DIET

Sattvic Dietary Principles For Everybody

Sattvic foods are foods that are abundant in *prana*—the universal life force that gives life to all sentient beings in both the plant and animal kingdoms. The ancient criteria for foods to be considered Sattvic were quite simple: foods were to be grown on good soil, far removed from waste sites, protected from animals; foods were to be of attractive appearance, have a form that is normal for that particular species, and be harvested at the correct time of year. Today, we must add to these criteria for Sattva several other modern concerns. Sattvic foods should be grown without pesticides, herbicides, chemical fertilizers, hormones, enzymes, irradiation or anything unnatural. Foods should be *whole foods* and be as unrefined as possible. Minor refinements are permissible such as making ghee from butter by heating or extracting sesame oil from sesame seeds by maceration. However, the modern use of refinement processes and chemical additives, besides actually adding toxic substances to our foods, depletes foods of their *prana* (life force) and hence renders them heavy, impotent and lifeless.

Sattvic Foods: General Description

Sattvic foods in contrast are of the highest quality available, fresh, light in quality, naturally colored, and full of prana. You can comprehend the difference by visualizing in your mind two different foods: a slice of pizza and a fresh, crisp, lightly steamed carrot. I think you get the idea.

The Sattva Program® is a ***lacto-vegetarian diet*** and it emphasizes complex carbohydrates of the highest quality.

Its food categories include: grains, vegetables, fruits, nuts, seeds, dairy products (although very limited), legumes, and spices. Flesh foods are included for those who feel they must continue to include these items. All foods are consumed immediately after preparing them, must be cooked to perfection, and must not ever be too oily. Spices are generally used according to the Ayurvedic Constitutional Type of the individual and will be detailed under each specific Type. In addition, Ayurveda emphasizes the importance of the state of mind of the cook: he or she should be happy, emotionally stable, enjoy cooking, and have a loving attitude towards those being fed. In fact, Ayurveda gently suggests only consuming food prepared by one's parents, grandparents, siblings, spouse, close relatives, or very dear friends.

Complex Carbohydrates

Since The Sattva Program lays emphasis on the proper use of complex carbohydrates, let us briefly define what we mean by this term. Let's start with the question: "What exactly is a carbohydrate?"

Carbohydrate Structure

Carbohydrates are organic compounds composed of carbon (C), hydrogen (H), and oxygen (O). Along with proteins and fats, they are one of the three classes of foods essential to the human physiology. The name *carbohydrate* was invented because in the late 19th century they were all thought to be combinations of C, H, and O which suggested compounds of carbon and water (H_2O), hence the contraction: carbohydrate was used. The general formula was given as:

$$C_n (H_2O)_n$$

We now know that the ratios of C:H:O not only occur as ratios which give carbon and water, but numerous other compounds as well and the general formula is now simply:

$$(CHO)_n$$

Carbohydrates are used by the body as a source of energy and heat—any excess is stored in the body as fat. It is interesting that no appreciable amount of carbohydrate is found in the human body (or any animal body) at any one time. The range of the blood glucose level for most animals is approximately 0.05 to 0.1%. However this tiny amount of glucose, which is constantly being replenished by breaking down glycogen to glucose in the liver, is sufficient to supply the energy for maintaining heat and powering all physiological processes including those of the brain. It is really quite astounding how life is so dependent on this one simple carbohydrate. Stored glycogen in the liver accounts for approximately only 5-7% of the organ's total weight.

Carbohydrates play a rather cosmic role in the entire scheme of life when you think about it. Consider the fact that carbohydrates are formed from combining the energy of the sun with carbon dioxide and water. The process is of course known as *photosynthesis*:

$$6\ CO_2\ \text{(carbon dioxide)} + 6\ H_2O\ \text{(water)} + \textbf{sunlight} =$$
$$C_6H_{12}O_6\ \text{(glucose/carbohydrate)} + 6\ O_2\ \text{(oxygen)}.$$

An estimated 100 billion tons of carbohydrates are synthesized by plants each year via the harnessing of photons of sunlight reaching earth. They are the link between the cosmic energy of the sun and human life. On the average most plants consist of approximately 75% carbohydrates that forms the leaves, stems, saps, and woody structures as well as the seeds, roots, and rhizomes.

Complex and Simple Carbohydrates

Carbohydrates occur in a wide array of forms that are classified into two large groups, simple and complex. Table 1 shows the current classification in use.

TABLE 1
CLASSIFICATION OF CARBOHYDRATES

SIMPLE			COMPLEX				
Monosaccharides			**Oligosaccharides**		**Polysaccharides**		
Pentoses	Hexoses	Disaccharides	Trisaccharides	Tetrasaccharides	Pentosans	Hexosans	Mixed
$(C_5H_{10}O_2)$	$(C_6H_{12}O_6)$	$(C_{12}H_{22}O_{11})$	$(C_{18}H_{32}O_{16})$	$(C_{24}H_{42}O_{21})$	$(C_5H_8O_4)n_2$	$(C_6H_{10}O_5)n_2$	
Arabinose	Fructose	Lactose	Maltoriose	Stachyose	Araban	Cellulose	Agar
Ribose	Galactose	Maltose	Melezitose	Maltotetrose	Xylan	Dextrins	Alginic
Xylose	Glucose	Sucrose	Raffinose			Glycogen	acid
	Carrageenan	Mannose	Trehalose			Inulin	Chitin
						Mannan	Gums
						Starch	Pectin
						(amylose,	
						amylopectin)	

Simple carbohydrates are monosaccharides or single sugars, which are only rarely found free in nature. Rather they constitute the building blocks of the complex carbohydrates.

Simple carbohydrates are classified according to how many carbon atoms make up each molecule. Although smaller ones exist, the 5-carbon simple carbohydrates (pentoses) and the 6-carbon simple carbohydrates (hexoses) are the most important. Glucose, the most important carbohydrate of all, is a hexose.

Complex carbohydrates are long chains of simple carbohydrates (monosaccharides). For convenience they are classified as *oligosaccharides* if they are chains of 2 to 10 monosaccharides or *polysaccharides* if they contain more than ten monosaccharides.

The Evils of Sugar

Is it an exaggeration to call sugar evil? It certainly is not. Sugar abuse is one of society's least recognized and most harmful habits. Close behind alcohol and tobacco, processed cane sugar is one of the most destructive substances consumed by mankind. This is particularly true in the United States where we become more or less addicted to sugar from childhood and by the time we reach adulthood each of us is consuming an average of 150 pounds of cane sugar per year! Judicious use of sugar, however, is probably not harmful; like all things it's a matter of proper measure and common sense.

Sugar, or *sucrose*, originally was derived from the *sugarcane* plant, *Saccharum officinarum*, a bamboo-like wild grass common to India and other tropical parts of Asia. The pure, unprocessed juice of the sugarcane plant is a useful medicine and is in fact only mildly sweet. It is not until this juice gets processed and desiccated that it acquires its familiar taste and appearance. It also acquires its many harmful effects. Sucrose is a *di*saccharide that is composed of two glucose molecules linked together. Hence, sucrose is an extremely easy source for glucose—the simplest and most insulin-stimulating of all carbohydrates. Sugar apparently reached Europe by the early fourteenth century but did not become a popularly used commodity until well into the seventeenth century.

Sugar can be considered a kind of stimulant, although not in the strictly scientific sense. It does, however, give the user a transient, euphoric "high", which is generally followed one to two hours later by some degree of lethargy, depression, heaviness, and feelings of remorse. Chronic use of sugar places a great physiological strain on the pancreas and kidneys. It causes a tremendous secretion of insulin into the bloodstream, which in turn promotes the conversion of glucose into fat in the liver and other tissues. Sugar consumption, especially simple sugars, have a direct correlation to weight gain—in case you had any doubts. Fortunately, not all carbohydrates are as simply converted into glucose as is sucrose.

Why Complex Is Better Than Simple

Despite the overwhelming variety of carbohydrates that exist in nature, over 95% of plant carbohydrates occur in one form: starch. You can find this very important carbohydrate in Table 1 modestly tucked away in the <u>hexosan</u> list of polysaccharides. Now, everybody has heard of starches and you probably have a negative view of them—we all know that bread and pasta are loaded with them and these are foods that make us fat. However, this is not the entire story, nor is the "starch equals fat" myth entirely true.

There are two types of starch:

1) amylose—a straight-chained complex of repeating glucose molecules, and

2) amylopectin—a highly-branched structure of glucose molecules

The amount of amylose and amylopectin in starch varies in different foods but on the average starch is approximately 73% amylopectin and 27% amylose. Furthermore, although starch appears to the naked eye as a white powder, under the microscope it actually consists of individual tiny granules that vary in size and shape according to the source. When starch is heated in water during cooking, the chemical bonds (hydrogen bonds) holding the granules together weaken, which allows water to enter. This causes the starch granules to swell, lose their shape, rupture and release amylose and amylopectin, which are then more vulnerable to enzymatic digestion. Due mainly to the distinctive shapes and physical characteristics of their starch granules, starch from rice, potato, wheat, corn, oats and every other food source will be digested at different rates. Ultimately all starch is broken down into glucose. But the critical factor for us is how fast this process happens. The slower the better. The reason for this is described in the next section.

Simple carbohydrates and carbohydrates that have been maximally refined and stripped of their husks and other coatings are almost instantaneously absorbed from our small intestines and into the blood. In the blood, when glucose levels rise this quickly it causes a large and rapid compensatory rise in the insulin released into the blood. The insulin is necessary to transport the glucose from the bloodstream into the cells where it can be used as energy. Unfortunately, this large insulin bolus occurs every time you eat refined or simple carbohydrates (candy, cakes, cookies, pastries and sucrose). So if you have lots of this type of carbohydrate all day long, your average insulin levels will remain elevated all day. This will cause excess carbohydrate to be converted into fat.

However, whole foods such as fruits, vegetables, beans, legumes, and whole grains that contain *complex carbohydrates* require a more complex series of digestive enzymes to act on it, before it can be absorbed as glucose. This slower digestive process is key because it in turn causes a slower and reduced insulin response. The average insulin level stays below the critical level necessary for fat synthesis from carbohydrate.

Carbohydrates and Insulin: Modern Science Meets Ancient Wisdom

Insulin and Glucagon

Insulin is a hormone that regulates the storage or release of not only glucose, but all physiological fuels (glucose, amino acids, and free fatty acids). Insulin is produced by the beta cells of the islets of Langerhans pancreas and consists of a chain of 51 amino acids.

Healthy non-obese adults store about 200 U of insulin in their pancreas and secrete approximately 31 U insulin daily. Obese, non-diabetic adults, because of insulin resistance, secrete approximately 114 U insulin daily. Type I diabetics secrete only 0-4 U insulin daily, whereas Type II diabetics secrete about 14 U insulin daily.

What does insulin have to do with weight loss? After a meal, insulin levels rapidly rise in response to component monosaccharides and amino acids. These nutrients arrive, via the portal vein, at the pancreas and stimulate insulin secretion. Sugars and amino acids that enter the liver with high ambient insulin immediately undergo glycogen synthesis, protein synthesis, and fatty acid synthesis. Muscles and adipose tissues receive the largest proportion of glucose and amino acids from any meal. Insulin causes both glucose and amino acids to rapidly enter muscle cells and glucose only to enter fat cells. In the muscles, the glucose goes into the glycogen pool and the amino acids serve as precursors for protein synthesis. In fat cells, the glucose that enters as a result of high insulin levels is converted into triglyceride and stored. The high insulin levels increase the activity of an enzyme named lipoprotein lipase, which promotes the deposition of triglycerides into fat cells. Insulin also inhibits enzymes that break down fats. In other words, insulin causes increased storage of all three fuels (carbohydrates, proteins, and fats) in the body.

Glucagon that is secreted by the alpha cells of the islets of Langerhans of the pancreas has several effects that are diametrically opposite to those of insulin. The three main effects of glucagon that are important to know are that it stimulates:

1) the breakdown of glycogen into glucose (gylcogenolysis)
2) the synthesis of new glucose from amino acids (gluconeogenesis)
3) the breakdown of adipose tissue

So glucagon, a peptide hormone, like insulin, but containing only 29 amino acids, is secreted in response to low blood glucose concentrations. Its most dramatic effect in the body is to cause a rapid breakdown of glycogen into glucose in the liver.

Now with regard to weight loss, you should know that overweight individuals have chronically elevated insulin and lipoprotein lipase levels. Lipoprotein lipase is an enzyme that powerfully promotes the storage and protection of fat. Obese people who eat foods with lots of refined carbohydrates can have insulin levels that remain elevated throughout their waking hours and fall only during sleep, which is basically a fast. This short sleep fast is not enough time for significant amounts of fat to be broken down. Thus you can see that overweight individuals are always metabolically geared towards storing fuel and fat at every meal. One key to weight loss is very simply to eat foods that do not produce a lot of insulin release into the blood.

Glycemic index

How can we know which foods will not cause a large secretion of insulin into the body? Since carbohydrates are the main stimulus for insulin secretion we need to address the question of whether we should just avoid all carbohydrates in our diet? The answer is absolutely not! Carbohydrates differ greatly in their capacity to induce insulin secretion. Today, carbohydrates are classified according to their *glycemic index*. The glycemic index of a food is simply the capacity of 100 grams of that food to raise the blood glucose level as compared to 100 grams of glucose.

The glycemic index is determined over several days. First, on a given morning after fasting all night, healthy test subjects are given 50 grams of pure glucose by mouth. Their blood glucose levels are measured beforehand and every half hour after drinking the glucose for three hours. The resulting blood glucose values are plotted on a graph. On another day, under the same conditions, the test subjects are given 50 grams of a specific "test food" and the resulting blood glucose values plotted on the same graph for comparison. This graph is known as the glycemic response curve for that food. The area under the glycemic response curve is then mathematically expressed as a percent of the area under the curve for glucose. Thus the glycemic index, using pure glucose as a baseline, is determined. The test food is usually given several times and the average taken to obtain the accurate glycemic index.

Although there are slightly different glycemic index values published for the same foods tested by different researchers, they are basically similar. For example, our own study found a sweet potato to have a glycemic index of 58, while in another published study it is valued at 54. White bread tests between 69 and 73 in independent studies. These variations are probably due to differences in the food itself. The amylose to amylopectin ratio of a food (different types of starches) can account for these small inter-study differences. Amylose is a non-branched form of starch that is harder to digest, releases glucose molecules more slowly, and therefore has a lower glycemic index. Amylopectin is a branching starch and is more prone to digestion at those branch sites and gives a higher value of glycemic index when it is predominant.

Also slight differences in how much a food has been processed will affect the observed glycemic index. The smaller the starch particles, due to very complete grinding, the higher the glycemic index; the more intact and whole the particles remain, the lower the glycemic index. Also depending on how a food is cooked, the glycemic index can change to a small degree.

The presence of soluble fiber, such as occurs in beans and certain whole grain cereals, tends to form a somewhat viscous coating around the accompanying starch and this physical barrier can slow down the digestive process. This effect probably contributes to the lower glycemic indexes seen in these foods.

GLUCOSE (reference food)

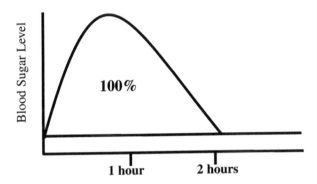

BASMATI RICE

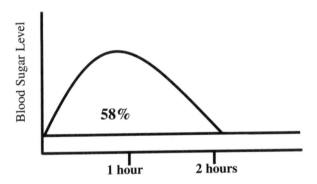

Figure 1. The effect of pure glucose (50 grams) and basmati rice (50 grams carbohydrate content) on blood sugar levels

The clinical relevance of the glycemic index has been shown in many studies where the quantity of carbohydrates, proteins, and fats in the diet have remained unchanged, but the type of starchy carbohydrate in the diet has been altered. A low glycemic diet has been shown to promote weight loss, to reduce serum triglycerides in hypertriglyceremic subjects, to reduce insulin secretion, to improve blood glucose control in both Type I and Type II diabetics, and to reduce insulin and glucose levels in cirrhosis; in addition some evidence exists that low glycemic foods may promote earlier satiety during meals, and enhance athletic performance.

As previously explained, the glycemic index of a carbohydrate is greatly influenced by its physical features and particle size. In general, the coarser and more whole a food is, the lower its glycemic index will be. Not only particle size, but the shape and form of the granules also affect the glycemic index. As previously described, starch particles consisting of amylose and amylopectin begin to swell when they are cooked in water. This eventuates the rupture of the granules, exposing these molecules to enzymatic breakdown—until all the amylose and amylopectin has been broken down to glucose. The faster this occurs, the higher the glycemic index and therefore the insulin response. What unfortunately is observed to dramatically speed up this breakdown of starch is modern food processing. These processes include adding dilute acid or oxidizing agents to produce syrups, addition of enzymes, canning, puffing, thermal extrusion, milling and grinding.

The Sattva Program food lists include foods that have undergone the least amount of processing and therefore naturally have the lowest glycemic indexes.

The following scale is the current guideline to distinguish low-, intermediate-, and high-glycemic index foods.

GLYCEMIC INDEX SCALE
(Glucose = 100)

Low Glycemic Index Foods . . . . less than 55

Intermediate Glycemic Index Foods 55-70

High Glycemic Index Foods . . . . greater than 70

The Sattva Program Food List

The Sattva Program diets described in this book will promote weight loss and balance for individuals of all constitutional types, although as we will see in the next chapter, it is imperative that the basic food list be modified for Vata, Pitta, and Kapha dominant people, respectively. The foods included in the general list below will give you an idea of just how vast and *unrestrictive* Sattvic diets are. This food list will not actually be the appropriate list for most individuals. (It actually is the list for the rare individuals with a constitution of exactly equal proportions of V, P, and K). It is rather offered as a preview of the types of foods that are included in a Sattvic diet. In Chapter nine we will refine this all-inclusive list into more specific lists for Vata, Pitta, and Kapha constitutional types.

Sattvic food should be organically grown whenever possible. These foods are all simple, pure foods that are light and cleansing in nature. Some foods have a cooling effect and some a warming effect in the body. This list is intended to *exclude* foods that are grown with chemical fertilizers or insecticides and those that cause harm to any living beings. The main feature of a Sattvic food is that it is rich in *prana*—the vital energy of all living beings.

Over the years, my patients have been pleasantly surprised at the wide variety of delicious foods that are recommended on the Sattva Program. Even today we still receive at least ten phone calls a week asking: "Can I really have (specific food)?"

The Sattva Program is one of abundance and not restriction. One point to bear in mind is that we do not necessarily intend that you should go out and buy every single item mentioned in this list. This is not a list of absolutely required foods. Rather, regard the list as a way to help guide you towards foods that you may perhaps have forgotten or never tried. On the other hand, you may find yourself perfectly nourished by only a few common foods listed here. In general, *the simpler the meals the better*, so don't worry about eating only a few items. We will talk more about the benefits of simple meals in the next section on Food Combining and debunk the notion of nutritional deficiencies from such a diet.

The Sattva Program Food List

FRUITS

Apples	Kiwi	Prunes
Apricots	Loquat	Tangerines
Bananas	Lychee	Pomegranate
Cantaloupe	Mango	Papaya
Cherries	Melons	Nectarines

Cranberry
Grapefruits
Grapes
Guava

Honeydew
Watermelon
Peaches
Pears

Oranges
Pineapples
Plums
Persimmon

VEGETABLES

Artichokes
Mustard Greens
Endive
Bok Choy
Broccoli
Brussels Sprouts
Cabbage
Carrots
Celery
Common Morels
Maitake
Shitake

Eggplant
Asparagus
Fennel
Garlic
Green Beans
Kale
Leeks
Mushrooms
Chanterelles
Squash
Butternut
Acorn
Pumpkin
Chinese

Lettuce
Arugula
Chicory
Iceberg
Radicchio
Romaine
Lima Beans
Spinach
Sprouts
Corn
Dandelion Greens
Sweet Potatoes
Watercress

Beets
Onions
Parsnips
Peas
Potatoes
Radishes
Shallots
Cauliflower
Chard
Daikon
Turnips
Yams

GRAINS

Amaranth
Barley
Buckwheat
Cracked Wheat (Bulgur)
Millet
Quinoa
Rice
Basmati
Brown
Wild
Rye

BEANS

Aduki
Black-eyed Peas
Garbanzo
Kidney
Lentils
red
brown
Lima
Mung
Navy
Pinto
Split Peas
tofu

OILS

Olive
Safflower
Sesame
Sunflower

SPICES

Asafoetida (Hing)
Basil
Black Pepper

Coriander
Cumin
Fennel seed

Horseradish
Nutmeg
Parsley

SPICES *(Cont'd)*

Cardamom   Fenugreek
Cinnamon
Clove

Garlic
Ginger

Turmeric

DAIRY
Low-fat cow's milk
Goat's milk
Soy milk*

NUTS/SEEDS
Brazil Nuts
Pumpkin Seeds
Sunflower Seeds
Walnuts

*Soy milk is not actually a dairy product but is listed here for practicality.

SWEETENERS
Gur (Unrefined cane juice)
Raw Honey
Stevia (*Stevia rebaudiana*)
Barley malt
Rice syrup

The Ten Features That Determine Healthy Foods

By this time you must have realized that the Ayurvedic physicians were much more than merely prescribers of medicines and surgeries, as we often find today. They were in fact known as *vaidyas* meaning "wise ones". The ancient physicians deeply contemplated the connections between the individual and the environment and often understood intuitively how to proceed to promote self-healing. Nowhere more than in the insights they have left us concerning food do they live up to this appellation. Although it is certainly beyond the scope and relevance of this book to detail all of the food-related principles they recorded, a few particularly useful recommendations will be given here.

The classic Ayurvedic textbook, the *Charaka Samhita*, describes ten factors that will determine if a particular food article or a meal is healthy or unhealthy for a given individual. Only if *all* ten factors are satisfactorily satisfied is a food or meal healthy.

Almost every single one of these important factors enumerated by the ancient Indian physicians is discussed at various appropriate places throughout this book. The one that is not discussed elsewhere, and which has particular significance for us is the last one, the principles of proper food intake.

In the *Charaka Samhita*, the author describes ten recommendations with regard to the proper way to take in food. Keeping in mind that these guidelines were written approximately two thousand years ago, it is astounding to see their relevance and importance in current times. I have translated both the rule and the short comment which follows each one as literally as possible from the original Sanskrit to preserve the flavor (no pun intended):

Nature of the food articles	*Climate or habitat*
Method of processing & preparation	*Season; time of day*
Method of cooking	*Doshic constitution of the individual*
Combinations	*State of mind of the individual*
Quantity	*Principles of proper food intake*

The Ten Principles of Proper Food Intake

The following principles are stated almost verbatim in the *Caraka Samhita*, in the chapter entitled Vimanasthana, section 1:24.

1. *Food should primarily be eaten when it is warm.*

When properly cooked and eaten warm, food is delicious and it is better able to stimulate the factors concerned with the digestion of food.

2. *Food should be slightly unctuous (i.e. moist and oily) when taken.*

When unctuous, food is delicious and awakens diminished powers of digestion.

3. *Food should be taken in proper quantity.*

Food taken in proper quantity promotes long life; the opposite causes short life.

4. *A meal should be started only if the previous meal is completely digested.*

If one eats more food before the complete digestion of the previous meal, the incompletely digested food juice of that previous meal mingles with the subsequent meal causing the strong aggravation of all three doshas.

5. *Foods taken at the same meal should not have strongly opposite potencies.*

Strongly heating foods should not be combined with strongly cooling foods at the same meal.

6. *Meals should be taken in a quiet, comfortable room that is used only for dining, equipped with all the proper serving and eating utensils.*

Like sleeping in the bedroom, eating should only take place in the proper place.

7. *Food should not be taken too quickly.*

If taken hastily, food is not properly digested by each portion of the digestive system; its wrong components enter the wrong channels and toxins are created.

8. *Food should not be taken too slowly.*

If taken too slowly, there will not arise satisfaction in the mind of the individual.

9. *Food should be taken with full concentration; there should not be excessive talking, laughing or emotion during meals.*

The mind must be fully engaged in the pleasure of eating and the attention should be focused on this activity.

10. *One should take food in a prescribed manner with regard for one's specific needs.*

Knowledge of the qualities of food articles and their utility or non-utility for ourselves is the hallmark of longevity.

Food Combining

Food combining is one of the most important features of *The Sattva Program.*

The order in which we eat different classes of foods and the amounts we consume will determine how well we digest and assimilate our vital nutrients. The better we digest and assimilate our foods, the less likely we are to accumulate excess fat and crave unhealthy substances.

CHAPTER 8. THE SATTVIC DIET

It is important to understand that there is one and only one major factor that determines the completeness and efficiency of digestive processes: the proper production and secretion of digestive enzymes. Very little else really matters when it comes to digesting the foods you eat. Therefore, if you can optimize the function of this multi-faceted system of digestive enzymes you can utilize all the healthy foods listed above in a way that will not only keep you healthy, but will also keep you thin.

Ayurveda emphasizes the proper combinations of foods to be taken together because of early observations that certain combinations of foods caused many physical and mental problems.

These problems include excess intestinal gas, constipation, diarrhea, abdominal pain, urinary retention, digestive fermentation, lethargy, sleep disorders, depression, anxiety, a confused mind, and ultimately a decrease in the function of the entire physiology. These were the *direct observations* made by the ancient Indian physicians. Today we know that different classes of food require their own specific digestive enzymes. This may seem like an obvious fact to anyone who has taken high school biology, yet as a society we seem to have missed the vitally important implication of this fact. By consuming many different types of food at a single meal we place a demand on our digestive glands to manufacture and secrete many different digestive enzymes simultaneously.

For an individual who enjoys optimal health and is maintaining physiological homeostasis reasonably well, it is no problem to produce these myriad enzymes in just the appropriate amounts at every meal no matter how complex. However, for the individual who is not at an ideal weight, whose diet has been inconsistent, and who has even minor health imbalances, the digestive enzyme system will not be able to execute its function optimally. In Ayurveda we say that the body lacks the full and unerring intelligence with which it was born; it has become confused and overwhelmed.

So what happens to the food in the intestines of the poor soul who eats a meal consisting of a variety of foods despite not having an optimum complement of digestive enzymes available? Fortunately the body has developed a back-up method for breaking down foods that are not broken down completely by our digestive enzymes. The intestines contain *bacteria* that are capable of digesting all classes of foods through intracellular fermentation and other metabolic processes. Unfortunately, this method of digestion is slower and also produces associated by-products of fermentation, which can cause many of the problems previously listed. Whereas the digestion of carbohydrates, proteins, and fats via bacterial degradation produces acetic acid, alcohols, lactic acid, and other toxins, normal enzymatic digestion produces only simple sugars, amino acids and free fatty acids.

The principles of food combining that are discussed below are very similar to the eating habits of our early ancestors according to written information left us in the ancient writing of the Indian physicians living around 100 AD. The basic difference from how we are used to eating today is that they only ate two or three different types of foods at any one meal. We tend to have at least six or seven (if not more) types of food at most meals. Foods should not be too fancy. Gourmet foods with rich, sweet tastes will influence even the most strong-willed, health-conscious person to overindulge. Foods should be simple and naturally delicious. For thousands of years mankind has prepared natural and unprocessed foods in simple ways—it is these foods that our physiology needs to function best and maintain its ideal weight. For those of us who have become stressed and gained weight, returning to a more simple dietary style is the key to health and weight loss. It's also the best way to maintain health. Remember that eating only a few kinds of foods at each meal will not result in nutrient deficiencies if you eat a variety of foods based on what is in season in the country in which you live. The Food Lists provided will give anyone a sufficient variety of healthy, nutrient-rich foods for an entire lifetime.

PRINCIPLES OF FOOD COMBINING
ACCORDING TO MODERN AYURVEDA

Principle #1: Eat high-protein foods at the start of the meal.

High-protein foods need to be eaten at the beginning of the meal due to the need for extended contact with the important digestive *stomach* enzyme known as *pepsin.* The digestion of carbohydrates and fats require less time in the stomach because their main digestive enzymes are located further down the track in the small intestines. If starches and other foods are eaten first and then followed by a significant portion of protein, the stomach will already be releasing foods to the intestines and there will be insufficient time for the proteins to be digested by the pepsin into oligo- and dipeptides. Foods such as legumes and beans are eaten before grains.

Foods with the highest protein contents are legumes (beans) including soy products, nuts, and seeds.

Principle #2: Do not eat concentrated protein and starch at the same meal.

The human stomach is not able to completely digest two heavy foods simultaneously. While very acidic digestive enzymes are required for the digestion of proteins, a more alkaline environment is needed to digest starches. Therefore if both food types are present simultaneously, it results in the secretion of both acidic and alkaline juices that partially neutralize each other and retard the digestion of both foods. Fruits and non-starchy vegetables are not heavy and are efficiently digested in either alkaline or acid environments.

One exception to the rule is that rice and beans can be eaten together.

Principle #3: Eat only one or two starches at any meal.

Because each starch (i.e. potato, rice, corn) requires a different set and proportion of enzymes, a meal consisting of many different starches cannot digest well because the enzymatic environment cannot be optimum for all of them simultaneously. In fact, one starch per meal would definitely be optimum; however, for most people, two starches can be metabolized very well. So if a meal includes whole wheat bread and zucchini, it would not be healthy to also have corn at the same meal. The digestion and absorption of all three starches would be compromised, their respective nutrients would be inefficiently assimilated, and the unutilized carbohydrate converted into fat.

Principle #4: Green vegetables are eaten along with or right after proteins.

Vitamin A and beta-carotene, which are abundant in both leafy green and orange-yellow vegetables, play a co-enzyme role in protein synthesis and glycoprotein synthesis, both of which occur in the liver. Studies have demonstrated that Vitamin A deficiency adversely affects both of these important protein metabolic pathways. The best vegetables to eat with proteins are generally the relatively non-starchy, leafy varieties: dandelion greens, kale, collard greens, turnip greens, beet greens, watercress, arugula, mustard greens, and broccoli rabe, and to a lesser extent potatoes, carrots, and squashes (because they are all quite starchy). It is best to eat the more starchy items at a separate meal that doesn't contain large quantities of protein.

Principle #5: Most fruits should be eaten alone.

Fruits are readily digested into their constituent simple carbohydrates that engage and monopolize the digestive system, leaving the more complex carbohydrates, proteins and fats in the stomach to putrefy and ferment. In addition, many fruits tend to buffer the acid environment in the stomach, which is important for protein digestion. The ideal way to eat fruits, either raw or cooked, is as a small entire meal (e.g. breakfast) or as a between meal snack. It is however acceptable to have a moderate amount of fruit with lettuce salad at the end of a meal.

Principle #6: Acidic fruits combine well with proteins and leafy green vegetables.

This means that salads containing leafy greens and protein foods such as seeds, nuts, or yogurt can also contain lemon, lime, orange slices, grapefruit, pineapple, kiwi, tomato, strawberry, or pomegranate (the acidic fruits).

Principle #7: Salty foods are best eaten towards the beginning of the meal.

According to Ayurvedic energetics, salt consists of a combination of fire and water, and hence will stimulate the digestive fire to digest the subsequent remainder of the meal. If not medically contraindicated (high blood pressure, kidney disease, edema, or congestive heart failure) salt can be used as a condiment along with black pepper near the beginning of the meal to season the protein articles.

Principle #8: Always eat fruits in the melon family alone (cantaloupe, honeydew, watermelon).

Ayurveda also warns us against certain other food combinations:

TABLE 8.
UNHEALTHY FOOD COMBINATIONS

Do Not Combine...	With
Milk	Banana, melon, yogurt, fish, sour fruit, leavened bread
Yogurt	Milk, mango, cheese, melon, sour fruit, tea, seafood
Eggs	Cheese, milk, fruit, yogurt, potatoes
Starches	Milk, eggs, banana
Lemon	Yogurt, milk, eggs

However, the Sattva Program does encourage the combination of complementary proteins, which are digested well together and which increase the completeness, and therefore the quality, of the protein. The three main plant-based Food Categories that provide our protein are grains, legumes, and nuts/seeds.

TABLE 9.
COMPLEMENTARY PROTEINS

Food Category	Can Be Combined With These Proteins
GRAINS	
Rice	legumes, cheese, sesame seeds
Wheat.	legumes, soy, milk, peanuts
Barley.	legumes
Corn	legumes
LEGUMES	
Dhal	rice, sesame seeds, corn
Beans	rice, wheat, barley
Soybeans	rice, wheat, peanuts, barley
NUTS AND SEEDS	
Peanuts.	sesame/pumpkin/sunflower seeds, soy
Sesame seeds	peanuts, soybeans, wheat, dhal

Dietary Fiber

In the not too distant past, dietary fiber was deemed unimportant by most of the conventional medical establishment. Difficult as it may be to believe, fiber was actually removed from foods to give them a smoother consistency, a finer texture, and better blending characteristics.

We now understand that sufficient dietary fiber plays some very important roles in maintaining health. Fiber can increase transit time of stool through the bowels, which reduces the risk of certain forms of colon cancer, as well as constipation, varicose veins, hemorrhoids, anal fissures, diverticulosis, appendicitis, and spastic colon. Fiber accomplishes this through increasing the degree of fecal bulking. Fiber may also slow the rate at which glucose and other simple sugars enter the bloodstream, and in this way help the body to regulate blood sugar levels. Epidemiological studies have concluded that high-fiber diets that use cereals as the main fiber source decreases the prevalence of coronary heart disease in both men and women.*

Fiber also appears to play a role in increasing the production of short-chain fatty acids (SCFA) by healthy bacteria that colonize the colon. These short-chain fatty acids participate in local immune protection of the colon from free radicals and help reduce colorectal cancer, and also reach the liver where they decrease its production of LDL-cholesterol, thereby lowering the total serum cholesterol. One of the SCFA's called *butyrate* is being actively investigated for its cancer-protective role. Short-chain fatty acids also bind with bile acids and help excrete them, which is another way they help lower total cholesterol.

What is Fiber?

Fiber simply consists of the cell walls and structural materials of plants that support and give them scaffolding. Fiber is the non-starch, *polysaccharide* component of plants. Plant fiber generally cannot be digested by humans, but instead passes through the intestines exhibiting both "broom-like" and "sponge-like" actions. This means that fiber has the ability to both gently sweep materials through the colon and also to absorb certain others. In the past few years, literature has appeared which sought to classify fiber as either "soluble" or "insoluble" in water, which has led to great confusion. Do not bother with this distinction should you come across it because simply classifying fibers in this way is insufficient to explain their biological effects.

Today, other more sophisticated properties such as bile-acid binding capacity, particle size, microbial degradation, and water holding capacity are used, which are outside of this present discussion.

What you should know are the names and sources of some of the more common fibers found in foods so you can recognize them on labels and know where to find them in nature.

* Rimm EB, Ascherio A, Giovannucci E, et al. Vegetable, fruit, and cereal fiber intake and the risk of CHD among men. JAMA 275:447-451, 1996 and Wolk A, Manson JE, et al. Long-term intake of dietary fiber and decreased risk of CHD among women. JAMA 281:1998-2004, 1999.

TABLE 10: TYPES OF FIBER FOUND IN MAJOR FOOD GROUPS	
FOOD GROUP	**FIBER PRESENT**
Fruits and Vegetables	cellulose, hemicellulose, pectin lignin, xyloglucans, waxes
Grains and Cereals	cellulose, hemicellulose, lignin, beta-D-glucans
Nuts and Seeds	cellulose, hemicellulose, xyloglucans, pectin
Beans	cellulose, hemicellulose, gums, mucilage

Of all of these fibers, only *lignin*, which occurs in the smallest amounts in foods, is not a polysaccharide. I make specific mention of this type of fiber because of the considerable interest in it as a possible anticarcinogenic substance.

All plant-based foods contain mixtures of different types of fiber, depending on the maturity of the plant and its specific type (i.e. leaf, seed, fruit, etc.). The best formula for health is to simply eat a variety of all of these foods every day, to ensure adequate fiber intake.

How Much Fiber Is Enough?

Twenty-five years ago you could not find any recommendations for daily fiber intake. Today, this subject is still evolving. Much of our current information is based on the work of Denis Burkitt and Hugh Trowell, who were physicians working in Africa after World War II. They studied the difference in the amount of "undigested roughage" (today known as *fiber*) in the native African diet (high) versus that of the typical British diet (low) and correlated this with the prevalence of chronic disease. Although a clear association between amounts of fiber intake and incidence of chronic disease has never been firmly established, the evidence is certainly very, very suggestive. It has led governmental health organizations around the world to make recommendations for daily fiber intake. The problem is that nobody seems to know exactly how much fiber we should be eating.

The current recommendations in the United States are officially given in the indecipherable values of *grams of fiber per kilojoule*, perhaps to underscore the uncertainty of the data and the reluctance of authorities to give out iron-clad guidelines. Other groups simply make fiber recommendations in terms of the number of servings per day of fruits, vegetables and grain products, thus avoiding specific quantities of fiber altogether.

Having researched this area myself over the years, I have been able to conclude that the amount of fiber that normal, healthy adults should be consuming is between *20 and 30 grams per day.* For individuals trying to lose weight, I advise increasing this amount, but only modestly, up to *35 to 40 grams per day.*

TABLE 11: Fiber Content of Some Common Foods (grams/ounce)	
Food	**Fiber Content**
Apple, medium w/peel	3.73
Pear, medium w/peel	3.98
Orange, medium	3.14
Grapefruit, medium	2.60
Kidney beans, 1/2 cup	6.55
Parsley, 1/2 cup	1.00
Celery, medium stalk	0.70
Carrot, meduim	2.16
Broccoli, 1/2 cup	2.26
Cabbage, medim, 1/2 head	14.5
Oatmeal, 1 cup	4.33
Whole Wheat Bread, 1 slice	1.93
Whole Wheat Flour, 1/2 cup	7.32
White Rice, 1/2 cup	0.31
Brown Rice, 1/2 cup	1.75
Barley, 1/2 cup	6.80
Millet, 1/2 cup	1.60
Almonds, three	0.50

Can Too Much Fiber Create Problems?

The only potential problem with fiber reported in the medical literature involves the taking of fiber *supplements*. In those rare cases, individuals developed intestinal obstruction and decreased mineral status. I want to emphasize that only when people were taking *isolated fiber supplements* did any problems arise, and these were very rare. Generally, mineral status is increased when the diet includes fiber-rich foods. Including foods containing dietary fiber as part of a balanced, varied diet can only improve your health and will also support your weight loss efforts.

With regard to *The Sattva Program*® for Weight Loss, we have found that dietary fiber plays a role, albeit a minor one, in weight reduction. Fiber is useful due to the following effects that it exerts:

1) Fiber requires an increased need for chewing and therefore slows the eating rate. This allows the brain to receive satiety signals accurately throughout the meal.
2) Improves glucose tolerance.
3) Increases the amount of calories excreted in the stool.
4) Provides a bulking action of the stool that increases a feeling of fullness and satiety.
5) Promotes proper gastrointestinal function, including the secretion and mixing of digestive juices.

Although it is much more preferable to obtain your fiber from foods, I have found dietary fiber can safely be added to your diet in a small quantity as a supplement in two forms:

1) Guar gum (Indian Cluster bean; Cyamopsis tetragonoloba). 1-3 grams before meals.
2) Apple pectin. 1-3 grams before meals.

These are both natural sources of fiber and should only be used in the dosage ranges indicated above. See Appendix for suppliers.

CHAPTER 9.

DETERMINING YOUR SATTVIC ENERGY NEEDS

Step 1. Determine Your Frame Size.

*E*xtend your dominant arm and bend your forearm at the elbow to make a 90-degree angle. Have the palm of the hand facing towards the body. Place the thumb and index finger of the other hand on the two prominent bones on either side of your elbow. Carefully measure this length against a ruler or tape measure; you can also mark the distance between your fingers on a piece of paper and then measure it, if this is easier for you.

Compare your measurement with the measurements in Table 1, "Elbow Breadth For Medium-Framed Men and Women". A smaller measurement indicates a small frame; a larger measurement indicates a large frame.

TABLE 1.
ELBOW BREADTH FOR MEDIUM-FRAMED MEN AND WOMEN

Height In 1" Heels	Elbow Breadth
Men	
5'2" to 5'3"	2 1/2" to 2 7/8"
5'4" to 5'7"	2 5/8" to 2 7/8"
5'8" to 5'11"	2 3/4" to 3"
6'0" to 6'3"	2 3/4" to 3 1/8"
6'4"	2 7/8" to 3 1/4"
Women	
4'10" to 5'3"	2 1/4" to 2 1/2"
5'4" to 5'11"	2 3/8" to 2 5/8"
6'0"	2 1/2" to 2 3/4"

Step 2. Determine Your Estimated Ideal Body Weight

Now that you know your frame size, use the height and weight table below to determine your *approximate* "desirable weight". The most accurate of these tables is provided by the Metropolitan Life Insurance Company. The one given here is the most recent and was compiled in 1983. This table gives weight ranges for men and women at one-inch increments of height for small, medium and large frames.

TABLE 2.
1983 METROPOLITAN LIFE HEIGHT AND WEIGHT TABLE

Height	Small Frame	Medium Frame	Large Frame
MEN			
5'2"	128-134	131-141	138-150
5'3"	130-136	133-143	140-153
5'4'	132-13	135-145	142-156
5'5"	134-140	137-148	144-160
5'6"	136-142	139-151	146-164
5'7"	138-145	142-154	149-168
5'8"	140-148	145-157	152-172
5'9"	142-151	148-160	155-176
5'10"	144-154	151-163	158-180
5'11"	146-157	154-166	161-184
6'0"	149-160	157-170	164-188
6'1"	152-164	160-174	168-192
6'2"	155-168	164-178	172-197
6'3"	158-172	167-182	176-202
6'4"	162-176	171-187	181-207
WOMEN			
4'10"	102-111	109-121	118-131
4'11"	103-113	111-123	120-134
5'0"	104-115	113-126	122-137
5'1"	106-118	115-129	125-140
5'2"	108-121	118-132	128-143
5'3"	111-124	121-135	131-147
5'4"	114-127	124-138	134-151
5'5"	117-130	127-141	137-155

5'6	120-133	130-144	140-159
5'7"	123-136	133-147	143-163
5'8"	126-139	136-150	146-167
5'9"	129-142	139-153	149-170
5'10"	132-145	142-156	152-173
5'11"	135-148	145-159	155-176
6'0"	138-151	148-162	158-179

Weight for adults aged 25 to 59 years, based on lowest mortality. Weight in pounds according to frame size including indoor clothing (5 pounds for men and 3 pounds for women) and shoes with 1-inch heels.

Step 3. Correct For Age

It is well established that in Western society weight gradually increases in both men and women between the ages of 20 and 60. As a person ages, a small increase in weight is acceptable and not harmful. Therefore, after finding your desirable weight in the above table, increase this figure by the following amounts as indicated in Table 3.

TABLE 3.
Weight Corrected For Age

AGE	Amount of Weight to Add To Determine Desirable Weight (lbs.)
Men	
55-59	6-8
60-64	7-10
>65	10-16
Women	
55-59	7-10
60-64	7-12
>65	12-18

The weight corrections are the lower amount for small frames and the higher amount for large frames; an intermediate amount is the correction for medium frames.

Step 4. Correcting For Your Ayurvedic Constitutional Type

This is the next step in determining your caloric needs. It has to do with the dominant dosha in your Ayurvedic Constitutional Type. You determined this earlier by answering the Ayurvedic Questionnaire.

Multiply your age and activity corrected caloric sum by the following factor for each of the following Ayurvedic Constitutional Type

TABLE 4.
CALORIC REQUIREMENT CORRECTION FOR
AYURVEDIC CONSTITUTIONAL TYPE

Dominant Dosha Of Your Ayurvedic Constitutional Type	Multiply Your Age- and Activity-Corrected Caloric Sum By This Factor
Vata	0.97
Pitta	1.00 (no correction)
Kapha	1.04

Step 5. Determination Of Caloric Requirement Based On Activity Level

This is the last step in determining your daily Ayurvedic Caloric Requirement. Now that you have determined your age-corrected estimated desirable weight you can calculate your optimum caloric requirement based on your usual Activity Level. Simply multiply your age- and type-corrected desirable weight by the following number of calories, according to your general Activity Level:

TABLE 5.
CALORIC REQUIREMENT BASED ON ACTIVITY LEVEL

Very little physical activity:	14 calories
Light physical activity:	15 calories
Moderate physical activity:	17 calories
Heavy physical activity:	20 calories

Examples of each Activity Level:

Very little physical activity: no formal exercise plan, sit more than 70% of the work day.

Light physical activity: no formal exercise plan, but sit no more than 50% of the work day; golf, light housekeeping, cumulative walking 30-60 minutes a day.

Moderate physical activity: formal exercise 3-4 times a week for 30 minutes that includes walking, slow jogging (outdoors or on a treadmill), use of light free weights or exercise machines, slow swimming, dancing, tennis, gardening, vacuuming, general housekeeping.

Heavy physical activity: lifting heavy objects, digging with a shovel, or other strenuous labor throughout the day, any of the following activities 4 to 5 times a week for one hour each session: moderately-paced jogging, free weight-training program, nautilus machine-training, shoveling snow, swimming laps.

Example:

If you are a 5'4" 160 lb. 58 year old woman with a Kapha-Pitta Ayurvedic Constitution who has a busy lifestyle that includes only light physical activity, your optimum daily Ayurvedic Caloric Need is determined as follows:

Step 1. Determine Your Frame Size. Let's say your measurement of elbow breadth is 2 1/2 inches. This means you have a *medium frame.*

Step 2. Determine Your Estimated Conventional Desirable Weight. Use Table 2 on page 134 to determine that for a 5'4" woman of medium frame your estimated conventional desirable weight is 124-138 lbs. Let's choose to use the approximate average figure of *130 lbs.*

Step 3. Correction For Age. Since you are older than 55 years, refer to Table 3 on page 135 to find the appropriate correction. According to that Table, add 7 to 10 lbs. to your desirable weight. Let's use 7 lbs. as the correction bringing the sum at this stage to *137 lbs.*

Step 4. Correction For Ayurvedic Constitutional Type. Now we refer to Table 4 on page 136. Since you are a Kapha-Pitta individual, your *dominant* dosha is Kapha. Therefore, multiply 137 lbs. by the Kapha factor of 1.04 to obtain your corrected desirable weight of *142 lbs.*

Step 5. Determination Of Caloric Requirement Based On Activity Level. Refer to Table 5 on page 137. Since you know your activity level fits into the Light Activity category, simply multiply your desirable weight of 142 lbs. by 15, the factor for Light Activity. Your daily Ayurvedic Caloric Requirement is now accurately determined: *2130 calories per day.*

What Do I Do With This Information?

Now that you know your daily Ayurvedic Caloric Requirement, you can use the Sattvic Diet appropriate for your Constitutional Type and Calorie Level to help you consume the appropriate amounts and quality of carbohydrate, fats, protein, fiber and calories.

Your daily Ayurvedic Caloric Requirement is the number of calories needed by your body to perform all of its functions and maintain your desirable weight. ***In order to lose weight, you must consume approximately this amount of energy daily.*** Although proper exercise is important for many reasons to be explained, the amount of calories you can burn off with physical activity is significantly less important than how many calories you consume. The most important requirement for anyone wishing to lose weight is to consume fewer calories for an extended period of time than your body needs to maintain its current weight. It is no use trying to change this fact of life, and other programs that try to circumnavigate this physiological fact are misleading you. However, weight loss is not only a matter of consuming fewer calories. Depending on your constitution, the *type* of diet you should be eating, the herbal supplements you use, and the lifestyle choices you adopt are of utmost importance and vary considerably, as you shall see.

For each Ayurvedic Constitutional Type we make it very simple by telling you how many *servings* to have each day of fruits, vegetables, breads, grains, legumes and so on. For each Type, not only is the number of servings of each of these foods different, but the actual food items in each food group are also distinct, according to Ayurvedic energetic principles.

Furthermore, for each Constitutional Type there are four distinct Sattvic Diets given for four different levels of caloric need: 1200 calories, 1500 calories, 2000 calories, and 2500 calories. We recommend that you choose a diet that approximates your calculated Ayurvedic Caloric Requirement and at the same time is about **500 to 1000 calories less** than your current caloric intake. For every 3500 calories that you are in deficit, you will lose one pound of body weight. Therefore, if you make your caloric deficit 500 calories per day, you will lose approximately 1 lb. per week (500 kcal x 7 days = 3500 kcal); if you make it 1000 calories you will lose approximately 2 lbs. per week. Do not try to lose weight at a rate faster than 2 lbs. per week. You don't have to know anything about the caloric value of any food—this has all been calculated for you. We do not recommend diets that furnish less than 1200 calories per day since these diets are rarely nutritious or satisfying.

For each Ayurvedic Constitutional Type there are lists of all the appropriate foods organized into seven separate categories:

Category 1: Vegetables
Category 2: Fruits
Category 3: Cereals, Starchy Vegetables, Grains
Category 4: Legumes

Category 5: Fats
Category 6: Dairy
Category 7: Meat, Cheese, Fish, Eggs

Why do we divide food into seven different groups? The reason is because foods in each category contain remarkably similar amounts of carbohydrate, protein, fat, and calories. On the other hand, foods in different categories differ greatly in their nutritional composition. Strictly speaking, *The Sattva Program* recommends against meat and fish unless there is an overriding medical reason why these foods must be included. A long history of recorded observations by knowledgeable and objective physicians has led to the consensus that consuming animal flesh does cause toxicity in the mind and body over one's lifetime. We include it in all our lists, however, for those individuals who wish to continue to eat moderate amounts of these flesh foods. The following table shows the average amount of these nutrients in one serving:

TABLE 6.
NUTRIENT CONTENT OF THE SEVEN AYURVEDIC FOOD CATEGORIES
(one serving)

Food Category	Carbohydrate (g)	Protein (g)	Fat (g)	Calories (kcal)
Fruit	15	–	–	60
Vegetable	5	2	–	25
Cereal/ Starchy Veg./ Grain	15	3	trace	80
Legumes	14	2	–	65
Fats	–	–	5	45
Dairy	12	8	trace-8	90-160
Meat/Cheese/ Fish/Eggs	–	7	3-5	55-75

You will create your own diet by referring to the Chapter on your specific Ayurvedic Constitutional Type and selecting the level of caloric intake that is right for you (1200, 1500, 2000, or 2500 calories). Under each calorie level you will find recommendations for how many servings of each category of food you should eat each day. We have included diets that include both (omnivore) and exclude (lacto-vegetarian) animal products. Then simply refer to the place in that Chapter on your Type that lists the specific foods you can choose from. Each Food Category contains foods that have been grouped together because they contain similar proportions of carbohydrates, proteins, fats, and calories. They also are Ayurvedically similar in their energetic effects on the doshas. Portion sizes are included for each food. Within each Category, you can substitute any food you like because their nutritive and energetic value are equivalent. It's simple, it's fun, and it works very, very well.

Today, there are many so-called weight loss experts who believe that sweet and starchy foods like potato, rice, whole-grain pasta, and of course sugar are exclusively the cause of obesity. Up until recently, almost every published weight-loss diet plan advocated the restriction of these carbohydrate-rich food articles from the diet. One of the reasons that this approach was quickly embraced and followed by many was the fact that a low-carbohydrate diet will result in fairly rapid *water weight loss.* In other words if you restrict carbohydrates and eat a primarily protein-rich diet, you will lose weight initially. The big problem is that what you lose is primarily *water,* not fat. This is because the body begins to break down the existing carbohydrate stores because it requires it for energy for the muscles, brain, kidneys, and other vital organs. In breaking down its stored carbohydrates, energy is released and water is formed in large amounts (remember that carbohydrates are basically combinations of carbon and water—hence the name *carbohydrate).* This increase in fluid is eventually excreted and the "weight" that corresponds to all of this fluid is "lost". This process normally lasts for seven to ten days, during which time seven to ten pounds of water weight will be lost.

Because the stored carbohydrates have come from the muscles throughout the body and from the liver, depletion of these important and necessary carbohydrate (glycogen) stores are *replaced* as soon as possible by the body. These carbohydrate stores are what makes it possible for our muscles, heart, and brain to function normally, so the body needs to maintain these stores. It does so by taking whatever carbohydrate is left in the diet and storing it (along with water) back in the muscles and liver. Restriction of the carbohydrate content of the diet results, at best, in only a temporary reduction in water weight. But that is not even the only problem with long-term low-carbohydrate restrictive diets. These diets will also make physical exercise more exhausting and difficult, due to the depletion of glycogen. This results in an inability to maintain a satisfactory resting metabolic rate and renders weight loss nearly impossible. Exercise also makes our muscles more efficient at using fat as a source of energy rather than protein, because it improves the way insulin works and reduces the amounts secreted. In fact, both exercise and carbohydrates (those with a low glycemic index) reduce the amounts of insulin in the body which, in turn, makes fat much easier to break down and much harder to store. The foods that are recommended in the Sattvic Diets for all the Ayurvedic Constitutional Types contain primarily carbohydrates with low glycemic indexes and will naturally promote loss of body fat in a permanent, safe, and continuous manner.

Current medical evidence does not support the notion that it is starchy food or sugar that causes overweight and obesity in most individuals. Rather it is the calorie-dense fatty food in our diet that should be reduced. Studies have found that obese people prefer and consume a higher-fat diet than people of healthy weight. The over-consumption of fatty food—and not carbohydrates—is strongly associated with the development of obesity. As we have stated throughout this book, to lose weight you need to consume *fewer* and burn *more* calories. People who consume a diet high in fats by definition will also be eating a high calorie diet because fat contains more calories per gram than either carbohydrate or protein.

TABLE 15.
THE CALORIC CONTENT OF FOODS

The Caloric Content Of Foods

The caloric content of a food is a measure of how fattening it is. The table below gives the number of calories (kcal) per gram of the three basic nutients and alcohol.

Carbohydrate . . . . 1 gram = 3.40 kcal per gram
Protein . . . . 1 gram = 4.00 kcal per gram
Fat
    Long Chain . . . . 1 gram = 9.00 kcal per gram
    Medium Chain . . . . 1 gram = 7.80 kcal per gram
Alcohol . . . . 1 gram = 7.00 kcal per gram

To find the caloric content of a six ounce glass of wine use the formula below:

Calories in Wine = 0.8 (2 x % alcohol) x ounces

Example: A six ounce glass of wine containing 12.5% alcohol would have a caloric content of 0.8 (2 x 12.5) x 6 = *120 kcal.*

Chapter 10.

Sattvic Excercise

The Physiology of Movement

Although overeating is the most important cause of overweight and obesity, physical activity and the amount of daily energy expenditure is also a factor. The human body is constructed for physical activity. Deep in the development of our species we are programmed for movement and physical exertions, which once-upon-a-time were necessary for our very survival. The need to exercise is therefore a natural and healthy impulse and one that must be honored as simply as we honor all of our other natural impulses to eat, drink, sleep, and enjoy sexual pleasure. The simple satisfaction in physical movement is poignantly witnessed in the manner in which any group of young children play. In less complicated times, this innocent playfulness was easily transformed into adult activities including farming, walking, carrying, and other requirements of survival, householding, and earning a living. Unfortunately, now as we become older in our modern Western society, there is much less physical activity required of us due to modern contrivances that eliminate—unnaturally—the need for physical work.

This modern sedentary lifestyle threatens more than just weight issues. We now know that lack of physical exercise is an independent risk factor for skeletal strength (bone density) in men and women, circulatory health, immune deficiency, and insulin resistance. Recently another correlation was made between sedentariness and the common disease gallstones. Researchers at the Harvard School of Public Health studied 60,290 women between the ages of 40 and 65 years old for ten years. (New England Journal of Medicine, 341, 777-784, 1999) The women kept track of how much time they spent in physical activities, including walking, yoga, swimming, gardening, and various other forms of exercise. During the decade-long study 3,257 of the women underwent gallbladder surgery due to gallstones. The study found that women who spent 41 to 60 hours per week sitting, whether at work or home, were 42% more likely to develop gallstones than those who sat for less than 6 hours per week. More realistically, the study found that women who exercised 2 to 3 hours per week lowered their risk of gallstones by 20%. Ayurveda has always taught that the best way to avoid gallstones is to maintain an ideal body weight, reduce great fluctuations in weight, and eat a diet appropriate for your Ayurvedic constitution that contains sufficient fiber. Now we can confidently add the preventative measure of moderate exercise.

This decrease in physical activity is also a contributing factor in the maintenance of excess weight, but is not a significant cause of primary weight gain in most overweight individuals between the ages of adolescence and forty. However, the ten to twenty pound weight gain that is often seen between the ages of forty to sixty may be more directly related to the decrease in physical activity. Nevertheless, for reasons that will be explained, exercise has a significant role in any weight reduction program at any age. Although it is true that even moderately vigorous exercise does not lead to enough of an increase in energy expenditure to significantly increase initial efforts at weight loss, regular exercise can produce important long-term caloric expenditure and weight reduction. For example, a daily increase in caloric expenditure of 300 kcal. over a four month period could produce a 13.7 lb. weight loss. Most practically, exercise is instrumental in maintaining weight loss accomplished from the primary and preeminent intervention of caloric restriction. To illustrate the approximate value of exercise in consuming calories acquired by eating, Table 9 shows the caloric value of some common foodstuffs and the time required to "burn it off" using different forms of exercise. This table should make it clear in your mind that even vigorous exercise alone cannot be relied upon to control weight—it simply would require an unrealistically enormous amount of time and energy. It is the other side of the equation, energy input, where we need to focus.

TABLE 9.
Time (minutes) Required To Expend Calories From Common Foods With Various Types Of Exercise*

Food	Energy Value (kcal)	Walking	Bicycle Riding	Swimming	Running	Reclining
Apple, large	101	19	12	9	5	78
Bacon, 2 strips	96	18	12	9	5	84
Beer, 8 oz.	114	22	14	10	6	88
Bread & butter	78	15	10	7	4	60
Soda, 8 oz.	106	20	13	9	5	82
Carrot, 1 (raw)	42	8	5	4	2	32
Cottage ch., 1 tbs.	27	5	3	2	1	21
Chicken, fried (breast)	232	45	28	21	12	178
Choc. chip cookie	51	10	6	5	3	39
Egg, fried, 1	110	21	13	10	6	85
Ham, 2 slices	67	32	20	15	9	128
Hamburger	350	67	43	31	18	269
Ice cream, 1/6 qt.	193	37	24	17	10	148
Mayonnaise, 1 tbs.	92	18	11	8	5	71
Milk, skim, 8 oz.	81	16	10	7	4	62
Milk shake	421	81	51	38	22	324
Orange, 1	68	13	8	6	4	52
Pancake w/syrup, 1	124	24	15	11	6	95
Peas, 1/2 cup	56	11	7	5	3	43
Pizza, 2 slices	180	35	22	16	9	138
Potato chips, 1/2 C.	108	21	13	10	6	83
Sherbert, 1/6 qt.	177	34	22	16	9	136
Tuna sandwich	278	53	34	25	14	214

Walking, 70 kg person = 5.2 kcal/min.
Bicycle riding = 8.2 kcal/min.
Swimming = 11.2 kcal/min.
Running = 19.4 kcal/min.
Reclining = 1.3 kcal/min.
*modified from Harrison, et. al.

A Moving Experience: The Mind-Body Interface

The purpose of exercise according to Ayurveda is precisely articulated in the *Charaka Samhita*, widely regarded as the most comprehensive Ayurvedic textbook. In it, the author states: "From physical exercise one obtains lightness, capacity to work, elimination of impurities from the body, firmness of the body, efficiency of digestion, and balance of the metabolism." However, it is also clearly argued that not only too little but also excessive exercise is potentially harmful. Furthermore, as with all treatments, exercise should be prescribed differently for individuals of different Ayurvedic constitutional types. Ayurveda reminds us that exercise should make us feel strong, stable, and energetic; if your exercise regimen makes you feel tired, miserable, and sore chances are you are not exercising suitably for your particular body type.

Sattvic exercise differs from conventional models of exercise in its simultaneous emphasis on physical, mental, and energetic bodies. Properly performed, exercise is intended to not only burn calories and increase muscle mass, but also to improve flexibility, coordination, balance, breathing, posture, strength, and most importantly, self-awareness, mental agility, self-image, and self-sufficiency.

What promotes these multi-faceted benefits of physical exercise and distinguishes Sattvic from conventional exercise programs is that Sattvic exercise is performed in a quiet, self-aware state. Although self-aware exercise is difficult to precisely define, it should be regarded as physical exercise performed with an inward focus. This means that during exercise, one should remain continuously aware of the signals being given by the body and mind. This is in distinction to exercise performed that is exclusively focused on the body. All forms of exercise can integrate some degree of self-awareness into the physical activity, even fast-paced, competitive sports. However, this technique works particularly well in relation to individual activities. Specifically, your attention should include breathing, posture, muscle sensations, joint sensations, secretions, thoughts, emotions, and all aspects of physical and mental function. According to Ayurveda, exercise can be used to strengthen you both within and without. Exercise creates the following internal challenges for us to experience:

- Can I maintain a calm and quiet mind during exercise?
- Can I allow my awareness to expand to include the entire body?
- What are the feelings arising in different areas of the physical body?
- Can I become aware of the beginning and end of each movement?
- Can I maintain an awareness of the breath without interfering with it?
- Can I use my mind to direct activity to a specific region of the body?

Self-aware exercise implies an inclusion of the entire physiology into the field of awareness, without allowing the attention to be "captured" by any single sensation. Self-aware exercise has another subtle, yet important, effect. As we exercise, it powerfully reorients our consciousness to the potent natural energies within us and gives us a sense of personal empowerment. Exercise then seems to happen with no effort and our minds become anchored in the present moment. It is this sense of empowerment and effortless movement that is the true hallmark of Sattvic exercise.

Practically speaking, this means that exercise should be done without the external distraction of a blaring television, radio, or Walkman. Exercise executed in this manner is essentially a way to cultivate a deep and lasting connection between the mind and body. As we have said before, an important consequence of Sattvic exercise is that it takes the emphasis away from the future and places it in the present moment. Hence, we no longer focus on fat-burning, muscle-building, or weight-reduction but rather cue in on our breathing, physical responses, and sense of well-being during the exercise period. This is a much saner attitude to foster regarding exercise and one that results in long-term adherence and benefits.

Are You Ready to Rumble?

With regard to exercise, people who have not established this behavior as an established part of their lives are psychologically at different levels of readiness to begin. Understanding where you are can help you figure out what your next step in the right direction should be.

A five-stage model has been developed to help you. It categorizes people with various problem behaviors into one of five stages:

Stage 1. Precontemplation. These are individuals who do not recognize that they have a problem. They do not feel that any change in their behavior is necessary.

Stage 2. Contemplation. These are individuals who have begun to recognize that their behavior is unhealthy and that they should take action, but they have not decided that they will take action. Simple suggestions by others to start exercising, quit smoking, stop drinking, etc. are doomed to failure because at this stage a person has not realized the full necessity for change. Often people are protecting themselves against embarrassment, shame, low self-esteem, or hopelessness. This is the beginning of the decision-making process.

Stage 3. Preparation. The decision to take action has been made. However no action has yet taken place. This is the stage at which encouragement and support from others is very helpful.

Announcing your decision to exercise to family and close friends can help crystallize your mental movement into physical movement.

Stage 4. Action. At this stage you have begun to change your behavior—started to exercise.

It is necessary to monitor yourself, assess your progress, and set realistic goals. Now a quiet and personal resolution should be made to stay with the program you have started.

Stage 5. Maintenance. Acknowledge for yourself the benefits your new behavior has brought to the body and mind. Establish exercise as something that is no longer a chore that you somehow fit into your schedule, but rather is a natural activity like bathing, sleeping, or brushing your teeth.

TABLE 7.
THE FIVE STAGES OF CHANGING EXERCISE BEHAVIOR

Which statement most accurately describes YOU?

Precontemplation—I do not exercise and have no plans to begin.

Contemplation—I plan to begin exercising in the next 6 months.

Preparation—I plan to begin exercising in the next month.

Action—I have been exercising consistently for 2-6 months.

Maintenance—I have been exercising consistently for > 6 months.

*consistent exercise means 3 or more times per week for at least 20 minutes.

The Practical Pearls of Exercise for All Types

Let's examine some of the features of a Sattvic Exercise Program that apply to all three body types.

- The weight-loss benefits of exercise are most associated with frequency, not long duration or high intensity.

Walking or jogging around the park once a week will bring no benefit; doing the same every day and including weight training two days a week will, however, have a noticeable and significant effect on your weight and total body fat.

- Low-intensity, moderate-duration exercise programs are the best for promoting weight loss and maintenance.

Short, intense workouts cannot be sustained long enough to burn off enough calories to make a difference. The point, in any case, is not to worry about "how many calories per hour" are expended. The intent of the Sattva Program is to use exercise to reset your metabolism so that your body expends energy at a higher, more normal rate, even when you are not exercising. This is called your resting metabolic rate, which is known to be up-regulated when an individual performs low-intensity, moderate duration exercise at regular and frequent intervals.

- Perform exercise that is pleasurable to both the body and mind.

The true benefits of exercise come as much to the mind as to the body. If we desire to have healthy effects in one realm (body), we cannot subject the other realm (mind) to stress and misery. Avoid thinking about exercise as a bothersome obligation, which you force yourself to endure. Avoid overly vigorous and straining types of exercise that inflict pain. Reframe your thinking and make exercise a greatly-anticipated part of each day.

There are specific types of exercise that are most appropriate for each Ayurvedic Constitutional Type. See the next point below as well as the Chapter on your type for more details.

- Exercise to <u>fifty percent</u> of your maximum capacity.

This is an excellent guideline for all body types. If you can perform a particular free weight exercise one time with 150 lbs., begin to exercise with 75 lbs.; if you can jog on a treadmill for 60 minutes with your maximum effort, use 30 minutes as your initial duration. Exercise at fifty percent of our maximum capacity will not exhaust our energy supply, but rather add to it. After two weeks you should re-test your maximum effort, which will increase with time. Always maintain your exercise level at fifty percent of your maximum effort as it changes.

- Do not over-exercise.

Over-exercising not only predisposes you to injury, it depletes the energy stores of the entire physiology and can actually slow the metabolism as the body reacts by adopting an energy-conserving mode. Likewise, it has unsettling effects on the mind and can destabilize healthy behaviors (i.e. eating behaviors) that you have been developing.

- During menstruation keep exercise to a minimum, especially during the days of heaviest bleeding (Days 1 and 2).

Acknowledge and respect the body's need to rest during this time. Light exercise is fine, but additional rest is always a good idea, because the body expends extra energy in cleansing and rejuvenating itself during this time. Normal exercise during the pre and post menstrual periods can be continued.

Exercise For the Three Different Constitutional Types

It is important to try and choose forms of exercise that are appropriate for your Ayurvedic Constitutional Type. This is one of the most unique aspects of the Sattva Program. The tables below are a general guide to which forms of exercise are best for the three different body types.

TABLE 10A.
EXERCISES FOR VATA TYPES

These are exercises that incorporate slow, synchronized movements that will not cause exhaustion or unnecessary mental disturbance.

Aerobics, low-impact	Horseback Riding
Archery	Ice skating (indoors)
Badminton	Judo
Baseball	Sailing
Bicycle (leisurely)	Step-training
Bowling	Swimming
Dancing	Tai Chi
Golf	Table tennis
Gymnastics	Walking
Hiking	Yoga

TABLE 10B.
EXERCISES FOR PITTA TYPES

These are exercises that balance the fire element, are somewhat (but not excessively) competitive, and draw on speed, strength, stamina, and concentration.

Basketball
Bicycling (moderate)
Field hockey
Football
Gymnastics
Ice hockey
Ice skating (in/outdoors)
Kayaking
Karate
Mountainbiking
Mountain climbing
Rollerblading

Skiing (downhill/cross country)
Soccer
Sprinting
Tennis
Surfing
Water skiing
Windsurfing
Yoga
Walking/Jogging
Weight lifting

TABLE 10C.
EXERCISES FOR KAPHA TYPES

These exercises take advantage of a great capacity for strength and endurance while often having a stimulating and intense nature.

Aerobics
Basketball
Bicycling
Bowling
Calisthenics
Cross country skiing
Football
Gymnastics
Ice skating
Jogging

Racquetball
Rockclimbing
Rollerblading
Rowing
Shot put
Skiing
Stairclimbing
Tennis
Walking/Jogging (long distance)

Remember that any individual can enjoy any type of exercise—in fact, enjoyment itself is the only strict criteria to observe.

Surya Namaskar (Salutation to the Sun)

In addition to the wide variety of common forms of exercise listed above, Ayurveda also highly recommends Yoga postures (or asanas) as a part of one's daily exercise routine. Yoga exercises benefit us in much more than merely a physical way. Because these exercises involve breathing in a specific way during each posture, yoga is truly neurorespiratory and neuromuscular in its physiological effect. A regular and properly performed yoga practice can help integrate the muscles, tendons, nerves, hormones, and mind into a synchronized unit with a powerful, healthy momentum.

Surya Namaskar, or The Salutation to the Sun, is a simple yet profound series of twelve flexion and extension postures that recruits activity in all of the major large muscles and joints of the body. It creates flexibility, strength, and balance of the body... and the mind.

Instructions on the performance of these traditional postures are given below and I encourage all of you to incorporate them into your exercise routine. They can be performed in fifteen or twenty minutes each day. Regardless of the name, feel free to do them in the evening if that is more convenient.

General Instructions for Surya Namaskar (Salutation to the Sun)

1. The illustrations below show one "cycle" of Surya Namaskar, which consists of twelve postures. Begin your practice with as many cycles as is comfortable and increase every few weeks to a maximum of twelve.

2. Perform this exercise at least 30 minutes before a meal or three hours after a meal. If you are performing some other form of exercise in the same period, Surya Namaskar can be done either before (as a warm up) or after (as a cool down).

3. Hold each posture for approximately five seconds. The only exception to this is posture #6, which is only held for 1-2 seconds.

4. As mentioned above, there is a specific sequence of breathing that is used for each posture of the cycle. You will be instructed to inhale during extension postures and exhale during flexion postures. This is because inhalation fills the lungs and helps straighten and lengthen the spine, while exhalation facilitates softening, folding and flexing of the body.

5. Note that there are several postures that repeat themselves in every cycle (postures #1 and 12; postures #2 and 11; postures #3 and 10; postures #4 and 9; postures #5 and 8). There are in fact actually only seven different postures in Surya Namaskar.

6. With reference to postures #4 and 9 (Equestrian Pose): Use the same knee forward during the same cycle. Then switch to the opposite knee for the next cycle and continue to alternate. Always perform an even number of cycles so that both sides of the body are exercised symmetrically.

7. Each cycle should take between one and two minutes. Do not rush through these postures and realize that performing them slowly optimizes their effects.

8. Do not stretch more than what is comfortable and feels good. These illustrations depict an idealized form for each pose, but you may need to modify some of them. Suppleness and range of motion develop over time. Discomfort or pain during these exercises means that you are over-stretching or that you have an injury that may require medical evaluation.

9. After finishing Surya Namaskar, lie down on your back with your arms at your side, palms facing upward, eyes closed, for two minutes (Shivasana). Allow your attention to rest on the sensations coming from your body.

10. It is advisable to drink a cup of room temperature water after any session of exercise.

Instructions For Performing One "Cycle" of Surya Namaskar (Salutations to the Sun)

1. Standing Posture. Begin the Salutation to the Sun by standing with your feet parallel and your weight balanced over your feet. Place your hands together at chest level and breath gently for a period of five seconds.

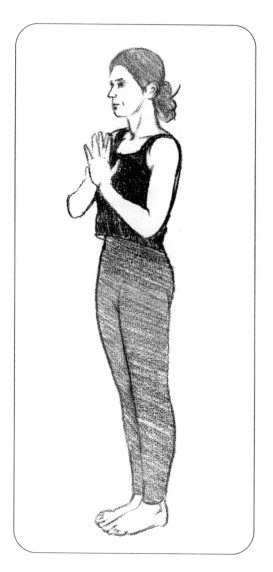

2. Hands Up Posture. As you inhale more deeply, raise both arms over the head and look upward. Feel the spine lengthening and extending.

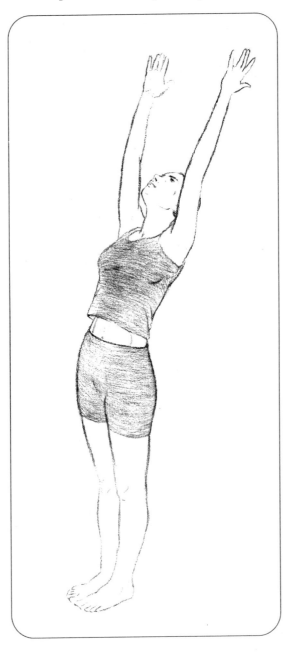

3. Forward Bend Posture. As you exhale, bend forward at the waist, allowing the knees to bend a little. The head and hands should be allowed to hang effortlessly or, if possible, the hands can touch the floor as shown.

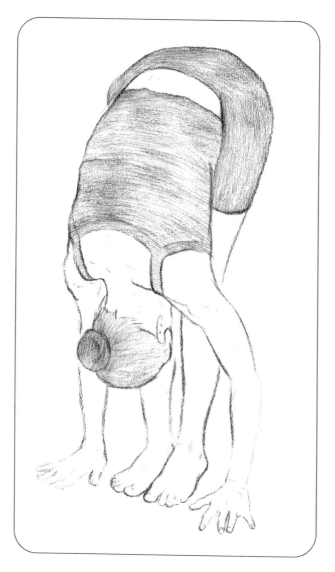

4. Lunge Posture. With the next inhalation, extend your right leg back, knee touching the floor. Let the left leg bend with the knee coming toward the chest. The left foot should stay flat on the floor. The head and neck should gently lengthen and stretch upward.

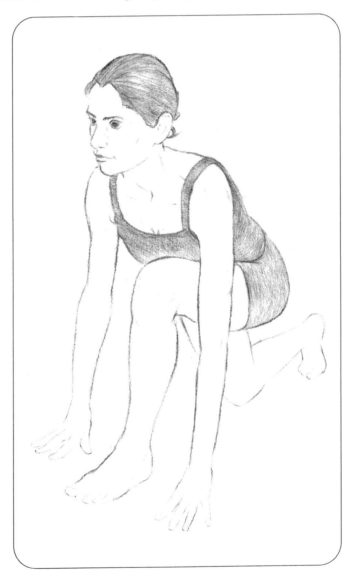

5. Downward-facing Dog Posture. As you exhale, move the right leg back, even with the left leg. Both legs can bend a little at the knees. Push the hands into the floor and raise the buttocks upward. The body should form a triangle with the floor.

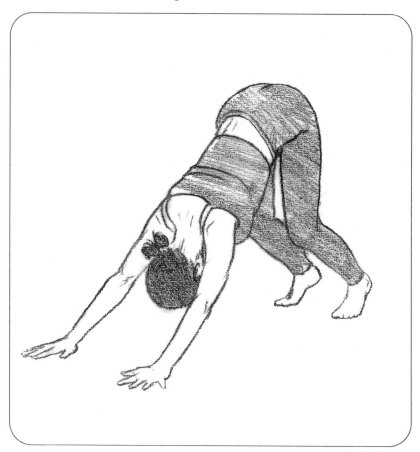

6. Stick Posture. Lower the chest and knees to the floor and briefly
   allow your chin to touch the floor also. The pelvis and buttocks are
   slightly raised off the floor. Maintain the exhalation and do not
   inhale until the next position. Hold this posture for only one or two
   seconds before proceeding to the next posture.

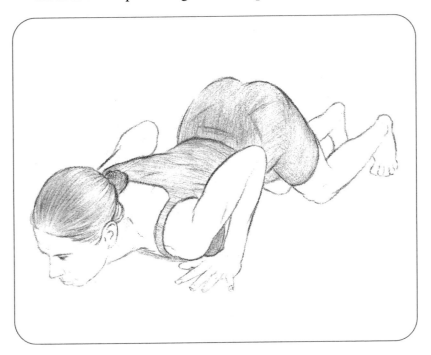

7. Cobra Posture. As you now inhale lift the head and chest up while pressing down into the floor with your hands. Keep the elbows in close to the body. Start the movement with the spine and allow the spine to then raise the head.

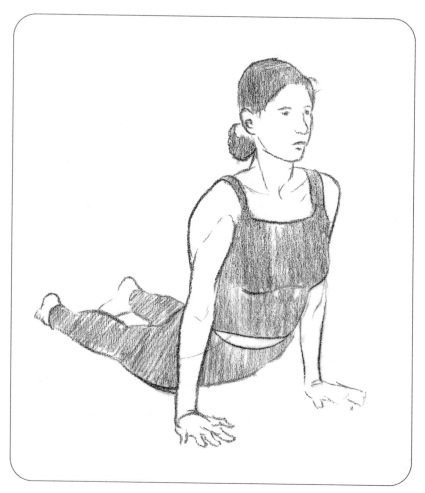

8. Downward-facing Dog Posture. Exhale and flex the hips as you raise the buttocks upward. This is a repeat of posture #5.

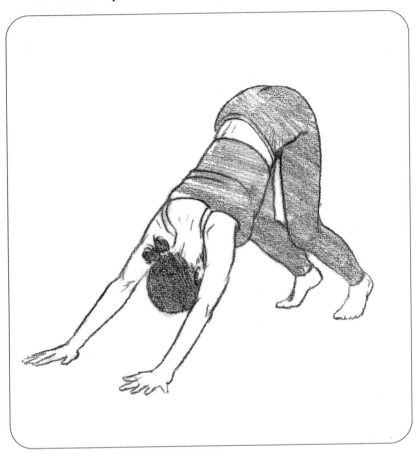

9. Lunge Posture. As you inhale, bring the left leg forward and place the left foot flat on the floor between your hands; this is a repeat of position #4. Extend the right leg backward, allowing the knee to touch the floor.

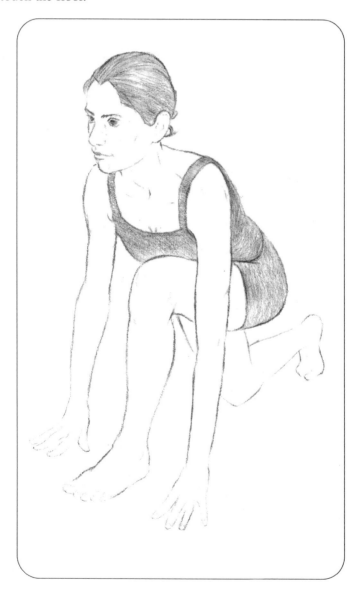

10. Forward Bend Posture. As you now exhale, bend forward and down into a flexion position, allowing the knees to bend slightly. This is a repeat of posture #3.

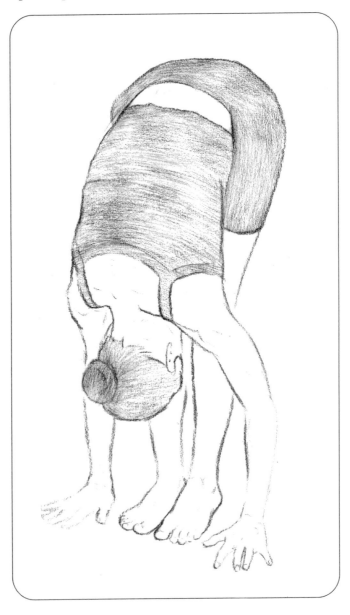

11. Hands Up Posture. Inhale and raise the arms and hands over the head as the spine stretches and lengthens upward. This is a repeat of posture #2.

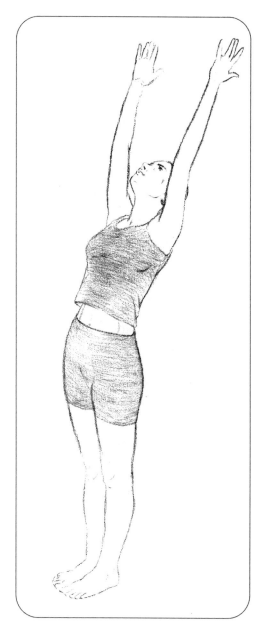

12. Standing Posture. Exhale and assume position #1 with the hands together in front of the chest. Breathe naturally for five seconds in this posture and begin the next cycle. (Note that position #12 becomes position #1 of the next cycle.)

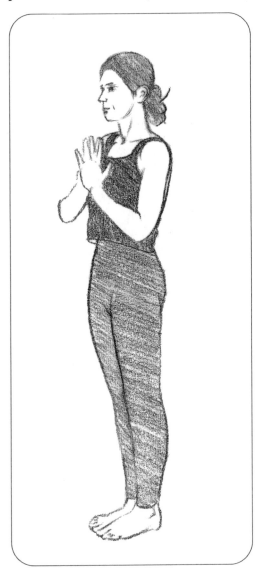

Surya Namaskar: Sequence of the Postures

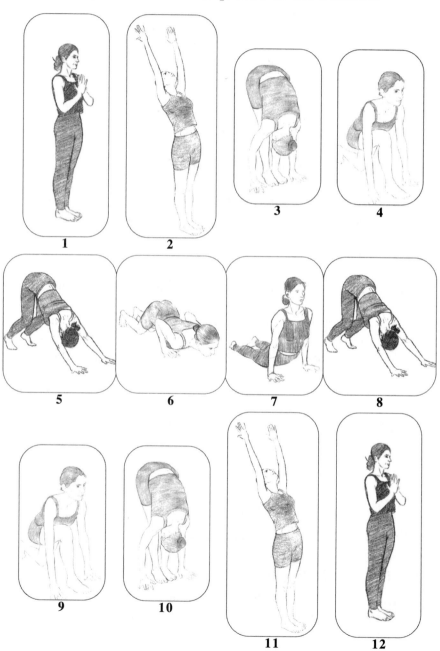

Model Sattvic Walking Program

The following is the program that I have prescribed for many of my patients over the past several years to help them begin a daily walking regimen. Although it is appropriate for almost all people of any Constitutional Type, it can be modified to meet your individual level of fitness.

This program requires a minimum of three periods of exercise each week. If possible, work up to seven days a week.

The Sattvic Walking Program

Week	Warm Up (Slow walking)	Brisk Walking	Cool Down (Slow walking)	Total Time
Week 1	5 minutes	5 minutes	5 minutes	15 minutes
Week 2	5 minutes	10 minutes	5 minutes	20 minutes
Week 3	5 minutes	12 minutes	5 minutes	22 minutes
Week 4	5 minutes	15 minutes	5 minutes	25 minutes
Week 5	5 minutes	20 minutes	5 minutes	30 minutes
Week 6	5 minutes	24 minutes	5 minutes	34 minutes
Week 7	5 minutes	28 minutes	5 minutes	38 minutes
Week 8 and...	5 minutes	30 minutes	5 minutes	40 minutes

Medical Self-Evaluation

Everyone should take the following survey before initiating any exercise program. This will help you assess if you need to consult with your physician before getting started.

Medical Self-Evaluation Survey

1. Has a physician ever told you that you have any type of hearing problem?

2. Do you currently take medication to lower your blood pressure or have you taken such medication in the past?

3. Has any close relatives (parent, sibling, child) had a heart attack before the age of 50?

4. Have you ever had:

   a) pain, pressure, or tightness in the chest caused by exertion?
   b) an episode of severe dizziness or passing out?
   c) an irregular heart beat?
   d) shortness of breath after climbing one flight of stairs?
   e) diabetes, high blood sugar, or low blood sugar?
   f) a blood test that indicated high cholesterol or "lipids"?

5. Do you currently smoke more than 1 pack of cigarettes per day?

6. Do you currently have joint pain or arthritis?

7. Do you have osteoporosis?

8. Are you more than 50 pounds overweight?

9. Are you over the age of 65 and not currently exercising regularly?

10. Do you have any reason not mentioned here to see a doctor before beginning an exercise program?

If you answered "yes" to any of these questions, you must speak to your personal physician before starting any exercise plan. Even if you answered "no" to all of these questions, it is still always a sound idea to check with your physician before significantly increasing the intensity or duration of your exercise regimen. Answering "no" to these questions does mean, however, that you are reasonably healthy and ready to exercise on a regular basis.

ATP: The "Energy Currency" of the Human Physiology

It would be useful for us to understand something about how the body turns our foods into a useable form of energy. First, all the foods that we eat are broken down into their basic components. Carbohydrates and starches (which are complex carbohydrates) are converted into glucose, proteins are converted into amino acids, and fats into fatty acids. These basic nutrients then enter into the various cells of the body where they react with specific enzymes and oxygen. These enzymes essentially break down these basic nutrients even more by breaking the chemical bonds that hold glucose, amino acids, and fatty acids together.

The energy released from the breaking of these chemical bonds is used to form a molecule called adenosine triphosphate, or ATP. Its chemical structure is shown below. Note that it is composed of three distinct parts: the nitrogen-containing base adenine, the five-carbon (pentose) sugar, ribose, and three phosphate (PO_4) groups. Further, it is important to note that the last two phosphate groups are connected by high-energy phosphate bonds, designated by the "~" symbol. These bonds contain about 8000 calories of energy per mole of ATP, which is much greater than the average chemical bonds of other organic compounds. These high-energy phosphate bonds are also able to release their stored energy instantly whenever a need arises. When ATP releases energy by splitting off one or both of its terminal phosphate groups, it becomes adenosine diphosphate (ADP) or adenosine monophosphate (AMP), respectively. By then using energy from our foods, these molecules recombine with phosphoric acid to form ATP once again. Thus, ATP is a reusable energy source that can be continuously used and remade over and over.

FIGURE 1.
The Chemical Structure Of ATP (Adenosine Triphosphate).

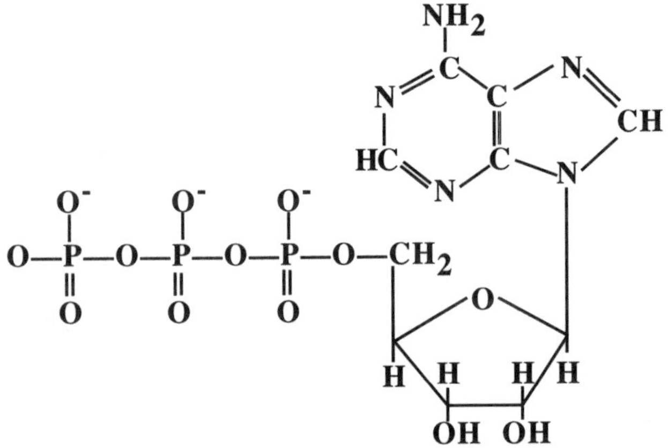

ATP is without a doubt the most important naturally synthesized chemical in the human body and that is why I feel it is important to at least mention its place in the general scheme of weight management. Everyone working in the nutritional sciences acknowledges that it is excess calories that result in the accumulation of excess body weight, but technically speaking, it is excess ATP that is at the root of it all. After all, foods have their caloric values calculated from a knowledge of how much ATP is created from it in the body and then released in the form of heat. A calorie is simply the amount of heat needed to raise the temperature of one gram of water 1 degree Centigrade. You can appreciate the power of ATP when you consider that each of its two high-energy phosphate bonds provide 8000 calories or 16,000 calories per molecule.

ATP is used as the energy source for every physical, mental, endocrine, nervous, secretory, and any other process or function in the physiology. It is perhaps useful to mention a few of the more specific processes that ATP makes possible. It is used for the synthesis of new proteins by forging new peptide bonds between amino acids. It is used to synthesize nerve tissue, hormones, enzymes, and all metabolically active substances of the body. It is used to make the waste product urea, which is how the body rids itself of the extremely toxic metabolite ammonia. In addition ATP makes possible the many instances of active transport across cell membranes against electrochemical gradients, without which life could not be maintained. It is used to propagate nerve impulses in our brains and nervous system. It makes possible the fertilization of the ovum by the sperm and the continuation of our species. And perhaps most appropriate to present during our discussion of exercise, ATP is the energy source for the contraction of our muscles—which points to its fundamental significance in utilizing exercise to promote energy expenditure in the Sattva Program for weight loss.

Exercise and the Mind

Because the state of one's emotions and mental balance is so influential on the success of any weight loss program, I want to focus for a moment on the mental health benefits associated with a regular exercise program. Centuries ago, exercise was recognized as a therapeutic intervention to promote mental well-being. It is inexpensive, can be practiced by almost anyone, can be modified to any individual's needs, is extremely effective, and has very few side effects. Without a stable and calm mind, it is difficult to use The Sattva Program, or any program, to its fullest potential to manage weight issues.

Despite several study design limitations found in the literature, a significant body of evidence supports the ancient observation that exercise can improve mental health. The relationship between exercise and depression and exercise and anxiety has been most extensively studied. Both physiological and psychological theories have been proposed to explain why exercise affects emotional and mental states.

Physiological Theories

One theory is based on the observation that exercise enhances the release and neurotransmission of dopaminergic, serotoninergic, and adrenergic nervous impulses, which results in mood modification. Another theory postulates that it is the release of the endogenous substances endorphin and enkephalin that creates the psychological benefits. Other researchers have shown that the increase in body temperature that results from exercise causes the brain stem to program a more synchronized electrical activity pattern in the cerebral cortex, subjectively experienced as a more restful state of mind. Temperature increases in the brain stem has also been shown to decrease muscle spindle activity, which reduces the antagonistic tension in muscles throughout the body and contributes to generalized relaxation. Finally, exercise is known to increase the production and release of endogenous steroidal compounds (i.e. cortisol) from the adrenal glands that help mitigate against the effects of stress.

Psychological Theories

In addition to the proposed physiological mechanisms through which exercise exerts its influences on the mind, numerous psychological theories have been advanced. Among these is one that observes that both exercise and anxiety have similar physical effects of increased heart rate, perspiration, increased systolic blood pressure, increased respiratory rate, and increased levels of arousal. Anxiety has one feature that exercise does not, and that is emotional distress. Therefore, the absence of emotional distress in exercise conditions the mind to not automatically exhibit that distress when the other accompanying physical symptoms occur. Other studies have shown exercise to improve a sense of self-control and improved self-image. Another theory proposes that exercise simply distracts an individual from negative thoughts, emotions and behaviors. An interesting investigation by one researcher concluded that perceived fitness was more closely correlated with psychological improvement than actual fitness (as measured by VO_2 max exercise testing). A growing number of researchers are validating what the ancient Ayurvedic physicians told us long ago. Proper exercise can play a major role in alleviating mental stress.

CHAPTER 11.

AYURVEDIC HERBAL MEDICINES USED TO SUPPORT WEIGHT LOSS

*O*n any given day, over 75% of the medicines taken by the people of our planet will be herbal medicines. In what seems to be an astonishing oversight, modern medical science has until now largely dismissed herbal medicine as primitive and inadequate to address modern health issues. There may now finally be a reversal taking place in the medical community as an increasing number of reports appear in scientific journals around the world documenting the efficacy and safety of many herbal medicines. This new popularity of herbal medicine is based in large part on the ability of researchers to dissect and isolate biologically active components, with the help of powerful new analytic tools. Our modern "alternative" community seems to embrace an herbal remedy only after reports come out of its "active component". These active components are then shown in clinical studies to neutralize, activate, or in some way effect various tangible aspects of human physiology. More and more, the modern herbal ideal is becoming distorted into an effort to pharmacologically target our remedies—in almost the exact same way as conventional medicine uses antibiotics, monoclonal antibodies, and prescription medicines. This is not in accord with the Ayurvedic view of herbal therapy, as we shall see.

Ayurveda sees the root of obesity and all diseases as disorders of energies that in turn disrupt the healthy function of the body, mind and spirit. If we accept this premise, then we can easily see how the use of herbs or medicines aimed at the physical dimension of a disease can be, at best, only partially effective and at worst may even exacerbate the disease further.

If we understand diseases to be simultaneously affecting the body, mind, and spirit as an integrated whole, then we really should be searching for an entirely new class of medicines—a class of medicine that promotes a self-corrective, homeostatic (i.e. balancing) action. This class of medicines would not depend, could not depend, on single active components with specific and limited actions; rather they would have wide-ranging supportive effects on many different systems simultaneously.

Fortunately, we do not have to search very far for this "new" class of medicines. They are our plant-based herbal medicines used for centuries around the world by sophisticated cultures that have used them extensively to prevent and cure disease.

Whereas modern medicine is obsessed with the notion of a tangible, identifiable "enemy", Ayurveda sees illness more as an imbalance in the constitution of the individual that allows disease to take root. We see the problem to be more a question of the soil than of the seed. So often today we hear about modern medicine identifying a virus, a bacteria, or a genetic mutation that is the "cause" of a specific malady. In very few cases is this single, materialistic "enemy" the true cause. There are so many examples of the flaw in this reductionist approach. One such example is our attempt to explain the cause of coronary artery disease, which can lead to heart attack. The conventional thinking on this issue has changed constantly over the past thirty years as we pass from one singular causative candidate to the next. First it was considered to be a result of increased total serum cholesterol which led to plaque formation. Then, scientists decided it was due to the proliferation of underlying intimal smooth muscle protruding into the blood vessel, then LDL-cholesterol oxidation, then lipoprotein-a, and then a mutation of a specific platelet fibrinogen receptor. It has also been hypothesized that the process begins not with accumulation of any substance but with injury to the endothelial lining of the coronary vessels. Some researchers have even pointed to a specific bacteria (Chlamydia pneumoniae) as the cause as well as a number of other putative infectious agents. Most recently, a substance known as homocysteine has been offered as yet another possible cause of myocardial infarction.

Clearly, we still do not know what causes coronary artery disease, asthma, arthritis, hypertension, depression or any disease. We will never identify that elusive physical "enemy" because all diseases are the result of multifactorial imbalances at the level of body, mind and spirit. Even in "holistic" circles I witness the exact same reductionist approach, especially among the newest breed of poorly trained "holistic practitioners", "educators", "counselors", and the like. In the place of the virus they do little more than substitute a new enemy, which they label stress, depleted qi or another term. They then perpetuate the medical illusion of control and protection by plying their patients full of supplement after supplement in a misguided effort to build a stronger physical fortress.

Ayurveda contains a well-established and effective knowledge base of herbal medicines that promote and maintain detoxification, general balance and weight reduction. Herbs can be combined in literally hundreds of formulations to support lipid metabolism, blood cleansing, tissue cleansing, thermogenesis, or to strengthen the function of the immune system. In addition to herbal materials, Ayurveda also uses common but very medicinal spices to help direct and intensify the effects of the treatment. We do not abandon the achievements of medical science but rather bring it into line with our timeless truths and forge an intellectually vigorous and intuitive synthesis of ancient and modern knowledge.

The following are the most important herbs and spices used in Ayurvedic Medicine to promote weight loss. Please refer to the Appendix for a complete profile on each of these herbs.

HERBS

Triphala
Guggulu (*Commiphora mukul*)
Citraka (*Plumbago zeylanica*)
Vidanga (*Embelia ribes*)
Katuki (*Picrorrhiza kurroa*)
Garcinia cambogia (*Malabar Tamarind*)
Gurmar (*Gymnema sylvestre*)
Pushkarmula (*Inula racemosa*)
Agnimantha (*Premna mucronata*)
Punarnava (*Boerhaavia diffusa*)
Arjuna (*Terminalia arjuna*)
Ativisa (*Aconitum heterophyllum*)
Patala (*Steroespermum suaveolens*)
Tea (*Camellia sinensis*)

SPICES

Ginger (dry)
Garlic
Black Pepper
Cayenne Pepper
Parsley Leaf
Cardamom seed
Turmeric
Cinnamon
Coriander

For convenience, at the beginning of this chapter, the make-up of the Sattva Basic Formulation is given. I strongly urge you to continue reading the remainder of this chapter that gives important information regarding the Ayurvedic concept of herbal medicine.

All individuals, regardless of Ayurvedic Constitutional Type, should take the *Sattva Basic Formulation*, which consists of a combination of the following herbs found in the two lists above. Dosages of each component are given. Weigh and combine all ingredients and put into "00" veggie caps. Take two capsules twice a day 30-60 minutes before breakfast and dinner.

Guggulu (standardized to 2.5% guggulsterones) . . . . . . 125 mg. (1 part)
Citraka . . . . 500 mg. (4 parts)
Punarnava (standardized to 25% alkaloids) . . . . 125 mg. (1 part)
Garcinia (standardized to 10% hydroxycitric acid) . . . . 125 mg. (1 part)
Triphala powder . . . . 500 mg. (4 parts)
Ginger . . . . 250 mg. (2 parts)
Cayenne Pepper . . . . 250 mg. (2 parts)
Black Pepper . . . . 250 mg. (2 parts)

Obtain these herbs and spices in powdered form from a reputable source of Ayurvedic herbs. For recommendations of reputable suppliers, see Appendix.

If you do not have a scale, simply combine the herbs by parts as indicated above. For example, combine one teaspoon of Guggulu, four teaspoons of Citraka, one teaspoon of Punarnava, etc. Mix very well. Obtain "00" veggie caps from your local pharmacy, health food store, or supplier (see Appendix) and fill them yourself.

Dosage: 2 "00" capsules twice a day 30-60 minutes before breakfast and dinner.

The other herbs and spices in the above lists should be added to the Basic Formulation according to your Ayurvedic Constitutional Type. See the specific recommendations for each Type that are given in the chapter entitled "Recommendations for Specific Constitutional Types".

Ayurvedic Herbology

Although a complete review of Ayurvedic pharmacodynamics is outside the scope of this book, it is relevant to include some information on the fundamental principles of the Ayurvedic materia medica. I think you will find it fascinating and helpful.

You already know that the basic foundation of Ayurvedic science rests upon our understanding of the five elements, which are considered the physicochemical cause of the human body and the whole of nature, including our foods and herbs. We have previously described how the ancient physicians saw that in living systems the five elements generate the three doshas, or tridoṣa. The three doshas enable us to understand the physiological functions of the body as well as the features of health and disease through an assessment of their state of balance or imbalance. Furthermore, we have seen that the primary objective in Ayurvedic Medicine is the restoration and maintenance of doshic equilibrium, which is accomplished through knowledge of the principle of "like increases like". In other words, substances with similar elemental compositions will increase those elements and those with dissimilar elemental compositions will decrease those elements.

It must by now be clear that Ayurveda is not oriented primarily to administering herbs or drugs as the main therapeutic approach. Nevertheless drug therapies continue to be the chief tool in western medicine. As a result of the growing interest in Ayurveda over the past twenty years, many pharmaceutical companies are today attempting to exploit the ancient materia medica in an effort to develop contemporary "natural" medicines. While there is no debate that Ayurveda should be revisited and supported from a modern technological viewpoint, we must be extremely cautious about applying technology and over-analysis where it does not belong.

The fact is that Ayurvedic medicines are much more closely related to foods than to drugs.

Both foods and medicines exert their effects on the human biology in much the same way; the laws that govern these effects are the same. Ayurvedic herbal "drugs" are understood to consist of specific nutrients for different tissues and organs. They act at the molecular level within cells in an essentially non-pharmacological manner by restoring health and normalizing function. Their observed actions are explained more accurately by holistic nutritional dynamics rather than by classical pharmacodynamics. Thus, it should not surprise you that Ayurvedic scientists did indeed develop a complete and insightful system of Ayurvedic Pharmacology, which is holistic and allows us to understand the actions of both herbal medicines and foods in our bodies. This system of Ayurvedic Pharmacology is known as Principles of the Qualities of Substances and it includes seven aspects:

Principles of the Qualities of Substances

1. Dravya	Substance or material
2. Guṇa	Qualities or attributes
3. Rasa	Taste
4. Vīrya	Potency
5. Vipāka	Long-term action
6. Prabhāva	Unique action
7. Karma	Biological action

Let us briefly define each of these seven concepts.

Dravya means the actual substance that is being used as a medicine or food.

Guṇa(s) are the physical properties, or qualities, of an herb or food article. These qualities include ten pairs of opposites, e.g. hot/cold, soft/ hard, oily/dry, etc. and were discussed in Chapter 5. Rasa refers to the taste of a substance, which is in turn determined by its elemental composition. Taste is perceived by the tastebuds on the tongue. Rasa, i.e. taste, exists only for the time that a given substance is in contact with the tongue and ceases to exist as an attribute as the herb or food is transformed during the subsequent stages of digestion.

Vīrya is often translated as the potency of an herb, but this definition has caused confusion among many students of Ayurveda so I will try to perhaps clarify this term a little more. Vīrya is essentially the biological action that a plant possesses due to its particular guṇas (qualities). It is this very biological action that must be carefully preserved through the proper collection, handling, drying, and processing of any herb, which must take place in the proper season and when the plant has aged appropriately. In other words, vīrya is the innate power of a plant derived from its constellation of qualities. There are six types of vīryas:

THE SIX TYPES OF VĪRYAS

Heavy

Light

Hot

Cold

Oily

Dry

Vipāka refers to the post-digestive "taste" of a food or herb after it has been consumed, metabolized and absorbed into the body. However, vipāka is not truly a perceived "taste" but rather is an indirect taste inferred from its long-term effect on the doshas and tissues of the body.

Vipāka is of three kinds:

THE THREE VIPĀKAS

Sweet

Sour

Pungent

After a particular rasa (i.e. taste) has been consumed over a period of weeks or months, the action of the vipāka of that taste becomes apparent. The tastes (rasa) become post-digestive tastes (vipāka) according to the following pattern:

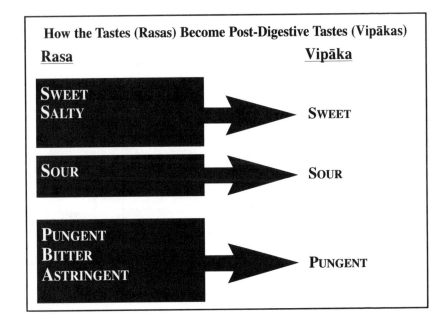

How the Tastes (Rasas) Become Post-Digestive Tastes (Vipākas)

The sweet and salty tastes become sweet in their effect on the body tissues; sour taste remains sour in its effect; and the pungent, bitter, and astringent tastes all exert a post-digestive pungent action on the body tissues. This concept of vipāka is a concept unique to Ayurveda.

Prabhāva is another fascinating aspect of Ayurvedic pharmacology theory. This term refers to any unique action of an herb (or food) that is not predictable from a knowledge of its taste, qualities, constituents, or other factors. Whereas the vīrya of a substance is always predictable from its taste, qualities, and elemental composition, prabhāva is the unique and specific action of that substance. Examples would be the analgesic effects of chili peppers (*Capsicum annum L.*) or the putative anti-tumor effects of aloe vera (*Aloe barbadensis Mill.*)

Finally, **karma** refers to the predominant action of a substance on the mind-body of the individual who is using it. Ayurvedic texts list fifty groups of herbal medicines based on their actions. We will not include the entire list here but give just a few examples of herbal actions (karmas): anti-itch, laxative, anti-cough, fatigue-reducing, weight-reducing, cardioprotective, analgesic, febrifuge, promoting fertility, expectorant, anti-arthritic, anti-asthmatic, aphrodisiac, diuretic, etc.

Compound Herbal Formulations

Once the qualities and actions of individual herbs are understood, we can begin to comprehend the principles of herb combining, which has been brought to a very high art in Ayurveda. Ayurvedic medicine uses a true holistic science in prescribing herbal medicines. Ayurveda never uses "herbal extracts" or other forms of isolated active ingredients. Ayurveda only uses the whole crude plant or plant part, which contains many constituents. Some of these constituents are biologically active, some mitigate against undesired side effects, some act as co-factors, some are enzymes, some are nutrients, some promote assimilation, some are synergistic, and some may be inert. It is this entire and unique combination of organic components that has given life to that plant and endowed it with its strength and structure. Thus, technically, even a single herb is in reality a multitude of substances. Yet, Ayurvedic physicians take this further in creating complex mixtures of many plants and plant parts. The herbal formulations recommended in this book to help promote weight loss and maintenance are classical formulations observed for centuries to produce the desired therapeutic effect when used correctly by the appropriate individual who also incorporates the other features of the Sattva Program.

If you have further interest in the theory and practice of Ayurvedic pharmacology and herbology, please see the bibliography for additional references.

Allopathic Medicines for Weight Loss

With the failure of the conventional dietary approach to weight loss in many obese patients in the 1960's came the appearance of different powerful pharmacologic agents that were prescribed for this purpose. This brief section is not meant to be an exhaustive review of the allopathic drugs used in obesity, but rather an examination of several very common agents used today for weight control. I think the story of the ineffectiveness of these few drugs will make the point that allopathic diet pills of any kind will, at best, result in meager, temporary benefit and, at worst, cause life-threatening consequences.

When weight loss was noted as a side effect of dextroamphetamine, it wasn't long before pharmaceutical companies began manufacturing this synthetic drug for this indication and doctors began prescribing it without much discrimination. By the 1970's it became obvious that amphetamines are associated with serious problems including dependence, tolerance, and a significant number of deaths which resulted in a decrease in their use. Although several drugs in this class remained in use through much of the1980's (e.g. phentermine and mazindol) medical reports of their serious adverse effects and ineffectiveness has fortunately finally led to their rejection by mainstream medicine and most consumers.

But the general paradigm of using drugs as a simple solution to the multifactorial problem of obesity somehow survived. In the early part of the 1990's the weight-loss consciousness of the nation was once again captured by two dramatic events. I say dramatic only because the media coverage that was afforded both of these events made them so. One was the discovery of leptins, which was touted as the key to understanding the genetic basis of obesity. The second, more ominous event, was the publication of a single clinical trial that showed the success of the now infamous drug phen-fen (a combination of phentermine and fenfluramine) in reducing weight in obese individuals. You probably know the rest of the story. Within a year, the disturbing discovery of heart valve abnormalities in users of this drug, as well as a high incidence of primary pulmonary hypertension, resulted in its mandated withdrawal in 1997.

Since that time several other new agents have been approved for use by the Food and Drug Administration (for example, orlistat, a fat absorption blocker, and sibutramine, an appetite suppressant) but physicians are now reluctant to prescribe drugs for weight loss after the phen-fen debacle.

Sibutramine was initially created as an antidepressant and weight loss was noted as a side effect. Sibutramine is both a seratonin and noradrenaline re-uptake inhibitor. To date several trials have typically shown anywhere between 5-9% weight loss in obese subjects over 9-12 months. Adverse effects include increases in blood pressure and heart rate, among others.

Orlistat is a drug in a class called lipase inhibitors that supposedly works by reducing the intestinal absorption of dietary fat. It doesn't get absorbed into the body and remains in the gastrointestinal tract. Several (six) studies have shown a modest increase in weight loss by using this drug. The problem is that orlistat causes loose stools, oily stools, abdominal bloating, and underwear spotting. These effects are particularly troublesome if fat is the source of 30% or more of a person's calories. Orlistat is absolutely contraindicated for individuals with chronic malabsorption syndromes, colitis, irritable bowel syndrome, or cholestasis. Also, because it blocks fat absorption, it reduces the absorption of the important fat-soluble vitamins A, D, E, and K, as well as the carotenes.

You can see neither of these two newer drugs are particularly effective and their safety is questionable as well. I do not understand why scientists persist in this narrow-minded quest for the imaginary magic obesity bullet.

This is also probably a good place to comment on the so-called "herbal supplements" being promoted to achieve weight loss. Herbs can be as dangerous, ineffective and expensive as conventional medicines. One of the best examples of one of these hoaxes is the many products that combine caffeine and ephedrine. These "natural" products commonly derive their ephedrine content from the Chinese herb ephedra (also known as Ma Huang) and their caffeine content from the Brazilian herb guarana. They typically also contain Siberian ginseng, stinging nettles, chromium, damiana leaf, and even vitamin E and bee pollen for good measure. These latter ingredients will neither give any clinical benefit in weight loss nor protect from the adverse effects of caffeine or ephedrine. Ephedrine acts as a sympathomimetic and is presumed to stimulate the metabolic rate by causing increased release of norepinephrine from sympathetic nerve endings. It is thought to act as both an appetite suppressant and a thermogenic (heat increasing) agent. Ephedrine is structurally similar to adrenaline and methamphetamine but has fewer side effects because it doesn't reach the cerebral circulation as efficiently.

Caffeine, a methylxanthine, is chemically similar to theophylline. It is a mild central nervous system stimulant as everyone knows and is also a diuretic. Ephedrine has a half-life in the body of about six hours while caffeine ranges between three and six hours.

The side effects of caffeine are well known to most and are generally benign, unless an individual is particularly sensitive to it (approximately 10% of the population). Caffeine may cause insomnia, nervousness, anxiety, tremors, palpitations, acid reflux, heartburn and restlessness.

The side effects of ephedrine are more serious. It can cause significantly increased blood pressure, chest pain, tachycardia (increased heart rate), palpitations, coronary artery spasm, tremors, psychotic episodes, vertigo (sensation of the room spinning), headache, perspiration, urinary retention, dry mouth, nervousness, insomnia and acute anxiety. It is definitely contraindicated in people with high blood pressure, heart disease of any type, and hyperthyroidism. In addition it is potentially dangerous (relatively contraindicated) to use if you happen to have any of the following conditions: diabetes, glaucoma, pregnancy, seizure disorder, benign prostatic hypertrophy, or a history of anxiety.

Yet with all of these potential adverse effects and paltry benefits, dozens of products containing combinations of ephedrine and caffeine (as Ma Huang/Guarana) continue to be sold. Because "food supplement" advertising and labeling regulations have been relaxed in recent years, the consumer has to be careful—really careful. As in the world of conventional obesity medications, in the arena of herbal medicines it is also buyer beware.

CHAPTER 12.

RECOMMENDATIONS FOR SPECIFIC CONSITUTIONAL TYPES

*D*iets and general programs that are appropriate for each of the three major constitutional types are considered in detail in this chapter. In Chapter 2 we defined *constitutional type* as the proportion of Vata, Pitta, and Kapha energies with which we were born. It is this proportion which influences our physical appearance, our biological strength, and our mental and emotional tendencies. Every food, herb, and activity in nature is characterized by different attributes. For example, a food can have attributes like soft, hard, hot, cold, etc.; an herb can be light, heavy, oily or dry; an exercise activity can be relaxing or vigorous. All of these attributes are known in Ayurveda as *gunas*, or qualities. Substances and activities that are similar in qualities to our constitutional type tend to increase or aggravate it, while those with opposite qualities to a particular dosha decrease and control it. For example, Kapha dosha tends to be heavy, moist, and solid. A food like avocado is also heavy, moist, and solid. A person of Kapha constitution who eats too much avocado will aggravate Kapha and promote excess water and earth element in the body resulting in water retention, mucous production and weight gain. Conversely, foods like asparagus or apple have qualities opposite to those of Kapha and will reduce this dosha.

The idea behind the Sattva Program is to consume foods and engage in activities that will calm and control the main dosha in your constitution.

The Sattva Program For Kapha Types

Sattva Program Diet For Kapha Types

Many of the general principles of the Sattva Program outlined in the previous chapters apply to Kapha Types and should be incorporated. If you've skipped to this section and haven't read those chapters yet, I strongly suggest you do so. However, some of these general principles need to be modified to best suit individuals of Kapha constitutional type. These modifications are the subject of this chapter. Since the *diet* is the most important of these modifications, we will begin there.

Because Kapha-type people tend towards *tamas*, it will be useful to briefly review this mental tendency. Tamas is described as a mental imbalance that brings about *stagnation and inertia*. There is an attraction towards darkness and obsession with dull and destructive pastimes. These people generally develop heaviness and congestion of body and mind. They have difficulty initiating and then maintaining relationships because of their tendency for self-regard and inability to extend concern for others. They are somewhat greedy and overly concerned with personal finances. Usually there is degeneration first of the emotional and ethical foundation of the mind which is wrought with depression followed sometimes by nervous and circulatory disease. Chronic fatigue, arthritis, cancer, cysts, heart disease, and general metabolic imbalances will often follow, according to genetic predisposition. Rather than being of service to mankind, tamasic individuals prefer to be served and entertained; they suffer from "sedentarism" and find it difficult to be active. Most of all tamas destroys discrimination and discipline and leads to overeating and overindulgence in unevolved behaviors. Tamas leads to cravings for rich-tasting, sweet, processed foods devoid of prana as well as meat and intoxicants which further dull the mind.

Therefore, Kapha type individuals will do best with a diet that is somewhat more spicy and stimulating than the other two doshic types. Also, Kapha types benefit most from a diet that is light, warm, and dry. They should greatly reduce foods that are oily, heavy, dense, and cold.

As you will see from the list below, the Kapha Diet favors foods with the *pungent, bitter, and astringent* tastes and reduces foods with the sweet, sour and salty tastes. Because by definition most foods are somewhat sweet in taste, it follows logically that to reduce the sweet taste Kapha individuals need to eat less food in general. On the other hand herbs, which are usually bitter and/or astringent in taste, can be used to great advantage in people of Kapha constitutional type.

THE KAPHA DIET

How to use this list

One of the most unique facets of Ayurvedic dietetics is that different foods from each food group are recommended for different Ayurvedic Constitutional Types. In Chapter 8 a general Sattvic food list was provided. The list that follows has been developed according to Ayurvedic principles and is specific for individuals of Kapha Constitution.

In using the following lists, eat mainly from the "Often" and "In Moderation" lists and only infrequently or on special occasions from the "Seldom" list.

"Often" in this context means consuming these foods every day would be fine.

"In Moderation" means that you should consume approximately **one-third to one-half** the amount of these foods as you do the "Often" foods. These foods are an important part of your diet, are not unhealthy for you and should definitely be included in your diet *in the proper amounts.*

"Seldom" means about once a month.

The Sattvic Kapha Shopping List

Please use this list as a convenient shopping list to assist you in shopping intelligently at your local supermarket and natural food stores. We suggest that you purchase organically grown products as much as possible. This will ensure that you will not be exposed to pesticides, insecticides, hormones and other harmful chemicals. If you cannot obtain organic produce, make sure you follow the suggested produce-washing procedure outlined on page 195. Once you have assembled a variety of the appropriate food items listed here, we will explain when and how much of each to eat. As you will see, the Sattva Program is simple and easy. It requires little in the way of strict discipline and becomes a uniquely individualized program of health that you help to create.

THE KAPHA DIET

FRUITS

Often	In Moderation		Seldom
Apples	Oranges	Strawberries	Bananas
Pears	Grapefruits	Raspberries	Dates
Pomegranate	Pineapple	Papaya	Mango
Cranberries	Grapes	Lemon	Coconut
Persimmons	Cantaloupe	Lime	Avocado
	Figs (raw)	Cherries	Raisins
	Passionfruit	Plums	Prunes
	Peaches	Loquats	Honeydew
	Lychees	Nectarine	
	Guava	Blueberries	
	Apricots		

VEGETABLES

Often		In Moderation	Seldom
Green Peppers	Lettuce (all)	Beets	Tomatoes
Red Peppers	Watercress	Potatoes	Squash (all)
Asparagus	Celery	Pumpkin	Corn
Cauliflower	Collards	Mushrooms	Okra
Artichoke (Globe)	Dandelion		Sweet potatoes
Garlic	Fennel		Yams
Artichoke (Jerusalem)	Horseradish		Cucumbers
Bamboo Shoots	Kale		Pickles
Green Beans	Leeks		
Peas	Mustard Greens		
Lima Beans	Onions		
Mung Beans	Parsley		
Bean Sprouts (all)	Parsnips		
Cabbage	Chili peppers		
Brussels Sprouts	Radishes		
Carrots	Shallots		
Spinach	Swiss Chard		
Turnips			

GRAINS

Often	In Moderation	Seldom
Barley	Basmati rice	Wheat
Millet	Brown rice	Semolina
Rye	Oats	Wild rice
Buckwheat		White rice
Amaranth		Corn
Arrowroot		Sorghum
Quinoa		

LEGUMES

All legumes and beans without exception are good for Kapha types. Consider them all to be "Often" foods.

Adzuki beans	Soybeans
Common Beans	Mung beans
Tofu	Peas
Miso	Split peas
Tempeh	Lentils
Lima beans	Chickpeas (Garbanzo beans)
Broad beans	Jackbeans
Kidney beans	

NUTS AND SEEDS

Although nuts and seeds are an excellent protein source and need not be strictly avoided, they are dense, heavy, and oily and are best used in moderation.

Often	In Moderation	Seldom
None	Alfalfa seeds	Brazil nuts
	Pumpkin seeds	Cashew nuts
	Sesame seeds	Coconut
	Almonds	Filberts (Hazelnuts)
	Chestnuts	Macadamia
	Flaxseeds	Peanuts
	Pinenuts	Pecans
		Pistachio nuts
		Sunflower seeds
		Walnuts

193

FATS AND OILS

All fats and oils are best used in strict moderation.

Often	In Moderation	Seldom	
None	*Unrefined* Flaxseed oil	Corn oil	Butter
	Unrefined Olive oil	Soy oil	Tahini
	(extra virgin only)	Sunflower oil	Olives
	Unrefined Sesame oil	Safflower oil	Mayonnaise
	Ghee	Canola oil	
		Almond oil	
		Peanut oil	
		Cottonseed oil	
		Palm kernel oil	
		Coconut oil	

In ancient times, there was no concept of "calories" as we know it today. Modern Ayurvedic Medicine recognizes the usefulness of this concept and incorporates it into the context of a holistic approach to weight loss and management. However, Ayurveda shuns the idea of selecting foods solely on the basis of their caloric value. This type of diet typically leads to dietary deficiencies, energetic imbalances at the doshic level, and a high rate of non-compliance.

Rather, the Sattva Program—Ayurveda's answer to weight problems—advises us to select a proper amount of foods from each of the various food groups so that we take in a nutritionally balanced diet. The trick is to have enough of these highly nutritious foods to be physically and emotionally satisfied, yet little enough to keep the energy content of the diet sufficiently low to promote weight loss.

Ayurveda elegantly solves this problem by offering diets consisting of foods from the seven Food Categories that are recommended in different quantities, depending on the calorie level you are observing. Simply choose the specific foods from the *Kapha Sattva Shopping List* (or the Vata or Pitta shopping lists, according to your Ayurvedic Constitutional Type), and observe the recommendations for daily servings (see section entitled "What Is A Serving" at the end of this chapter).

Chapter 12. Recommendations For Specific Constitutional Types

Produce-Washing Procedure

Non-organic raw vegetables and fruits often contain pesticides, parasites and other microorganisms not visible to the naked eye. Through my own experimentation I have found that the following simple procedure effectively removes these substances and organisms:

Soak all fruits, vegetables, greens roots, and other produce which you want to eat raw in a dilute solution of apple cider vinegar and 3% hydrogen peroxide for 15 to 30 minutes. Then rinse in clean, cold water. Use one tablespoon of each per gallon of water. In practical usage this means about two tablespoons of each added to the average sink full of water (assuming approximately two gallon capacity). The apple cider vinegar is effective for disrupting the cell membranes of many microorganisms and the hydrogen peroxide can effectively break down the amino acid structure of most pesticides. This procedure does *not* affect the taste or smell of the foods in any way.

It is worth noting here that we all harbor a great number of organisms in our bodies. The person who establishes a high level of health and balance usually is not affected by these organisms in an adverse way. Normally the digestive enzymes are concentrated enough to destroy harmful organisms and denature poisonouos substances. However, it certainly is wise to follow this procedure regardless of your state of health.

Kapha Sattva Diets For Different Calorie Levels

Choose foods from the above Kapha Sattva Shopping List and enjoy them in the quantities indicated below according to the calorie level you wish to utilize.

1200 Calorie Lacto-Vegetarian Diet For Kapha Types

Category 1: Fruits	3 servings/day
Category 2: Vegetables	5 servings/day
Category 3: Cereals, Starchy Vegetables, Grains	6 servings/day
Category 4: Legumes	2 servings/day
Category 5: Fats	3 servings/day

Category 6: Dairy   1 serving/day
Category 7: Meats, Cheese, Fish, and Eggs   –

Carbohydrate calories:	71%
Fat calories:	14%
Protein calories:	15%
Total Protein content:	52 g
Dietary fiber content:	38-72 g

Recommended Meal Design

Breakfast
1 Fruit serving
2 Cereal/Starchy Vegetable/Grain servings
1 Fat serving
1 Dairy serving

Lunch
2 Vegetable servings
2 Cereal/Starchy Vegetable/Grain servings
2 Legume servings
1 Dairy serving
1 Fat serving

Mid-Afternoon Snack
1 Fruit serving

Dinner
3 Vegetable servings
2 Cereal/Starchy Vegetable/Grain servings
1 Fat serving
1 Fruit serving

1200 Calorie Omnivore Diet For Kapha Types

Category 1: Fruits	3 servings/day
Category 2: Vegetables	5 servings/day
Category 3: Cereals, Starchy Vegetables, Grains	4 servings/day
Category 4: Legumes	1 serving/day

Category 5: Fats   3 servings/day
Category 6: Dairy   1 serving/day
Category 7: Meats, Cheese, Fish, and Eggs   2 servings/day

Carbohydrate calories: 66%
Fat calories: 18%
Protein calories: 16%
Total Protein content: 59 g
Dietary fiber content: 28-55 g

Recommended Meal Design

Breakfast
1 Fruit serving
1 Cereal/Starchy Vegetable/Grain servings
1 Fat serving

Lunch
2 Vegetable servings
1 Cereal/Starchy Vegetable/Grain servings
1 Dairy serving
2 Meat/Cheese/Fish/Egg servings
1 Fat Serving

Mid-Afternoon Snack
1 Fruit serving

Dinner
3 Vegetable servings
2 Cereal/Starchy Vegetable/Grain servings
1 Legume serving
1 Fat serving
1 Fruit serving

1500 Calorie Lacto-Vegetarian Diet For Kapha Types

Category 1: Fruits   3 servings/day
Category 2: Vegetables   5 servings/day
Category 3: Cereals, Starchy Vegetables, Grains   8 servings/day

Category 4: Legumes   3 servings/day
Category 5: Fats   5 servings/day
Category 6: Dairy   1 serving/day
Category 7: Meats, Cheese, Fish, and Eggs   –

Carbohydrate calories:	68%
Fat calories:	17%
Protein calories:	15%
Total Protein content:	61 g
Dietary fiber content:	33-68 g

Recommended Meal Design

Breakfast
1 Fruit serving
2 Cereal/Starchy Vegetable/Grain servings
1 Fat serving
1 Dairy

Lunch
2 Vegetable servings
3 Cereal/Starchy Vegetable/Grain servings
2 Legume servings
3 Fat servings

Mid-Afternoon Snack
1 Fruit serving

Dinner
3 Vegetable servings
3 Cereal/Starchy Vegetable/Grain servings
1 Legume
1 Fat serving
1 Fruit serving

1500 Calorie Omnivore Diet For Kapha Types

Category 1: Fruits   3 servings/day
Category 2: Vegetables   5 servings/day

Category 3: Cereals, Starchy Vegetables, Grains 4 servings/day
Category 4: Legumes 1 serving/day
Category 5: Fats 3 servings/day
Category 6: Dairy 1 serving/day
Category 7: Meats, Cheese, Fish, and Eggs 2 servings/day

Carbohydrate calories:	66%
Fat calories:	18%
Protein calories:	16%
Total Protein content:	76 g
Dietary fiber content:	28-75 g

Recommended Meal Design

Breakfast
1 Fruit serving
2 Cereal/Starchy Vegetable/Grain servings
1 Fat serving
1 Dairy serving

Lunch
2 Vegetable servings
2 Meat/Cheese/Fish/Egg servings
1 Fat serving

Mid-Afternoon Snack
1 Fruit serving

Dinner
3 Vegetable servings
2 Cereal/Starchy Vegetable/Grain servings
1 Legume serving
1 Fat serving
1 Fruit serving

2000 Calorie Lacto-Vegetarian Diet For Kapha Types

Category 1: Fruits 4 servings/day
Category 2: Vegetables 5 servings/day

Category 3: Cereals, Starchy Vegetables, Grains   10 servings/day
Category 4: Legumes   4 servings/day
Category 5: Fat   4 servings/day
Category 6: Dairy   1 serving/day
Category 7: Meats, Cheese, Fish, and Eggs   –

Carbohydrate calories:	69%
Fat calories:	16%
Protein calories:	15%
Total Protein content:	61 g
Dietary fiber content:	33-68 g

Recommended Meal Design

Breakfast
2 Fruit servings
2 Cereal/Starchy Vegetable/Grain servings
1 Fat serving
1 Dairy serving

Lunch
2 Vegetable servings
5 Cereal/Starchy Vegetable/Grain servings
2 Legume servings
2 Fat servings

Mid-Afternoon Snack
1 Fruit serving

Dinner
3 Vegetable servings
3 Cereal/Starchy Vegetable/Grain servings
2 Legume servings
1 Fat serving
1 Fruit serving

2000 Calorie Omnivore Diet For Kapha Types

Category 1: Fruits   2 servings/day
Category 2: Vegetables   5 servings/day

Category 3: Cereals, Starchy Vegetables, Grains	7 servings/day
Category 4: Legumes	2 servings/day
Category 5: Fats	5 servings/day
Category 6: Dairy	1 serving/day
Category 7: Meats, Cheese, Fish, and Eggs	2 servings/day

Carbohydrate calories:	65%
Fat calories:	18%
Protein calories:	17%
Total Protein content:	79 g
Dietary fiber content:	22-82 g

Recommended Meal Design

Breakfast
1 Fruit serving
2 Cereal/Starchy Vegetable/Grain servings
1 Fat serving
1 Dairy serving

Lunch
2 Vegetable servings
2 Cereal/Starchy Vegetable/Grain servings
2 Fat servings
2 Meat/Cheese/Fish/Egg servings

Mid-Afternoon Snack
1 Fruit serving

Dinner
3 Vegetable servings
3 Cereal/Starchy Vegetable/Grain servings
2 Legume servings
2 Fat servings
1 Fruit serving

2500 Calorie Lacto-Vegetarian Diet For Kapha Types

Category 1: Fruits	5 servings/day
Category 2: Vegetables	8 servings/day

Category 3: Cereals, Starchy Vegetables, Grains   13 servings/day
Category 4: Legumes   4 servings/day
Category 5: Fats   6 servings/day
Category 6: Dairy   1 serving/day
Category 7: Meats, Cheese, Fish, and Eggs   –

Carbohydrate calories:	69%
Fat calories:	15%
Protein calories:	16%
Total Protein content:	91 g
Dietary fiber content:	35-102 g

Recommended Meal Design

Breakfast
2 Fruit servings
2 Cereal/Starchy Vegetable/Grain servings
1 Fat serving

Lunch
4 Vegetable servings
6 Cereal/Starchy Vegetable/Grain servings
2 Legume servings
3 Fat servings
1 Dairy serving

Mid-Afternoon Snack
1 Fruit serving

Dinner
4 Vegetable servings
5 Cereal/Starchy Vegetable/Grain servings
2 Legume servings
2 Fat servings
2 Fruit servings

2500 Calorie Omnivore Diet For Kapha Types

Category 1: Fruits   3 servings/day
Category 2: Vegetables   7 servings/day

Category 3: Cereals, Starchy Vegetables, Grains   12 servings/day
Category 4: Legumes   2 servings/day
Category 5: Fats   7 servings/day
Category 6: Dairy   1 serving/day
Category 7: Meats, Cheese, Fish, and Eggs   3 servings/day

Carbohydrate calories: 65%
Fat calories: 18%
Protein calories: 17%
Total Protein content: 96 g
Dietary fiber content: 42-108 g

Recommended Meal Design

Breakfast
1 Fruit serving
2 Cereal/Starchy Vegetable/Grain servings
1 Fat serving
1 Dairy serving

Lunch
4 Vegetable servings
5 Cereal/Starchy Vegetable/Grain servings
3 Meat/Cheese/Fish/Egg servings
3 Fat servings

Mid-Afternoon Snack
1 Fruit serving

Dinner
3 Vegetable servings
5 Cereal/Starchy Vegetable/Grain servings
2 Legume servings
3 Fat servings
1 Fruit serving

What Is A Serving?

One serving is equal to any one of the following for each category of food.

Category 1: Fruits
- 1 medium hand-held piece of fruit
- 1/2 cup chopped, cooked or canned fruit
- 6 oz. fruit juice, any type
- 4 oz. nectar, any type
- 1/2 cup applesauce, unsweetened
- 2 small apricots
- 1/2 banana
- 3/4 cup berries (black, blue, straw, rasp)
- 12 cherries
- 1/4 cup cranberries (1.5 ounces)
- 4 dates
- 1 fig
- 1/2 grapefruit
- 15-20 grapes
- 1/3 cantaloupe
- 1/4 honeydew
- 2" slice of watermelon
- 2 cups watermelon (cubes)
- 1/2 mango
- 1/2 papaya
- 1 cup pineapple
- 2 small plums or prunes
- 1/3 cup prune juice
- 2 tbsp. Raisins
- 1 kiwi (4 oz.)
- 4 kumquats
- 2 dates

Category 2: Vegetables
- 1/2 cup cooked vegetables
- 1 cup of raw vegetables
- 1 cup raw leafy green vegetables
- 6" piece of corn on the cob
- 6 oz. vegetable juice

Category 3: Cereals, Starchy Vegetables, Grains
- 1/2 cup bran cereal
- 3/4 cup ready-to eat unsweetened cereal
- 1/2 cup cooked cereal

- 1 cup pasta (spaghetti, macaroni, ziti)
- 1/3 cup cooked rice
- 1/2 cup cooked kasha (buckwheat groats)
- 1 tbs. wheat germ
- 1 small baked potato or sweet potato
- 1 small yam
- 1/2 cup mashed potato
- 6" piece of corn on the cob
- 2 cups non-fat popcorn
- 1/2 cup corn kernels
- 1 slice bread
- 1/2 bagel or English muffin
- 2 pancakes (4" diameter)
- 1 chapati
- 1 dosa

CATEGORY 4: LEGUMES
- 1/2 cup cooked beans, peas, dals, or lentils
- 1/2 cup vegetarian chili

CATEGORY 5: FATS, NUTS, AND SEEDS
- 8 cashews
- 6 pecans
- 6 walnuts
- 20 peanuts
- 12 almonds (dry roasted)
- 3/4 tablespoon nut butter
- 3/4 tablespoon tahini
- 1 tbs. jam or preserves
- 1/4 cup seeds (pine, sunflower, pumpkin, sunflower)
- 1/4 avocado
- 10 small olives
- 1 tbs. salad dressing
- 1 tsp. mayonnaise
- 2 tbs. coconut, shredded
- 1 tsp. butter
- 1 tsp. ghee
- 1 tsp. vegetable oil

CATEGORY 6: DAIRY
- 1 cup skim milk (90 kcal)
- 1 cup 1/2% milk (100 kcal)
- 1 cup 1% milk (120 kcal)
- 1 cup 2% milk (135 kcal)
- 1 cup whole milk (160 kcal)

CATEGORY 7: MEATS, CHEESE, FISH, AND EGGS
- 2 oz. beef, pork, veal, poultry, rabbit, duck, or pheasant
- 4 oz. fresh fish fillet (salmon, swordfish, tuna, snapper, cod, halibut, mahi, flounder)
- 2 sardines
- 1/4 cup canned tuna, in water
- 1 small lobster tail
- 2 oz. scallops
- 4 pieces sushi (raw fish and rice rolled in seaweed)
- 1/4 cup cottage cheese
- 2 tbs. grated parmesan cheese
- 1 oz. all cheeses
- 1 egg
- 3 egg whites
- 4 oz. tofu

Remember that eating too much of any food article, even pure and simple sattvic foods, will sabotage your weight loss program. You must pay attention—close attention!—to serving size. Of course the most *im*practical approach to regulating your serving sizes would be to carry a scale around with you and weigh everything you eat. While this is *one* method, it is not the method of choice. You can get a theoretical idea of the proper serving size from the above list, and then a practical sense of what these quantities look like from the following Ayurvedic observations:

Your Closed Fist:	equals approximately 1 cup or 1 medium-sized fruit
Your Entire Thumb:	equals approximately 1 ounce of meat or cheese

Your 1/2 Thumb (including the knuckle):	equals approximately 1 tablespoon.
Your 1/2 Thumb (excluding the knuckle):	equals approximately 1 teaspoon.
Your Open Palm (excluding the fingers):	equals approximately 3 ounces of cooked tofu, meat, fish or poultry
Your Open Palm (including the nearest 1/3 of the fingers):	equals approximately 4 ounces of cooked tofu, meat, fish or poultry

Herbal Supplements For Kapha-Type Individuals

Ayurveda has for centuries understood the ability of certain combinations of herbs to promote detoxification and to assist in weight loss. Today there is extensive literature to support the safety and efficacy of these herbal medicines when used as recommended. The true value of herbal medicines lie not in their ability to treat specific disease entities, but rather in their ability to initiate and promote tissue cleansing and improved physiological function at many different levels.

As we mentioned in Chapter 11, all individuals, regardless of Ayurvedic Constitutional Type, should take the **Sattva Basic Formulation,** which consists of a combination of the following herbs. This formulation will support cleansing of the body's tissues and help up-regulate fat catabolism for people of all Ayurvedic Constitutional Types. For your convenience, here again is the Sattva Basic Formulation:

Guggulu (standardized to 2.5% guggulsterones) . . . . . . 125 mg. (1 part)
Citraka . . . . 500 mg. (4 parts)
Punarnava (standardized to 25% alkaloids) . . . . 125 mg. (1 part)
Garcinia (standardized to 10% hydroxycitric acid) . . . . 125 mg. (1 part)
Triphala powder . . . . 500 mg. (4 parts)
Ginger . . . . 250 mg. (2 parts)
Cayenne Pepper . . . . 250 mg. (2 parts)
Black Pepper . . . . 250 mg. (2 parts)

Kapha-type individuals should add the following herbal components to the Basic Formulation:

Gurmar . . . . .250 mg. (2 parts)
Pushkarmoola . . . . .125 mg. (1 part)
Arjuna . . . . .500 mg. (4 parts)
Parsley leaf . . . . .250 mg. (2 parts)
Cardamom seed (powdered) . . . . .125 mg. (1 part)

Mix all ingredients very well in a bowl and use the mixture to fill "00" veggie caps. Kapha individuals should start by taking two "00" veggie caps twice a day before breakfast and dinner for the first week. If well tolerated, you can increase to three times a day before breakfast, lunch and dinner.

It is safe to continue taking this herbal formulation for up to one year. However, every six to eight weeks it is recommended to stop taking the herbs for approximately one week, then resume as before.

Here is a brief summary of the medicinal uses of the herbs used in the Kapha formula.

Gurmar (Gymnema sylvestre R.Br.)

A common climbing plant found in central and western India whose leaves contains a glucoside known as *gymnemic acid*, which has been shown to reduce blood sugar and act as a mild diuretic (i.e. increases urine formation). Its name *gur-mar* means "sugar-destroying".

Pushkarmoola (Inula racemosa Hook f.)

A tall, stout herb found in northern India, the root of pushkarmoola is pungent, bitter, heating, and an excellent anti-Kapha herb. It helps remove mucous, excess fluid accumulations, phlegm, and is also anti-inflammatory. It is actually considered a specific remedy for asthma and congestive cough, but is useful for Kapha disorders of all types.

Arjuna (Terminalia arjuna Wight &Arn.)

A large deciduous tree whose bark extract exhibits blood pressure lowering effects and is a tonic for the heart. The bark is astringent in taste and also possesses detoxifying effects and is helpful in removing accumulated toxins from the liver, intestines and blood vessels.

Parsley leaf (*Petroselinum crispum* **Mill.**)

A basic member of every herb garden, parsley is renown as a gentle diuretic and blood purifier, attributable to its apiin and apigenin content. Its leaves do in fact have antimicrobial properties as well as a mild laxative effect. Parsley is a good source of calcium, vitamin A, C, and a small amount of iron.

Cardamom (*Ellettaria cardamomum* **Maton**)

The seeds of this common condiment are pungent, slightly sweet, drying and light giving it a tridoshic calming action. It is useful as a digestive corrective and as a remedy for flatulence and heartburn. It is an excellent general cardiac and digestive tonic.

Exercise For Kapha Individuals

As previously explained in the section on the general principles of the Sattva Program, an effective exercise program, like any other health-promoting activity or substance, is only effective when it suits the specific needs of the individual. Exercise that is done properly always creates vitality and energy; it does not destroy it.

Kapha individuals require the most exercise to achieve and maintain homeostasis. If you happen to be a bi-doshic (two doshic) type, for the purposes of exercise, refer to your overall physique to determine your type. If you are large, muscular, and thick, with joints well-covered with fat and tendon, and fleshy hands and fingers, consider yourself a Kapha type for matters of exercise.

Kapha individuals will benefit most from exercises that take advantage of their great capacity for strength and endurance and which have a stimulating and intense nature. Examples of Kapha-reducing exercises include:

Aerobics	Racquetball
Basketball	Rockclimbing
Bicycling	Rollerblading
Bowling	Rowing
Calisthenics	Shot put
Cross country skiing	Skiing

Football	Stairclimbing
Gymnastics	Tennis
Ice skating	Walking/Jogging (long distance)
Jogging	

In addition, remember that *walking is the best form of exercise for all types*. Kapha individuals benefit more from a vigorous style of walking that is sustained for thirty to forty minutes, twice a day. The main criteria for a successful exercise program for the Kapha individual is to exercise for a long, continuous period and not in a start-and-stop pattern. Kapha individuals should choose a form of exercise that they sincerely enjoy; Kapha types strongly resist that which is not inherently pleasurable to them. With regard to weight training, Kapha types need to recruit the use of the largest muscle group in the body through exercise such as squats, leg curls and extensions, rowing motions, and bench presses.

The word prāṇāyāma means "control or regulation of the breath". Breathing is a natural, automatic activity for almost everyone most of the time. Ayurveda emphasizes the connection between breathing correctly and the vital energy of an individual. In fact in the Sanskrit language the word for "breath" and the word for "life force" is the same: prāṇa. Some people do unfortunately develop breathing disorders or suffer from diseases which affect the breathing. These disturbances in breathing may affect the strength of an individual's will power, mental alertness, sleeping pattern and mental stability. You can understand, in light of this, why breathing is so vital to The Sattva Program for weight management. Fortunately, most people can learn to improve their breathing with very little effort. Later in this section, we will describe a useful specialized breathing technique to be used especially by individuals with a Kapha constitution. Later we will similarly describe other specific breathing techniques for people of Vata and Pitta constitutions. However, before moving into the practice of these specific techniques, I recommend that all people first master the Deep Breathing Technique described below. In Sanskrit this technique is known as *purakarechaka* (*puraka* means inhalation, *rechaka* means exhalation).

CHAPTER 12. RECOMMENDATIONS FOR SPECIFIC CONSTITUTIONAL TYPES

Despite the fundamental importance of breathing to the very existence of the human race, I have found to my amazement that most people have developed incorrect breathing habits. This is particularly true of overweight and obese individuals. Correct inhalation and exhalation is the basis for all advanced forms of breathing exercises, so the Deep Breathing Technique should be understood and practiced by everyone before learning the specialized techniques given for each constitutional type. To be certain, all the other prāṇāyāma techniques are merely variations upon this fundamental exercise.

This technique is nothing more than full, natural breathing through the nose. In natural breathing, inhalation causes the middle ribs, i.e. those located just beneath the breasts, to expand more than the upper and lower ribs. The abdomen expands too, but only slightly; the sternum moves out and away from the spine. Exhalation involves a relaxation of the muscles of inspiration. The diaphragm releases its tension and the outflow of air is not willfully modified by the respiratory muscles. Between inhalation and exhalation there is a brief interval during which there is no movement of air. Actually, there are two of these periods: one just after full inhalation and one just after full exhalation. The duration of these intervals is controlled unconsciously and should be manipulated only with extreme care.

Deep Breathing Technique (Purakarechaka)

1. Sit in a balanced, upright posture in a chair with a straight back. Feet should be flat on the floor about shoulder width apart; remove the shoes and socks. Place hands on the lap, palms up. Mouth should be closed. All breathing is through the nostrils.

2. Exhale whatever air is in the lungs.

3. Take a normal inhalation observing the following:

   a) the initial movement is that of the abdomen expanding slightly.
   b) the chest expands next starting in its lower zone, followed by the middle zone, and finally the upper zone.

c) do not constrict the throat in any way or make any sound during inhalation

d) the sternum (breast bone) moves out away from the spine.

e) do not strain to fill the lungs; the inhalation will stop naturally at the precise lung volume that is required. Observe this as it happens.

f) at the end of inhalation, a brief interval of no air movement occurs. Observe this without in any way interfering or prolonging it.

4. Exhale normally observing the following:

a) do not force the exhalation or use extra effort or undue haste.

b) as you observe the breathing the exhalation phase naturally becomes slightly longer and deeper than the inhalation phase. Allow this to occur.

c) relax the abdominal muscles as you exhale.

d) do not allow the head and chest to slouch forward during exhalation.

e) at the end of exhalation, a brief period of no air movement occurs. Observe this without in any way interfering or prolonging it.

5. This completes one cycle. It is recommended to complete 16 cycles per session.

Perform this exercise twice a day, morning and evening. It requires approximately 90 seconds to complete each session.

It is usual for most individuals to use this Deep Breathing Technique as their prāṇāyāma *exercise for six to eight weeks before advancing to the more specific exercises described for each constitutional type. This will be time well invested.*

Prāṇāyāma

Ayurveda borrows a number of highly specialized techniques from the Yoga tradition. One example of this is its use of specific breathing exercises for the different doshas.

CHAPTER 12. RECOMMENDATIONS FOR SPECIFIC CONSTITUTIONAL TYPES

The best breathing exercise for Kapha types is known as *kapalabhati*. Kapalabhati breathing is a vigorous cardiovascular activity comparable to engaging in ten or fifteen minutes of jogging. The true function of this type of breathing is to assist the body in eliminating waste materials. This is a very important function for people who are in the process of losing weight and who are producing increased loads of metabolic breakdown products.

The technique is very simple. It consists of a series of short, forceful exhalations, each followed by a passive and natural inhalation. Begin by sitting in a balanced and upright posture with your back straight, either on the floor or in a chair. The shoulders should not slump forward. Correct posture is the key to kapalabhati breathing because the abdominal muscles need to move with absolute freedom.

Once you have established a comfortable and upright posture, begin breathing through your nostrils in a deep and even rhythm. After a few seconds of this, as you exhale through the nostrils, contract your abdominal muscles quickly and forcefully. This will force air out of your lungs through the nostrils. The correct technique is to make these exhalations as complete as possible, using short, powerful actions. Immediately following this exhalation, relax the abdominal muscles and inhalation occurs naturally and passively—without any effort on your part. Another key to kapalabhati breathing is to develop the ability to completely relax the abdominal muscles following these strong exhalations, so that air can be passively inhaled. After every inhalation, follow with another forceful exhalation.

Start slowly and gradually increase the speed of your breathing. Visualize a locomotive chugging slowly at first and gradually gaining speed. Do no try to go faster than about two exhalations per second, at the most. The idea is not to perform kapalabhati as fast as you can but rather to concentrate on exhaling as completely as possible and then *relaxing the abdominal muscles with each inhalation.*

Do rounds of 30 to 40 when you are initially learning this technique. Rest approximately 60 seconds between rounds and perform 3 to 5 rounds in the morning and evening. Later, you can increase the number and duration of the rounds to 50 to100, 6 to eight rounds.

Massage Oils For Kapha Types

Kapha individuals benefit most from massage oils that are lighter in nature and somewhat warming. Ayurveda recommends a number of traditional massage oils that can be found in the ancient Ayurvedic formularies (see appendix for sources). In addition modern Ayurveda has recognized more readily available commercial oils which are also appropriate as massage oils for the various constitutional types. The oils listed below can be used individually or combined in any way. If you do combine two or more oils, its best to use only one of the traditional oils in your formula.

Kapha Massage Oils

TRADITIONAL OILS	MODERN OILS
Vranashodak taila	Sunflower
Vacha taila	Safflower
Citrakadi taila	Sesame
Nirgundi taila	Mustard
Saindhavadi taila	Corn

In general, individuals of Kapha constitutions benefit from a vigorous and stimulating massage technique. When using the self-massage technique known as *abhyanga*, the strokes should be quicker, shorter, and more forceful than the gentler and slower strokes given to a Vata individual. The rate of massage should be approximately twice the rate of your pulse rate. Thus, if we take the average pulse rate to be 72 beats per minute, twice this rate is 144 beats per minute. This equals about 2.3 beats per second. Therefore, Kapha individuals should use approximately two to three strokes per second. If you use this calculation as a guideline and simply use what seems to you to be "fast" strokes, you will do well.

It is also recommended that Kapha individuals not perform an oil massage every single day. Rather, consider alternating oil massage with *garshana* massage, every other day. As you recall from Chapter 7, garshana massage is a dry massage that is performed with a loofa glove or mitt. Any slightly rough material, such as raw silk, may also be used. The rough and dry qualities of the material are pacifying for Kapha energy and help to disperse it.

FASTING

There are many misconceptions and much misinformation being generated in the popular Ayurvedic literature regarding the value of fasting. Let us examine the facts about this subject and clarify its place in a weight management program.

Among the many approaches to the treatment of disease that Ayurveda has to offer are two distinct lines of therapies: shodhana and shamana. Shodhana refers to therapies which radically and in a reasonably short time eliminate toxins from the body. This is accomplished primarily through physical therapies known as panchakarma, which we will fully describe in Chapter 16. Shamana, on the other hand, refers to more gradual therapies that cause the eventual correction and subsidence of imbalances in the physiology. Included under this category of treatment are seven natural therapies:

1) Fasting from food
2) Fasting from food and water
3) Exercise, including yoga postures
4) Sunbathing for appropriate lengths of time
5) Exposure to wind
6) Increasing the digestive fire
7) Optimizing the metabolism

Thus, fasting is advocated as a *bona fide* approach to the treatment of disease when, like any other therapy, it is prescribed and supervised by an experienced physician. The fallacy being advanced in the current plethora of Ayurvedic books is that "juice fasting" or "light food fasting" brings benefit to all those wishing to lose weight. These types of eating (and they are types of *eating*—not fasting) do not always promote weight loss for all individuals. Absolute fasting, the voluntary abstinence from food and water is a medical procedure requiring guidance from a physician; it can be valuable for Kapha-type individuals and some Pitta-types. It is rarely indicated for Vata-types, who may become disoriented and weak from this type of fast. Water-fasting is somewhat less radical but also subject to possible adverse effects if not done properly. Probably because most popular authors are not experienced or knowledgeable about these more profound fasting techniques, they tend to dilute the information given on

FASTING (CONT'D)

fasting techniques by only advocating vegetable juice "fasting" or some other modification. Although these techniques may offer some nutritional and even health benefits, these "fasts" can be ineffective for many of us in the context of weight loss. Let us see why.

THE PHYSIOLOGY OF FASTING

As we all know, the primary purpose of our digestive and metabolic processes is to sustain a sufficient energy supply for our many necessary life processes. The single most important energy source for the cells of the human body is the simple carbohydrate, glucose. When we do not consume enough glucose, the liver breaks down *glycogen* (a chain of glucose molecules) into simple glucose to provide energy. However this liver reserve only lasts several hours. The brain, heart, nerves, and other tissues require a very precise concentration of glucose to function—even during fasting. So the body has devised several means of ensuring a continuous glucose supply after the liver glycogen stores have run out.

First, an enzyme known as *hormone-sensitive lipase* is released that breaks down body fat into free fatty acids and glycerol, which enter the bloodstream. The glycerol, but not the free fatty acids, is converted to glucose. The free fatty acids do form *ketone bodies*, which are an alternative energy source for the brain and other tissues. Ketone bodies include acetone, beta-hydroxybutyric acid, and acetoacetic acid

In addition, glucose is produced from amino acids, which come from muscle protein. Alanine is the main amino acid that is converted into glucose. Also, lactic acid from the muscle stores of glycogen are converted into glucose in the liver.

As fasting continues, fatty acid-derived ketone bodies assume a larger role and glucose a smaller role in energy supply. The maximum shift from glucose to ketone bodies as an energy source occurs after approximately 72 hours of fasting. People usually acquire a sweetish acetone odor to their breath at this time. In common terms, this indicates that the body is breaking down body fat and using it as an energy substrate. These changes are accompanied by a reduction in the secretion of thyroid hormone, which reduces the metabolic rate unless some form of exertion is undertaken. Individuals vary in their response to the relative hypoglycemia and hyperketosis that comes with fasting. Some may experience dizziness or fatigue after one day, while others may feel fine even after several days. Short term fasting—three days or less—can be endured with no harm and great benefit by healthy individuals under a physician's care.

Now it should be clear to you why "juice fasting" or "light food fasting" is not as beneficial. As soon as the body receives a sufficient bolus of glucose contained in carrot juice, beet juice, or any form of carbohydrate, it may immediately slow the fasting processes outlined above. Food of any kind and in any quantity in fact will cause the body to modify its fasting metabolic changes. The greatest benefits of fasting in a weight management program therefore come from true (i.e. absolute) fasting: abstaining completely from food for a period of time. However, absolute fasting is definitely not appropriate for all individuals (see following, Fasting for Kapha Individuals). If it is appropriate for you but you have a strong aversion to this kind of therapy or cannot find the proper medical supervision necessary, it is best to forego this particular modality. But if you are generally healthy and can meet the requirements, it can be an excellent boost to your weight loss and maintenance efforts.

CONTRAINDICATIONS FOR FASTING

Fasting can be a useful adjunct in the treatment of almost every health disorder which involves accumulation and excess. However, one should always exercise caution and seek competent medical guidance whenever possible.

Fasting should not be performed under the following circumstances:

- Pregnancy
- Lactation
- 20 < Age > 70
- Mental illness
- Underweight by 10 lbs. or more
- History of anorexia-bulimia syndrome
- Moderate to severe osteoporosis
- Extremely cold weather
- HIV-related illness
- Cancer, unless advised by a physician
- Within 2 months of a surgical procedure

Fasting for Kapha Individuals

Ayurveda recommends either a 2-3 day water fast or a 1-2 day absolute fast every month for people of Kapha constitution.

Absolute Fast

Sometimes referred to as an "air and sunshine" fast, this is indicated for individuals who suffer from water retention, excess body weight, mucous accumulation, lethargy, food addiction and sluggishness. Absolute fasting is recommended for individuals of Kapha, Kapha-Pitta, Pitta-Kapha, and, occasionally, for Pitta types. It should not be done by individuals with Vata as a component of their prakriti, by very thin individuals, or by those susceptible to becoming easily overheated or easily anxious.

The technique is a simple one. Starting at 6:00 p.m. on an auspicious evening when the mind is tranquil and settled, eat or drink nothing for 24 to 48 hours. Without close medical supervision it is unsafe to extend this type of fast beyond 48 hours.

This is a profound physical and psychological fast in which one abstains from all forms of food and water (water and earth elements) and is sustained by the three lightest elements: space, air and fire. Absolute fasting lends itself quite naturally to contemplative states of mind, meditation and reflection on the nature of one's life and of reality. During the fast you should go outside into the fresh air and sunlight at least twice a day. Although it is wise to rest and enjoy the quiet during this period, short walks or periods of yoga are strongly encouraged.

Water Fast

During this time one should drink between six and ten 12-ounce glasses of filtered water each day. A larger quantity is permissible if thirsty. Do not flavor with lemon or anything else. The water temperature should be slightly warm or at least room temperature; never drink cold water. During this period you will want to rest as much as possible. However, short periods of walking, yoga or other light forms of exercise are acceptable. Proceed with other activities as you would normally. Generally, with water fasting hunger will be noticeable intermittently during the first 24-36 hours and then recede. Because of the possibility of releasing large quantities of toxins, which could overwhelm the eliminatory organs, we recommend no more than a three-day water fast if it is not physician-supervised. This is an excellent fast for releasing accumulated fats, mucous, drugs, pesticides, toxins, infectious agents and acids.

Other Liquid Fasts for Kapha Types
Teas
There are many Ayurvedic herbal tea formulae that are known to promote detoxification. One formula is the Kapha Tea available through The National Institute of Ayurvedic Medicine which contains: Vasaka (*Adhatoda vasica*), Sounth, Pippali (*Piper longum*), Elaichi (*Elettaria cardamomum*), and Tulsi (*Ocimum sanctum*).

Other excellent fasting teas for Kapha types are:

1) Four parts tulsi (*Ocimum sanctum*), two parts tejpatra (*Cinnamomum tamala*), one part ginger (*Zingiber officinale*), one part cardamom (*Ellettaria cardamomum*)

2) Two parts citraka (*Plumbago zeylanica*), two parts saunf (*Foeniculum vulgare*), one part palasa (*Butea monosperma*), one part twak (*Cinnamomum zeylanicum*)

MAKING TEAS

There are many variations of this simple preparation found throughout the literature. In every case the procedure is based upon a common experience which we all have had, making tea. All of us have at one time in our lives placed a tea bag in a teacup and poured boiling water over it. This is also the basic way to make a tea used for medicinal purposes, as you will see. However, there are a few nuances which can help you make the highest quality herbal tea.

First, let's define how much herb and how much water to use. There is considerable variation in different herbal traditions, and it's really essentially empirical (i.e. a matter of trial and error and personal preference). In addition, if quantities are given in weight units (grams), as is common in many pharmacopoeias and textbooks, we encounter the fact that teas containing different proportions of roots, leaves, seeds, stems and flowers will have different weights. If we use volume measure however, we have another difficulty: the fineness or coarseness of the material will greatly alter the quantity that fits on a teaspoon. Despite these issues, in the Ayurvedic tradition the quantities are generally as follows:

Amount of herb: one level teaspoon (2-4 grams)
Amount of boiling water: 6 ounces (170 ml.)

Second, the water *must* be brought to a boil before pouring over the herbs.

Third, the tea must be allowed to "draw" for 5-10 minutes before drinking. During this time the teacup should be covered.

Degree of Comminution

Comminution means the degree to which the material has been mechanically ground to smaller and smaller fragment sizes. For example, teas can be coarsely chopped, moderately chopped, finely chopped, moderately powdered or finely powdered. What is the difference, you ask. The difference is that the smaller the fragment size of the tea (i.e. the more highly comminuted), the greater the release of its constituents into the water. Thus, logically, finely ground coffee beans will make a stronger brew than whole or only coarsely chopped coffee beans. In fact, this common sense observation has been scientifically well documented by many investigators. For example, a tea made from powdered senna leaves releases approximately 85% of its sennosides into the infusion, while one made from chopped leaves yields only 65%. With cascara sagrada, the yield of anthracene derivatives with the powdered and chopped forms are 90% and 30%, respectively!*

Therefore, although most westerners are accustomed to teas with a moderately chopped texture, from a scientific point of view a tea that is powdered to some degree is highly preferable. This creates the inconvenience of perhaps having some of the tea particles floating in the tea, but this can be solved by straining through a fine mesh stainless steel strainer or by just getting used to it. After all, those bits of herb are good for you too.

*Bisset, Norman (ed), Herbal Drug and Pharmaceuticals, Scientific Publishers, Stuttgart, 1994.

Specific Juices

As mentioned above, from a scientific point of view juice fasting may not be as effective as absolute or water fasts for the purpose of weight management. This is due to the carbohydrate content of all juices, which may spare liver glycogen and body fat. However, particularly for those transitioning from eating histories that have included animal products to a more vegetarian diet, juice fasting may be extremely useful. Although most appropriate for Vata- and Pitta-type individuals, the following vegetable juice formula is especially good for Kapha-types:

```
Carrot .................... 30%
Celery        ⎫
Cabbage       ⎪
Parsley       ⎪
Watercress    ⎬ ............. 40%
Beet root     ⎪
Beet greens   ⎪
Ginger root   ⎭
Water..................... 30%
```

In this formula approximately 30% of a glass should be filled with freshly juiced carrot juice, 40% should contain a combination of the other vegetable ingredients and the remaining 30% should be filtered water. One half to one beet root and 1/2 - 1 inch of ginger root should be used.

Kapha-type individuals should not use fruit juices for fasting purposes because of its excessively cooling energy and sweet taste which will tend to aggravate Kapha.

Guidelines for Breaking a Fast

Remember, the success of any fast depends on how well it is broken—not on how well it is performed. When ending any fast, the one most important principle to follow is to *not overeat*. After any length of fasting, the urge to binge can be over-powering. Obviously, giving in to such urges will neutralize any benefits derived from the process and toxins will quickly re-accumulate in the tissues.

An excellent rule-of-thumb is to end a fast gradually by taking one full day during which you eat lightly—about three-fourths of your capacity and never to the point of feeling full. Choose foods from the food groups listed in Table 11: Foods Used For Fasting. On the first day after your fast, try to choose foods only slightly less cleansing than the level of your fast. For example, if you have just completed a water fast consider breaking the fast with other liquids such as vegetable or fruit juices, soups, sprouts, or raw fruits and vegetables. Do not indulge in cooked root vegetables, grains or legumes on that first day.

After the first day it is generally safe to resume your normal diet,
but continue to eat moderate *amounts* of food for the next several days.

TABLE 11.
Foods Used For Fasting

Fasting Type	Food	Effect
Absolute	Air, sunlight	
Liquid	Water Alterative herbal teas Barley, Wheat grass juice Vegetable juice Vegetable broth Fruit juice	
Raw Food	Sprouts Vegetables Fruits	*More Cleansing*
Cooked Food	Non-starchy (leafy) vegetables Starchy (root) vegetables Grains (especially millet, quinoa, and amaranth) Legumes (especially mung beans)	*More Nourishing*
Non-fasting Foods	Seeds and nuts Cheese, milk, yogurt Fish Eggs Red meat, poultry	

Aromatherapy for Kapha Types

The Importance of Smell

Ayurveda defines disease as the result of a disturbance in the original proportion of the doshas for any given person. In the case of overweight or obesity, this is commonly the result of excessive Kapha dosha that has accumulated in the physiology. It is important to understand that Kapha accumulates not only in the belly and thighs, but throughout our entire physiology. Therefore Ayurveda utilizes many diverse methods of decreasing the excessive doshas. Some of these are direct and rational, e.g. eat more Kapha-reducing foods, do more Kapha-reducing exercise, and consume more Kapha-reducing herbal supplements and teas. But there are other approaches to balancing the doshas that happen to be very effective, even if they seem indirect and barely relevant to weight management. Aromatherapy falls into this category of Ayurvedic therapies.

Essential oils are highly volatile aromatic oils that are produced by plants in order to attract insects, discourage predators, and help avoid disease. There is a growing body of neurobiological evidence that supports the view that certain essential oils and their constituents exert *psychotropic* effects. A psychotropic effect is one that modifies brain physiology in such a way as to cause a change in emotions and behavior. These effects in humans are found to be mainly in the limbic area of the brain, which is known to influence our memory, libido, and emotions. For example, there are several reports in the literature citing nutmeg (*Myristica fragrans* Houtt.) as causing perceptual changes and mood elevation. Two components of nugmeg essential oil, myristicin and elemicin, are reported to be the principle psychoactive constituents. Other studies in the literature which report the central nervous system (CNS)-sedating effects of several essential oils including valerian, lavender, rose, melissa, clary sage, and marjoram. Olfactory stimulation is known to stimulate activity in both the olfactory and trigeminal nerves. There are, in addition, several studies in the scientific literature which report changes in electroencephalographic (EEG) activity in the brain upon exposure to certain aromas.

Essential oils can be used in various ways. They can be used in an aroma-diffuser pot, they can be added to massage oils, humidifiers, or vaporizers, they can be added to baths, they can be worn or carried in small amulets and inhaled throughout the day, or they can be diluted in carrier oils and applied to marma points of the body. Here are the essential oils that are used in Ayurveda to pacify Kapha dosha:

Essential Oils Recommended for Pacifying Kapha Dosha

Eucalyptus	Lemon
Tulsi	Peppermint
Basil	Sage
Rosemary	Frankincense
Camphor	Lemongrass
Nutmeg	Palmarosa
Chamomile	Clove
Bergamot	Cinnamon

To begin, try one or more of these Kapha-pacifying combinations:

1. Bergamot, Lemon, Rosemary
2. Eucalyptus, Frankincense, Clove, Basil
3. Peppermint and Lemon

Continue to experiment with different combinations and quantities of these essential oils. You will undoubtedly discover your own unique blends.

Kapha Behavioral Therapies

Just as we give attention to how we nourish our bodies, we must also be aware of how to properly nourish the mind. Like the physical body, what we bring into the mind through our five senses will eventually have its consequences over time. Therefore we must carefully protect the mind from unhealthy influences, just like we would with our young children. Individuals of each Constitutional Type have specific behaviors to be encouraged as well as avoided.

Behaviors to be Avoided by Kapha Types

- Lack of exercise
- Overindulgence in sweet foods and beverages
- Overindulgence in cold foods and beverages
- Lack of spices in the diet
- Excessive sleep, especially in the late morning and during the Spring season

- Excessive exposure to damp conditions
- Wearing clothing which is damp or wet
- Tendency toward excessive ownership and control of property and luxuries
- Attachment to people or objects
- Dependence upon the affection of others for our peace of mind

Behaviors to be Encouraged by Kapha Types

- Outdoor activities in warm and dry climates
- Hiking in the mountains, jogging, mountain biking
- Massage the body regularly with appropriate oils and powders
- Moderate exposure to wind
- Changing one's routine from time to time
- Use of spices of all kinds in the diet
- Fasting (see Fasting for Kapha Types)
- Use foods with the pungent, bitter, and astringent tastes
- Exposure to stimulating colors including: red, gold, yellow, orange, and purple
- Light and penetrating aromas including: eucalyptus, sage, cedar, myrrh, camphor, peppermint, and rosemary
- Selfless service to others, generosity, non-attachment

The Sattva Program For Pitta Types

Sattva Program Diet For Pitta Types

As I have suggested in the section on the Kapha program, if you have skipped to this section and haven't read Chapter 8 yet, I strongly suggest you do so. Many of the general Sattva recommendations apply for Pitta types; however some of these general principles need to be modified to best suit individuals of Pitta constitutional type. These modifications are the subject of this chapter. As with the other two doshas, the *diet* is the most important of these modifications.

The mind of the Pitta individual is dominated by *rajas*. You may recall that rajas is a mental energy which creates activity and disturbance in the mind. Rajas in the mind of a Pitta individual is not just random, wandering activity; it is usually activity with a purpose. Pitta people usually are mentally engaged and become powerfully directed toward a goal. While rajas in a balanced Pitta individual can be stimulating, it often becomes an overly intense, unbalanced drive characterized by a need for sensory pleasure from outside objects. Food is commonly one of these objects for the Pitta mind.

THE PITTA DIET

How to use this list

One of the most unique facets of Ayurvedic dietetics is that different foods from each food group are recommended for different Ayurvedic Constitutional Types.

In using the list below, eat mainly from the "Often" and "In Moderation" lists and only infrequently or on special occasions from the "Seldom" list.

"Often" in this context means consuming these foods every day would be fine.

"In Moderation" means that you should consume approximately **one-third to one-half** the amount of these foods as you do the "Often" foods. These foods are an important part of your diet, are not unhealthy for you and should definitely be included in your diet *in the proper amounts*.

"Seldom" means about once a month.

The Sattvic Pitta Shopping List

Please use this list as a convenient shopping list to assist you in shopping intelligently at your local supermarket and natural food stores. We suggest that you purchase organically-grown products as much as possible. This will ensure that you will not be exposed to pesticides, insecticides, hormones, and other harmful chemicals. If you cannot obtain organic produce, make sure you follow the suggested produce-washing procedure outlined on page 195. Once you have assembled a variety of the appropriate food items listed here, we will explain when and how much of each to eat. As you will see, the Sattva Program is simple and easy. It requires little in the way of strict discipline and becomes a uniquely individualized program of health that you help to create.

THE PITTA DIET

FRUITS

Often	In Moderation	Seldom
Apple (sweet)	Apples (sour)	Apricots (sour)
Apricots (sweet)	Bananas	Berries (sour)
Avocado	Cherries	Grapefruit
Berries (sweet)	Cranberries	Lemons Coconut
Grapes (green)	Oranges (sour)	Pineapples (sour)
Dates	Kiwi	Persimmon
Figs	Limes	Plums (sour)
Grapes (sweet)	Papaya	Rhubarb
Mango	Peaches	Soursop
Melons		Strawberries
Oranges (sweet)		
Pears		
Pineapples		
Plums (sweet)		
Pomegranates		
Prunes		
Quince (sweet)		
Raisins		
Watermelon		

VEGETABLES

Often	Often	In Moderation	Seldom
Acorn Squash	Mushrooms	Beets	Beet Greens
Artichoke	Okra	Carrots	Fenugreek Greens
Asparagus	Olives (black)	Daikon Radish	Garlic
Bell Pepper	Parsley	Eggplant	Horseradish
Broccoli	Parsnip	Leeks (cooked)	Green Olives
Brussels Sprouts	Peas	Spinach	Kohlrabi (cooked)
Burdock Root	Peppers (green)		Mustard Greens
Butternut Squash	Potatoes (sweet or white)		Onions (cooked & raw)
Cabbage	Rutabaga		Peppers (hot)
Fresh Corn	Scallopini Squash		Pumpkin (cooked)
Cauliflower	Spaghetti Squash		Radish
Cucumber	Sprouts		Tomatoes

Often	Often	Seldom
Celery	Summer Squash	Turnips
Green Beans	Watercress	Turnip Greens
Jerusalem Artichoke	Winter Squash	
Jicama	Yellow Crookneck Squash	
Leafy Greens	Zucchini	
(esp. Collards & Dandelion)		

GRAINS

Often	In Moderation	Seldom
Barley	Amaranth	Buckwheat
Oats (cooked)	Corn	Millet
Rice (basmati)	Oats (dry)	Oat Granola
Rice Cakes	Oat Bran	Quinoa
Rice (white)	Rice (brown)	Rye
Wheat		
Wheat Bran		
Wheat Granola		

ANIMAL FOODS

Often	In Moderation	Seldom	
Chicken or Turkey (white meat)	Egg Yolk	Beef	Pork
Egg White	Rabbit	Duck	Shellfish
Freshwater Fish	Shrimp	Lamb	Venison

LEGUMES (all are recommended "Often")

Aduki Beans	Kidney Beans	Soy Beans
Black Beans	Lentils	Soy Products
Chana Dal	Lima Beans	Soy Powder
Black Eyed Beans	Mung Beans	Split Peas
Black Lentils	Navy Beans	Tempeh
Garbanzos	Pinto Beans	Tofu
Kala Chana	Red Lentils	Urad Dal
White Beans		

NUTS

Often	In Moderation	Seldom
Coconut	Almonds	Black Walnuts
	Macadamia Nuts	Brazil Nuts
	Pecan	Cashews
	Pine Nuts	English Walnuts
		Filberts (Hazelnuts)
		Peanuts
		Pistachios

SEEDS

Often	In Moderation	Seldom
Psyllium	Flax	None
Pumpkin		
Sunflower		
Sesame		

SWEETENERS

Often	In Moderation	Seldom
Barley Malt	Fruit Juice Concentrate	Jaggery
Brown Rice Syrup	Honey	Molasses
Maple Syrup	Sugar Cane Juice	White Sugar
Syrup Fructose		
Sucanat		

CONDIMENTS

Often	In Moderation	Seldom
Black Pepper	Daikon (Radish)	Black Sesame Seeds
Coconut	Grated Cheese	Chili Pepper
Coriander Leaves	Lime	
Cottage Cheese	Yogurt (undiluted)	
Dulse (well-rinsed)		
Ghee		
Hijiki (well-rinsed)		
Kombu		
Lettuce		

Mango Chutney
Mint Leaves
Sprouts

SPICES

Often	Often	In Moderation	Seldom	Seldom
Fresh Basil Leaves	Neem Leaves	Allspice	Ajwan	Marjoram
Black Pepper	Orange Peet	Almond Extract	Amchoor	Mustard Seeds
Cardamom	Parsley	Anise	Asafoetida	Nutmeg
Tamarind	Peppernunt	Bay Leaf	Basil	Onion
Cinnamon	Rose Water	Fenugreek	Caraway	(esp. raw)
Tarragon	Saffron	Rosemary	Cayenne	Oregano
Coriander	Spearmint	Star Anise	Cloves	Paprika
Cumin	Turmeric	Thyme	Garlic	Pippali
Mint	Vanilla	Horseradish	(esp. raw)	Sage
Dill	Wintergreen		Poppy Seeds	Mace
Fennel			Ginger	
			Savory	

DAIRY

Often	In Moderation	Seldom
Unsalted Butter	Ice Cream	Salted Butter
Cottage Cheese	Hard Cheeses	Buttermilk (commercial)
Mild Soft Cheeses	Yogurt	Feta Cheese
Dilute Yogurt (1-3 pints water)	Sour Cream	
Ghee		
Cow's Milk		
Goat's Milk		

OILS

Often	In Moderation	Seldom
Coconut	Almond	Corn
Olive	Apricot	Sesame
Soy	Avocado	
Sunflower	Safflower	
Walnut		

BEVERAGES

Often

Almond Milk
Aloe Vera Juice
Apple Juice
Apricot Juice
Berry Juice (sweet)
Mixed Veg (fresh)
Carob
Coconut Milk
Cool Dairy Drinks
Fig Shake
Grape Juice

Peach Nectar
Pear Nectar
Pomegranate Juice
Prune Juice
Soy Milk
Vegetable Bouillon
Date Shake
Coconut Smoothies
Cherry Juice (sweet)
Goat Milk
Mango Juice

Grain Teas (Barley, Cafix, Pero, Roma)

Herb Teas   (Alfalfa, Bansha, Blackberry, Borage, Catnip, Chamomile, Chicory, Chrysanthemum, Cornsilk, Dandelion, Elder Flower, Fennel, Hibiscus, Hops, Jasmine, Lavender, Lemon Balm, LemonGrass, Licorice, Lotus, Marshmallow, Nettle, Oat Straw, Orange Peel, Passion Flower, Peppermint, Raspberry, Red Clover, Rose Flowers, Saffron, Sarsaparilla, Spearmint, Strawberry, Violet, Wintergreen)

In Moderation

Banana Shake or Smoothie
Caffeine
Carrot Juice
Carrot-Vegetable Combination
Coffee
Chocolate
Ginger (fresh)
Hawthorne
Herb Teas (Burdock, Comfrey)
Orange Juice
Rosehips
Wild Ginger

Seldom

Alcohol
Berry Juice (sour)
Carbonated Drinks
Carrot-Ginger Juice
Cranberry Juice
Grapefruit
Highly Salted Drinks
Ice Cold Drinks
Lemonade
Miso Broth (in excess)
Papaya Juice
Pungent Teas
Sour Juices and Teas

Tomato Juice
V-8 Juice

Herb Teas   (Ajwan, Basil,
Cinnamon, Cloves, Eucalyptus,
Fenugreek, Ginseng, Hyssop,
Juniper Berries, Mormon Tea,
Osha, Penny Royal, Red Zinger,
Sage, Sassafras, Yerba Santa)

Pitta Sattva Diets For Different Calorie Levels

Choose foods from the above Pitta Sattva Shopping List and enjoy them in the quantities indicated below according to the calorie level you wish to utilize.

1200 Calorie Lacto-Vegetarian Diet For Pitta Types

Category 1: Fruits	3 servings/day
Category 2: Vegetables	5 servings/day
Category 3: Cereals, Starchy Vegetables, Grains	6 servings/day
Category 4: Legumes	2 servings/day
Category 5: Fats	3 servings/day
Category 6: Dairy	1 serving/day
Category 7: Meats, Cheese, Fish, and Eggs	–

Carbohydrate calories:	71%
Fat calories:	14%
Protein calories:	15%
Total Protein content:	52 g
Dietary fiber content:	38-72 g

Recommended Meal Design

Breakfast
1 Fruit serving
2 Cereal/Starchy Vegetable/Grain servings
1 Fat serving
1 Dairy serving

Lunch
2 Vegetable servings
2 Cereal/Starchy Vegetable/Grain servings
2 Legume servings
1 Dairy serving
1 Fat serving

Mid-Afternoon Snack
1 Fruit serving

Dinner
3 Vegetable servings
2 Cereal/Starchy Vegetable/Grain servings
1 Fat serving
1 Fruit serving

1200 Calorie Omnivore Diet For Pitta Types

Category 1: Fruits	4 servings/day
Category 2: Vegetables	5 servings/day
Category 3: Cereals, Starchy Vegetables, Grains	3 servings/day
Category 4: Legumes	1 serving/day
Category 5: Fats	2 servings/day
Category 6: Dairy	1 serving/day
Category 7: Meats, Cheese, Fish, and Eggs	2 servings/day

Carbohydrate calories:	66%
Fat calories:	18%
Protein calories:	16%
Total Protein content:	59 g
Dietary fiber content:	28-55 g

Recommended Meal Design

Breakfast
1 Fruit serving
1 Cereal/Starchy Vegetable/Grain serving
1 Fat serving

Lunch
2 Vegetable servings
1 Cereal/Starchy Vegetable/Grain serving
1 Dairy serving
2 Meat/Cheese/Fish/Egg servings
1 Fruit serving
1 Fat serving

Mid-Afternoon Snack
1 Fruit serving

Dinner
3 Vegetable servings
2 Cereal/Starchy Vegetable/Grain servings
1 Legume serving
1 Fruit serving

1500 Calorie Lacto-Vegetarian Diet For Pitta Types

Category 1: Fruits	3 servings/day
Category 2: Vegetables	5 servings/day
Category 3: Cereals, Starchy Vegetables, Grains	7 servings/day
Category 4: Legumes	3 servings/day
Category 5: Fats	4 servings/day
Category 6: Dairy	2 servings/day
Category 7: Meats, Cheese, Fish, and Eggs	–

Carbohydrate calories:	68%
Fat calories:	17%
Protein calories:	15%
Total Protein content:	61 g
Dietary fiber content:	33-68 g

Recommended Meal Design

Breakfast
1 Fruit serving
2 Cereal/Starchy Vegetable/Grain servings
1 Fat serving
1 Dairy

Lunch
2 Vegetable servings
3 Cereal/Starchy Vegetable/Grain servings
2 Legume servings
2 Fat servings
1 Dairy serving

Mid-Afternoon Snack
1 Fruit serving

Dinner
3 Vegetable servings
2 Cereal/Starchy Vegetable/Grain servings
1 Legume
1 Fat serving
1 Fruit serving

1500 Calorie Omnivore Diet For Pitta Types

Category 1: Fruits	3 servings/day
Category 2: Vegetables	5 servings/day
Category 3: Cereals, Starchy Vegetables, Grains	4 servings/day
Category 4: Legumes	1 serving/day
Category 5: Fats	3 servings/day
Category 6: Dairy	1 serving/day
Category 7: Meats, Cheese, Fish, and Eggs	2 servings/day

Carbohydrate calories:	66%
Fat calories:	18%
Protein calories:	16%
Total Protein content:	76 g
Dietary fiber content:	28-75 g

Recommended Meal Design

Breakfast
1 Fruit serving
2 Cereal/Starchy Vegetable/Grain servings
1 Fat serving
1 Dairy serving

Lunch
2 Vegetable servings
2 Meat/Cheese/Fish/Egg servings
1 Fat serving

Mid-Afternoon Snack
1 Fruit serving

Dinner
3 Vegetable servings
2 Cereal/Starchy Vegetable/Grain servings
1 Legume serving
1 Fat serving
1 Fruit serving

2000 Calorie Lacto-Vegetarian Diet For Pitta Types

Category 1: Fruits	4 servings/day
Category 2: Vegetables	5 servings/day
Category 3: Cereals, Starchy Vegetables, Grains	9 servings/day
Category 4: Legumes	4 servings/day
Category 5: Fats	4 servings/day
Category 6: Dairy	2 servings/day
Category 7: Meats, Cheese, Fish, and Eggs	–

Carbohydrate calories:	69%
Fat calories:	16%
Protein calories:	15%
Total Protein content:	61 g
Dietary fiber content:	33-68 g

Recommended Meal Design

Breakfast
2 Fruit servings
2 Cereal/Starchy Vegetable/Grain servings
1 Fat serving
1 Dairy serving

Lunch
2 Vegetable servings
4 Cereal/Starchy Vegetable/Grain servings
2 Legume servings
1 Dairy serving
2 Fat servings

Mid-Afternoon Snack
1 Fruit serving

Dinner
3 Vegetable servings
3 Cereal/Starchy Vegetable/Grain servings
2 Legume servings
1 Fat serving
1 Fruit serving

2000 Calorie Omnivore Diet For Pitta Types

Category 1: Fruits	3 servings/day
Category 2: Vegetables	5 servings/day
Category 3: Cereals, Starchy Vegetables, Grains	7 servings/day
Category 4: Legumes	2 servings/day
Category 5: Fats	4 servings/day
Category 6: Dairy	1 serving/day
Category 7: Meats, Cheese, Fish, and Eggs	2 servings/day

Carbohydrate calories:	65%
Fat calories	18%
Protein calories	17%
Total Protein content:	79 g
Dietary fiber content:	22-82 g

Recommended Meal Design

Breakfast
1 Fruit serving
2 Cereal/Starchy Vegetable/Grain servings
1 Fat serving
1 Dairy serving

Lunch
2 Vegetable servings
2 Cereal/Starchy Vegetable/Grain servings
2 Fat servings
2 Meat/Cheese/Fish/Egg servings

Mid-Afternoon Snack
1 Fruit serving

Dinner
3 Vegetable servings
3 Cereal/Starchy Vegetable/Grain servings
2 Legume servings
1 Fat serving
1 Fruit serving

2500 Calorie Lacto-Vegetarian Diet For Pitta Types

Category 1: Fruits	5 servings/day
Category 2: Vegetables	8 servings/day
Category 3: Cereals, Starchy Vegetables, Grains	11 servings/day
Category 4: Legumes	4 servings/day
Category 5: Fats	6 servings/day
Category 6: Dairy	2 servings/day
Category 7: Meats, Cheese, Fish, and Eggs	–

Carbohydrate calories:	69%
Fat calories:	15%
Protein calories:	16%
Total Protein content:	91 g
Dietary fiber content:	35-102 g

Recommended Meal Design

Breakfast
2 Fruit servings
2 Cereal/Starchy Vegetable/Grain servings
1 Fat serving

Lunch
4 Vegetable servings
5 Cereal/Starchy Vegetable/Grain servings
2 Legume servings
3 Fat servings
2 Dairy servings

Mid-Afternoon Snack
1 Fruit serving

Dinner
4 Vegetable servings
4 Cereal/Starchy Vegetable/Grain servings
2 Legume servings
2 Fat servings
2 Fruit servings

2500 Calorie Omnivore Diet For Pitta Types

Category 1: Fruits	5 servings/day
Category 2: Vegetables	7 servings/day
Category 3: Cereals, Starchy Vegetables, Grains	10 servings/day
Category 4: Legumes	2 servings/day
Category 5: Fats	7 servings/day
Category 6: Dairy	1 serving/day
Category 7: Meats, Cheese, Fish, and Eggs	3 servings/day

Carbohydrate calories:	65%
Fat calories:	18%
Protein calories:	17%
Total Protein content:	96 g
Dietary fiber content:	42-108 g

Recommended Meal Design

Breakfast
1 Fruit serving
2 Cereal/Starchy Vegetable/Grain servings
1 Fat serving
1 Dairy serving

Lunch
4 Vegetable servings
5 Cereal/Starchy Vegetable/Grain servings
3 Meat/Cheese/Fish/Egg servings
3 Fat servings

Mid-Afternoon Snack
1 Fruit serving

Dinner
3 Vegetable servings
5 Cereal/Starchy Vegetable/Grain servings
2 Legume servings
3 Fat servings
1 Fruit serving

Herbal Supplements For Pitta-Type Individuals

In addition to assisting with a generalized detoxification process throughout the body, the Sattva Pitta Herbal Formulation is geared toward specifically up-regulating the cleansing processes in the liver, gallbladder, blood and skin. These are all areas where Pitta dosha tends to accumulate.

As we mentioned in Chapter 8, all individuals regardless of Ayurvedic Constitutional Type should take the **Sattva Basic Formulation** that consists of a combination of the following herbs. This formulation will support cleansing of the body's tissues and help up-regulate fat catabolism for people of all Ayurvedic Constitutional Types. For your convenience, here again is the Sattva Basic Formulation:

Guggulu (standardized to 2.5% guggulsterones) . . . . . . 125 mg. (1 part)
Citraka . . . . 500 mg. (4 parts)
Punarnava (standardized to 25% alkaloids) . . . . 125 mg. (1 part)
Garcinia (standardized to 10% hydroxycitric acid) . . . . 125 mg. (1 part)
Triphala powder . . . . 500 mg. (4 parts)
Ginger . . . . 250 mg. (2 parts)
Cayenne Pepper . . . . 250 mg. (2 parts)
Black Pepper . . . . 250 mg. (2 parts)

Pitta-type individuals should add the following herbal components to the Basic Formulation:

Katuki . . . . 500 mg. (4 parts)
Patala . . . . 125 mg. (1 part)
Turmeric . . . . 250 mg. (2 parts)
Coriander . . . . 250 mg. (2 parts)

Mix all ingredients very well in a bowl and use the mixture to fill "00" veggie caps. Pitta individuals should start by taking two "00" veggie caps twice a day before breakfast and dinner for the first week. If well-tolerated, you can increase to three times a day before breakfast, lunch and dinner.

It is safe to continue taking this herbal formulation for up to one year. However, every six to eight weeks it is recommended to stop the herbs for approximately one week. Then resume as before.

Here is some information about these additional herbs.

Katuki (also Kutki, Katki) consists of the dried rhizomes of the herb *Picrorhiza kurroa* Royale ex Benth., and it is among the most studied herbs in Ayurveda. It grows only in the northwestern region of the Himalayas at altitudes of about 10,000 feet. It has been found to be beneficial in improving liver function and enzymatic homeostasis in patients with infective hepatitis. Classically, it is recognized as a mild purgative, promoter of bile from the liver and gallbladder, and an anti-inflammatory agent used in insect bites and scorpion sting. It is primarily anti-Pitta in its action but also possesses anti-kapha properties.

Patala consists of the roots of *Stereospermum suaveolens* DC, and is a large tree found in the deciduous forests along both Indian coasts. It is cooling, bitter, astringent, and slightly sedative—all qualities which make it a good Pitta-pacifying herb. In addition to being used for obesity, it is also useful in diarrhea, hemorrhoids, water retention and blood disorders.

Turmeric (*haridra*, in Sanskrit) consists of the bright yellow rhizomes of *Curcuma longa* Linn., found throughout India and in many parts of the world. In classical Ayurvedic medicine turmeric is still used as a blood purifier, anti-parasitic, and as an anti-inflammatory in rheumatic diseases, as well as externally to treat certain forms of skin infections, eczema, and insect bites. Recently, the component responsible for the rhizome's yellow coloration, curcumin, was isolated and is receiving a lot of attention as an effective anti-inflammatory in joint disease. It is given with coriander in this formulation also to increase the assimilation of the other herbs.

Coriander (*dhanyaka*, in Sanskrit) is a well-known spice that comes from the plant known as *Coriandrum sativum* Linn.. It is an annual herb that grows to about two feet high and, most important to us, produces plenty of brown, oval-shaped seeds, which are the medicinal (and tasty!) parts. It is commonly used as a remedy for flatulence, indigestion, nausea and bilious complaints. Coriander seeds are powdered and added to the Pitta formulation to improve its assimilation into the body as well as to lend its Pitta-pacifying action.

Exercise For Pitta-Type Individuals

As previously explained in the section on the general principles of the Sattva Program, an effective exercise program, like any other health-promoting activity or substance, is only effective when it suits the specific needs of the individual. Exercise that is done properly always creates vitality and energy; it does not destroy it. Regular exercise is not only important for the Sattva Program and weight loss, but is an essential component for maintaining optimal function of the human organism. It is an imperative initial step to be implemented in any health promotion strategy.

Pitta individuals benefit most from exercise that balance, and do not tend to aggravate, the fire element. Pitta-friendly forms of exercise can include somewhat (but not excessively) competitive sports, and should draw on speed, strength, stamina and concentration. It is common for Pitta individuals to be so thoroughly engaged in the business side of life and their many pursuits that they often eliminate exercise from their routines. Pitta people therefore, by the time they reach the age of thirty, are commonly existing below or just at the minimum level of healthy physical activity. Regular exercise of an appropriate nature can help Pitta individuals balance their physiology and promote detoxification.

Examples of healthy exercise for Pitta individuals include:

Basketball	Skiing (downhill/cross country)
Bicycling (moderate)	Soccer
Field hockey	Sprinting
Football	Tennis
Gymnastics	Surfing
Ice hockey	Water skiing
Ice skating (in/outdoors)	Windsurfing
Kayaking	Yoga
Karate	Walking/Jogging

If you happen to be a bi-doshic (two doshic) type, for the purposes of exercise, refer to your overall physique to determine your type. If you have a medium frame, good solid musculature which is not too thick, average padding around the joints and over the hands and feet and not too "bony", and skin which is fair and/or freckled or contains many moles, consider yourself a Pitta type for matters of exercise.

Pitta individuals will benefit most from the forms of exercise listed above. In addition, remember that walking is the best form of exercise for all types. Pitta individuals benefit more from a moderately vigorous style of walking which is sustained for thirty to forty minutes, twice a day. Pitta individuals should definitely drink water during every period of exercise that exceeds thirty minutes. The main criteria for a successful exercise program for the Pitta individual is to make exercise a permanent part of their daily schedule. Pitta individuals, like Kapha types, should choose a form of exercise that they sincerely enjoy. Pitta individuals, both men and women, can benefit greatly from weight lifting provided they exercise in moderation, stay hydrated, and guard against over-exertion, which can be a strong tendency.

Pranayama For Pitta Types

One of the keys to health for people of Pitta constitution is to continuously release excess heat in both the mind and body to prevent its accumulation. The ancient sages who perfected yogic breathing exercises understood how to use the breath to both increase or decrease heat in the physiology. The technique that is described below will decrease heat and balance the fire element of the mind and body. Advanced students of pranayama will recognize this Cooling Breath Technique to be an amalgam and variation of two well-known exercises: nadi shodhana pranayama and sheetali pranayama.

The Cooling Breath Technique

1. Sit in a balanced, upright posture in a chair with a straight back. Feet should be flat on the floor about shoulder width apart; remove the shoes and socks. In this exercise the left hand rests on the lap, palm up, throughout the exercise. The right hand initially is in the same position as well.

(All references to the thumb and ring finger refer to the right hand, which is the only hand used in this technique).

2. Exhale whatever air is in the lungs.

3. Inhale through a curled tongue. If you are in the 15% of the population who cannot curl the tongue (it's a genetically determined feature—like blue eyes), then inhale "through your teeth". This is done by starting with your mouth in its normal, relaxed position with the upper and lower teeth slightly apart or lightly touching. Then simply part the lips, keeping the teeth still, and allowing the inhaled breath to flow through and around the teeth.

4. In both techniques, you will definitely perceive a coolness of the air as it traverses the tongue and teeth and into the respiratory passages.

5. Inhale until the lungs are comfortably filled, without straining or unnaturally filling the lungs.

6. Now, before exhaling, occlude the right nostril with the right thumb and exhale out of the un-occluded left nostril.

7. Keeping the right nostril occluded with the thumb, now inhale again using either the "curled tongue" or "through the teeth" technique. Note the coolness of the air as it flows over the moist surfaces.

8. Before exhaling, release the thumb from the right nostril and simultaneously occlude the left nostril with the right ring finger. Then exhale slowly and steadily through the un-occluded right nostril.

9. This completes one cycle. Do not release the right ring finger. Begin the next cycle by keeping the left nostril occluded with the right ring finger while inhaling through the curled tongue (or through the teeth). Now, before exhaling, release the right ring finger from the left nostril and again occlude the right nostril with the right thumb. Exhale slowly and steadily.

To summarize, in this exercise all inhalations are taken through the curled tongue and the exhalations are alternated between the left and right nostrils, while occluding the other.

10. It is recommended to complete 16 cycles per session. Perform this exercise twice a day, morning and evening. It requires approximately 90 seconds to complete each session.

Massage Oils For Pitta Types

Pitta individuals tend to become overheated and benefit most from oils that are of medium thickness and somewhat cooling in nature. Fortunately, nature has provided us with several oils that have these characteristics. What's more, almost any oil can be given Pitta-reducing qualities by combining it with appropriate herbal materials. The oils listed below can be used individually or combined in any way. If you do combine two or more oils, its best to use only one of the traditional oils in your formula.

Pitta Massage Oils

TRADITIONAL OILS	MODERN OILS
Chandanbala laxadi taila	Coconut
Guduchyadi taila	Sandalwood
Manjisthadi taila	Almond
Madhuyastyadi taila	Sunflower
Pinda taila	Pumpkin seed

Chapter 12. Recommendations For Specific Constitutional Types

In general, individuals of Pitta constitutions benefit from a moderately vigorous yet soothing massage technique. When using the self massage technique known as abhyanga, the oil should be room temperature or slightly warm. The strokes should be of moderate speed—at about the same rate as your pulse rate. The average pulse rate is approximately 72 beats per minute, which means the strokes should be about one stroke per second. Remember this is only a guideline to get you started. The best rate is the one that you intuitively adopt from your understanding of the term "moderate speed".

Pitta individuals also benefit from a massage technique that is somewhat deep and penetrating, except for the head massage, which should be done in a gentle manner that does not create excessive friction.

Fasting Techniques For Pitta Individuals

One of the prominent defining features of people with a significant proportion of Pitta dosha in their constitutions is the very sudden and intense onset of hunger, especially at lunchtime. The urge to eat can besiege the mind of Pitta individuals so strongly that it matters little what important tasks require attention. "Whatever needs to be done can wait until I come back from lunch." As one of my professors of physiology used to say, "It is imprudent and possibly unsafe to stand between a Pitta person and the door at lunchtime." Often you might observe Vata or Kapha types working right through lunch, if the matter is important and they become fully engaged. You will rarely, if ever, see this behavior in strongly Pitta people.

Given this tendency, you can understand the special challenge which fasting represents to the Pitta type. What makes fasting particularly interesting for Pittas is the other dominating feature of their personalities: they tend to be capable of disciplining themselves and carrying out plans. They tend to be good at ignoring distractions, if they are truly interested in the activity. Thus, in fasting we have a fascinating dynamic. Pitta people have that strong inherent urge to eat when hungry yet also have the equally strong discipline to follow a planned fast.

Understanding the Logic of Fasting

If you happen to be someone with a high proportion of Pitta dosha in your constitution, one of the best ways to ensure that you will follow through with your desire to fast is to understand the reason for fasting. The Pitta mind is actually balanced and satisfied when it can acquire detailed and specific information. Therefore, although it would be inappropriate to include an entire treatise on the physiology of fasting, a few interesting facts may help encourage not only you Pitta folks, but people of all constitutions as well. Also refer to the section on fasting for the Kapha individual for additional background.

To begin with, fasting is of course a time-honored and safe activity that has been performed by humans for literally thousands of years. Philosophers, scientists, and seekers have used fasting to promote purification, healing, and mental awareness. Socrates, Plato, Aristotle, Paracelsus, and the father of modern medicine, Hippocrates, all recommended fasting as an important healing tool. Certainly, within the Hindu tradition fasting has been utilized as both a medical and a spiritual method for at least two thousand years.

Medically, fasting technically begins when all of the nutrients from the last meal have been absorbed and metabolized into energy. At this point, there is a mandatory transition to endogenous fuel consumption. This transition occurs after the same amount of time in all people: twelve hours after the last meal. This is the time period that corresponds quite closely with the usual overnight fast. After this twelve hour period, the body obtains its energy through the breakdown of glycogen stored in the liver and from the oxidation and breakdown of fat. If unfed for periods exceeding three days, a contribution also comes from muscle protein. However, what you should realize is that during a one to three day fast the major source of fuel, in the absence of carbohydrate intake, is fat. In fact we know that approximately 65% of the energy during a fast does indeed come from fat sources. This is a good reason to consider fasting as a part of your approach to weight management.

Another physiological highlight of fasting involves the insulin to glucagon ratio. You will recall that insulin is a hormone responsible for the absorption of glucose into muscle and liver tissues, protein synthesis, and new fat biosynthesis. Glycogen promotes the opposite processes of glucose release from the liver and the breakdown of fats. When we fast, since there is no glucose to stimulate insulin secretion, our blood insulin levels decrease. This decrease in insulin drives two important reactions. First, low insulin levels cause free fatty acids to be mobilized from our adipose tissues throughout the body. Secondly, the lowered insulin levels cause a lowering of the insulin: glucagon ratio, which causes all of these newly liberated fatty acids to undergo oxidation (i.e. breakdown) in the liver.

We now have so much detailed information on the effects of fasting that it is difficult to choose only one or two features to discuss. But the point is that we now understand that periodic fasting is a safe and effective way to support a weight loss and maintenance program. Of course, you must be aware of the contraindications for fasting and avoid it entirely if you have any of them (see page 218).

Because a carbohydrate intake of as little as 150 grams per day can elevate the insulin level enough to inhibit the oxidation of fat, we should try to stay under that threshold. It's not that difficult if you have some idea of typical carbohydrate contents in food. Here are some examples of the carbohydrate content of some common foods:

> Orange juice, fresh (8 oz.) . . . . . . 26 g
> Carrot juice, fresh (8 oz.) . . . . 12 g
> Whole wheat bread (1 slice). . . . . 13 g
> Apple, medium . . . . 22 g
> Banana, medium . . . . 28 g

Once some knowledge has been acquired about the science of fasting, Pitta people need to immediately formulate a plan and make a resolution to adhere to it.

Absolute Fast

Although abstinence from food and water for short periods of time is recognized throughout India as an effective part of the therapy for obesity, exposure to toxins or chemicals, rheumatoid arthritis, allergies, edema, irregular appetite, disturbed eating patterns, psoriasis, and many other medical disorders, it is largely ignored by the Western medical culture.

Absolute fasting is most commonly used in people with some component of Kapha dosha in their constitution, however for Pitta individuals with a significant amount of water retention, mucous accumulation, and food addictions it is a safe and effective option. The duration of this type of fast should be limited to 24 hours. The method is quite simple.

I usually advise beginning an absolute fast at 6:00 p.m. on an auspicious evening when the mind is tranquil and settled. On that day, your lunch should consist of fresh fruits, herbal tea, soup, or steamed vegetables. Dinner should be similarly light and end at around 6:00 p.m. The fast starts after dinner, when you will eat or drink nothing for 24 hours, including water.

It is necessary to refrain from any strenuous activities and get as much rest as possible; even moderate exercise is discouraged. It is, however, perfectly fine to take short walks outside and to enjoy gentle yoga asanas or other stretching techniques. Be aware that during an absolute fast, core body temperature, pulse rate, respiratory rate, and blood pressure can all drop—reflecting a general slowing of the metabolism. Daytime napping is encouraged.

As with all fasts, it is important to reintroduce foods, even for a fast of only one-day duration, in moderate quantities. Remember to chew your food well, and not to drink anything cold for at least one day following the fast. Do not overeat; if you do you will most likely feel lethargic, slightly nauseous, and possibly develop a headache. Worse, you will have wasted your investment from the previous 24-hours and may disrupt your digestive system for as much as a week. Do not overeat.

Pitta Fruit Juice Fast

Juices for Pitta individuals work best for fasting when they are freshly prepared from raw organic fruits. Canned, frozen, or otherwise packaged fruit juices should be avoided. The juices of certain fruits are actually excellent for generalized cleansing, but must be minimized in the Sattva weight loss program, due to their relatively high caloric values. These include: apples, grapes, mango, and oranges. Juices that are more useful are grapefruit, lemon, cucumber, pineapple, pear, cantaloupe, cranberry, and watermelon.

I recommend the following recipes, although any combination of the fruit juices that are listed above may be used.

Pitta Fruit Juice Fast #1

Pineapple	1 cup, cubed
Watermelon	1 cup, cubed
Blueberry	1/4 cup
Water	1 cup

Pitta Fruit Juice Fast #2

Fresh Lemon Juice	1/2 cup
Cranberry	1/2 cup
Pear	1 cup, cubed
Water	1 cup

Pitta Fruit Juice Fast #3

Lemon	1 cup
Orange	1/4 cup
Pineapple	1/2 cup, cubed
Water	1/2 cup

Pitta Vegetable Juice Fast

As with fruits, we want to always use the freshest and most pesticide-free vegetables possible. They should be stored properly and cleaned well in warm water before use. Some Ayurvedic physicians recommend submerging vegetables into a pot of boiling water for 1-2 minutes before juicing. Vegetables that are not organic should be peeled, especially if they have a wax coat.

Remember that the juice of each vegetable has a specific nutritional composition and no doubt has numerous benefits throughout the physiology. Juices contain numerous vitamins and minerals in proportions which nature has evolved; they occur in association with other specific complex arrangements for good reason. The body recognizes these natural proportions as characteristic of "food", which it is designed to assimilate. Juices, of course, therefore have an efficient assimilation rate and yet do not require large amounts of work for their digestion.

Vegetables that are particularly appropriate for Pitta individuals include:

Carrot (in moderation), beets, beet greens, collard greens, kale, radish, cabbage, cucumber, spinach, parsley, green pepper and turnip.

Any of the above vegetables can be used to prepare juices for people with Pitta constitutions. Here are a few recipes that I find especially delicious.

This first one uses the most ingredients (total volume 8 oz.):

Carrot	**30%**
Spinach	
Cabbage	
Parsley	
Collard Greens	**40%**
Beet root	
Beet greens	
Radish	
Water	**30%**

In this formula approximately 30% of a glass should be filled with freshly juiced carrot juice and the remaining 70% should contain a combination of the other ingredients. One half to one beet root and 2-3 radishes should be used.

Another simple recipe for Pitta constitution (total volume 8 oz.):

Cucumber	**20%**
Spinach	**20%**
Cabbage.	**10%**
Green Pepper.	**10%**
Parsley	**10%**
Beet root	**10%**
Water.	**20%**

A third Pitta vegetable juice recipe is very basic yet satisfying (total volume 8 oz.):

Carrot	30%
Spinach	20%
Green Pepper	20%
Beet root	5%
Beet greens	5%
Water	20%

Teas *(also see "Making Teas" on page 220)*

Herbal teas consisting of ingredients that have blood cleansing, liver cleansing, alkalinizing and cooling effects will be effective in detoxifying Pitta individuals. There are many Ayurvedic herbal tea formulae that are known to promote gentle detoxification and are specifically good for weight loss programs.

One formula is the Pitta Tea available through The National Institute of Ayurvedic Medicine which contains: Amalaki (*Emblica officinalis*), Coriander (*Coriandrum sativum*), Bilva leaves (*Aegle marmelos*), rose petals, and Eranda (*Ricinus communis*).

Other excellent fasting teas for Pitta types are:

1) Four parts guduchi (*Tinospora cordifolia*), two parts cumin seed (*Cuminum cyminum*), one part neem leaf (*Azadirachta indica*), one part gokshura (*Tribulus terrestris*), one part bhumyamalaki (*Phyllanthus fraternus*)

2) Two parts tejpatra (*Cinnamomum tamala*), two parts fennel (*Foeniculum vulgare*), one part coriander seed (*Coriandrum sativum*), one part gotu kola (*Centella asiatica*), one part shyonaka (*Oroxylum indicum*)

Aromatherapy for Pitta

Here are the essential oils that are used in Ayurveda to pacify Pitta dosha:

Essential Oils Recommended for Pacifying Pitta Dosha

Sandalwood	Saffron
Rose	Jasmine
Lavender	Lotus
Gardenia	Vetivert
Niaouli	Jatamansi
Peppermint	Coriander

Here are three Pitta-pacifying blends that are cooling, relaxing, and easy to prepare.

1. Sandalwood, Lavender, Gardenia

2. Jasmine, Lavender, Coriander

3. Lotus, Sandalwood, Rose

Continue to experiment with different combinations and quantities of these essential oils. You will undoubtedly discover your own unique blends.

Pitta Behavioral Therapies

Both physical and emotional disorders are caused by imbalances in the three doshas (biological energies) as well as in the three gunas (mental energies). If the specific condition is of a more physical than mental nature, it is likely that the doshic imbalance is more important; if the specific issue is more mental/emotional than physical, it is probably more related to the gunas.

It is important to understand that dis-ease, both the physical and mental varieties, reflects a loss of balance between the forces and energies of nature and those of our individual self. Ayurveda counsels us about certain behaviors for each Constitutional Type that can help re-establish and maintain harmony among these energies.

CHAPTER 12. RECOMMENDATIONS FOR SPECIFIC CONSTITUTIONAL TYPES

Behaviors to be Avoided by Pitta Types

- Consumption of excessively spicy foods
- Excessive exposure to the sun in the Summer season
- Wearing inappropriately warm clothing in the warm seasons
- Excessive consumption of alcoholic beverages
- Insufficient consumption of pure, clean water
- Excessive number of quarrels, disagreements, and arguments
- Excessive criticism of self or others
- Lack of time spent outdoors in nature, especially near lakes, rivers, and fields
- Anger and jealousy
- Excessive ambition and competition
- Excessive time spent in uncertain or insecure relationships or partnerships
- Dealing with one's own tardiness or that of others

Behaviors to be Encouraged by Pitta Types

- Cool and quiet environments
- Soft music, especially wind instruments
- Use of cooling colors including green, blue, and white
- Placement of fresh flowers in the home
- Walking or sitting outdoors at night; looking at the moon
- Using turmeric, fennel, dill, and coriander but not other spices in excessive amounts
- Cooling aromas: sandalwood, rose, gardenia, lotus, vetivert
- Cultivating forgiveness, compassion and kindness
- Guarding against anger, jealousy, judgment and hatred
- Enjoy foods which are not piping hot and are bitter and astringent in taste
- Take a short nap or rest in the afternoon
- Recreational activity should balance work activity
- Meditation on a regular basis

The Sattva Program For Vata Types

Sattva Program For Vata Types

As I have suggested in the sections on the Pitta and Kapha programs, if you have skipped to this section and haven't read Chapter 8 yet, I strongly suggest you do so. Many of the general Sattva recommendations apply for Vata types; however, some of these general principles need to be modified to best suit individuals of Vata constitutional type. These modifications are the subject of this chapter. As with the other two doshas, the *diet* is the most important of these modifications.

Like Pitta types, the mind of the Vata dominant individual is also characterized by *rajas*, which creates a strong tendency toward movement and activity, though the mental activity is often less focused and more changeable. Vata individuals have interests in many things simultaneously but may have only superficial knowledge, due to a tendency to shift their attention before in-depth penetration of any subject can proceed. Their minds can be indecisive and their willpower can easily waver. Vata people are prone to anxiety and fear. They are very amiable and social but tend to overextend themselves and suffer from the consequent mental and physical fatigue. When balanced they are the most adaptable of all constitutional types, however excess Vata quickly renders them hypersensitive to even minor criticisms and they can lose self-confidence and stability.

Vata people do best with the sweet, sour, and salty tastes that ground the mind and body, especially if a moderate amount of appropriate spices is included. In contrast, foods with excessively pungent, bitter, and astringent tastes tend to aggravate Vata if taken in excess, so foods with these dominating tastes are reduced. Vata types should consume foods that are for the most part well-cooked and served very warm. However, food should never be taken when it is too hot or too salty, as these conditions are also excessively rajasic and stimulating.

THE VATA DIET

How to use this list

One of the most unique facets of Ayurvedic dietetics is that different foods from each food group are recommended for different Ayurvedic Constitutional Types.

In using the list below, eat mainly from the "Often" and "In Moderation" lists and only infrequently or on special occasions from the "Seldom" list.

"Often" in this context means consuming these foods **every day** would be fine.

"In Moderation" means that you should consume approximately **one-third to one-half** the amount of these foods as you do the "Often" foods. These foods are an important part of your diet in the proper amounts.

"Seldom" means about **once a month**.

THE VATA DIET

FRUITS

Often	Often	In Moderation	Seldom
Apricot	Mango	Apples	Dried Fruits
Avocado	Melons (sweet)	Soursop	Cranberries
Bananas	Oranges	Strawberries	Pears
Berries (all)	Papaya		Persimmon
Cherries	Peaches		Pomegranate
Coconut	Pineapples		Prunes
Dates	Plums		Quince
Figs (fresh)	Raisins (soaked)		
Grapefruit	Rhubarb		
Grapes	Watermelon		
Kiwi			
Lemons			
Limes			

VEGETABLES

Often	Often	In Moderation	Seldom
(cooked vegetables)	Radish	Broccoli	(frozen, dried, raw vegetables)
Acorn Squash	Rutabaga	Cauliflower	Beet Greens
Artichokes	Scallopini Squash	Fresh Corn	Brussels Sprouts
Asparagus	Summer Squash	Peas	Burdock Root
Beets	Watercress	Potatoes (white)	Cabbage
Butternut Squash	Winter Squash	Spinach	Celery
Carrots	Yellow Squash	Tomatoes	Eggplant
Cucumber	Zucchini	Leafy Greens	Jerusalem Artichoke
Daikon Radish			Jicama
Fenugreek Greens			Kohlrabi
Green Beans (well cooked)			Lettuce
Olives (black & green)			Mushrooms
Onion (cooked)			Parsnip
Potato (sweet)			Onions (raw)
Peppers			Parsley
Spaghetti Squash			Pumpkin
Sprouts			
Turnips			
Turnip Greens			

SWEETNERS

Often	In Moderation	Seldom
None	Barley Malt Syrup	White Sugar
	Brown Rice Syrup	
	Fructose	
	Most Fruit Juice Concentrates	
	Honey	
	Jaggery	
	Maple Syrup	
	Sucanat	
	Sugar Cane Juice	

CONDIMENTS

Often	Often	In Moderation	Seldom
Black Pepper	Onion (cooked)	Cardamom	None
Coconut	Orange Peel	Cayenne	
Coriander Leaves	Oregano	Cloves	
Cottage Cheese	Paprika	Parsley	
Grated Cheese	Peppermint	Poppy Seeds	
Daikon Radish	Pippali	Thyme	
Dulse	Rosemary	Neem Leaves	
Garlic	Rosewater		
Ghee	Saffron		
Ginger (fresh)	Sage		
Gomasio	Savory		
Hijiki	Spearmint		
Horseradish	Star Anise		
Kelp	Tamarind		
Kombu	Tarragon		
Lemon	Turmeric		
Lime	Vanilla		
Lime Pickle	Wintergreen		
Mango Chutney			
Mango Pickle			
Mint Leaves			

DAIRY

All dairy is acceptable in moderation.

Often	In Moderation	Seldom
Buttermilk	Goat's Milk (liquid)	Goat's Milk (powdered)
Cow's Milk	Ice Cream	Condensed Milk
Hard Cheese	Sour Cream	
Soft Cheese		
Goat Cheese		
Yogurt		

GRAINS

Often	In Moderation	Seldom
Amaranth	Barley	(cold, dry, puffed cereals)
Oats (cooked)	Corn	Buckwheat
Rice (all)	Wheat Bran	Millet
Wheat		Oats (dry)
		Granola
		Oat Bran
		Quinoa
		Rice Cakes
		Rye

ANIMAL FOODS

Often	In Moderation	Seldom
Beef	Freshwater Fish	Lamb
Blue Green Algae	Shellfish	Pork
Chicken	Shrimp	Rabbit
Mahi		Venison
Red Snapper		
Swordfish		
Turkey (white meat)		
Tuna		

LEGUMES

Often	In Moderation	Seldom
Adzuki Beans	Black Beans	Black Eyed Beans
Black Lentils	Common Lentils	Chana Dal
Mung Beans	Lima Beans	Garbanzos
Red Lentils	Soy Beans	Kala Chana
Soy Milk (liquid)		Kidney Beans
Tepery Beans		Navy Beans
Tofu		Pinto Beans
Tur Dal		Soy Flour
		Soy Powder
		Split Peas
		Tempeh
		White Beans

NUTS

Often		In Moderation	Seldom
Almonds	English Walnuts	Peanuts	None
Black Walnuts	Filberts (Hazelnuts)	Pine Nuts	
Brazil Nuts	Macadamia Nuts	Pistaschios	
Cashews	Pecans		
Coconut			

SEEDS

Often	In Moderation	Seldom
Chia	Psyllium	None
Flax		
Sesame		
Pumpkin		
Sunflower		

OILS

All oils are fine, especially sesame, olive and flaxseed.

BEVERAGES

Often

Almond
Apricot Juice
Banana Shake or Smoothie
Carrot Juice
Carrot-Veg Combinations
Carrot-Ginger Juice
Cherry Juice
Coconut Milk
Dairy Drinks (hot)
Date Shake
Grain Teas (Cafix, Roma, Pero)
Grape Juice
Grapefruit Juice
Lemonade
Mango Juice
Milk (hot, spiced)
Miso Broth
Mixed Vegetable Juice
Orange Juice
Papaya Juice
Peach Nectar
Pineapple Juice
Salted Drinks
Sour Juices & Teas
Soy Milk (well spiced & hot)
Herb Teas (Ajwan, Bansha w/ milk & sweetener, Basil, Catnip, Cinnamon, Elder Flowers, Eucalyptus, Fennel, Fenugreek, Ginger (fresh), Ginseng, Hawthorne, Hyssop, Juniper Berries, Lavender, Lemon Balm, Lemon Grass, Licorice, Lotus Marshmallow, Oat Straw, Orange Peel, Osha, Peppermint, Red Zinger Roseflowers, Rosehip, Saffron)

In Moderation

Alcohol
Aloe Vera Juice
Berry Juice
Chocolate
HerbTeas (Chamomile, Cloves, Comfrey, Jasmine,
Raspberry, Sage, Yarrow)

Seldom

Apple Juice
Pear Juice
Caffeine
Carob
Carbonated Drinks
Coffee
Cranberry Juice
Dairy Drinks (cold)
Ice Cold Drinks

Pear Juice
Pomegranate Juice
Prune Juice
V-8 Juice
Herb Teas (Alfalfa, Barley, Blackberry,
Borage, Burdock, Chrysanthemum,
CornSilk, Dandelion, Hibiscus, Hops,
Mormon Tea, Nettle, Passion Flower,
Red Clover, Strawberry, Violet,
Wintergreen, Yerba Mate)

Vata Sattva Diets For Different Calorie Levels

Choose foods from the above Kapha Sattva Shopping List and enjoy them in the quantities indicated below according to the calorie level you wish to utilize.

1200 Calorie Lacto-Vegetarian Diet For Vata Types

Category 1: Fruits	3 servings/day
Category 2: Vegetables	5 servings/day
Category 3: Cereals, Starchy Vegetables, Grains	6 servings/day
Category 4: Legumes	2 servings/day
Category 5: Fats	3 servings/day
Category 6: Dairy	1 serving/day
Category 7: Meats, Cheese, Fish, and Eggs	–

Carbohydrate calories:	71%
Fat calories:	14%
Protein calories:	15%
Total Protein content:	52 g
Dietary fiber content:	38-72 g

Recommended Meal Design

Breakfast
1 Fruit serving
2 Cereal/Starchy Vegetable/Grain servings
1 Fat serving
1 Dairy serving

Lunch
2 Vegetable servings
2 Cereal/Starchy Vegetable/Grain servings
2 Legume servings
1 Dairy serving
1 Fat serving

Mid-Afternoon Snack
1 Fruit serving

Dinner
3 Vegetable servings
2 Cereal/Starchy Vegetable/Grain servings
1 Fat serving
1 Fruit serving

1200 Calorie Omnivore Diet For Vata Types

Category 1: Fruits	3 servings/day
Category 2: Vegetables	5 servings/day
Category 3: Cereals, Starchy Vegetables, Grains	3 servings/day
Category 4: Legumes	2 servings/day
Category 5: Fats	3 servings/day
Category 6: Dairy	1 serving/day
Category 7: Meats, Cheese, Fish, and Eggs	2 servings/day

Carbohydrate calories:	66%
Fat calories:	18%
Protein calories:	16%
Total Protein content:	59 g
Dietary fiber content:	28-55 g

Recommended Meal Design

Breakfast
1 Fruit serving
1 Cereal/Starchy Vegetable/Grain servings
1 Fat serving

Lunch
2 Vegetable servings
1 Cereal/Starchy Vegetable/Grain serving
1 Dairy serving
2 Meat/Cheese/Fish/Egg servings
1 Fat Serving

Mid-Afternoon Snack
1 Fruit serving

Dinner
3 Vegetable servings
1 Cereal/Starchy Vegetable/Grain serving
2 Legume servings
1 Fat serving
1 Fruit serving

1500 Calorie Lacto-Vegetarian Diet For Vata Types

Category 1: Fruits	3 servings/day
Category 2: Vegetables	5 servings/day
Category 3: Cereals, Starchy Vegetables, Grains	6 servings/day
Category 4: Legumes	3 servings/day
Category 5: Fats	5 servings/day
Category 6: Dairy	2 servings/day
Category 7: Meats, Cheese, Fish, and Eggs	–

Carbohydrate calories:	68%
Fat calories:	17%
Protein calories:	14%
Total Protein content:	61 g
Dietary fiber content:	33-68 g

Recommended Meal Design

Breakfast
1 Fruit serving
2 Cereal/Starchy Vegetable/Grain servings
1 Fat serving
1 Dairy serving

Lunch
2 Vegetable servings
3 Cereal/Starchy Vegetable/Grain servings
2 Legume servings
3 Fat servings

Mid-Afternoon Snack
1 Fruit serving

Dinner
3 Vegetable servings
3 Cereal/Starchy Vegetable/Grain servings
1 Legume serving
1 Fat serving
1 Fruit serving

1500 Calorie Omnivore Diet For Vata Types

Category 1: Fruits	3 servings/day
Category 2: Vegetables	6 servings/day
Category 3: Cereals, Starchy Vegetables, Grains	3 servings/day
Category 4: Legumes	1 serving/day
Category 5: Fats	2 servings/day
Category 6: Dairy	1 serving/day
Category 7: Meats, Cheese, Fish, and Eggs	2 servings/day

Carbohydrate calories:	66%
Fat calories:	18%
Protein calories:	16%
Total Protein content:	76 g
Dietary fiber content:	28-75 g

Recommended Meal Design

Breakfast
1 Fruit serving
2 Cereal/Starchy Vegetable/Grain servings
1 Fat serving
1 Dairy serving

Lunch
3 Vegetable servings
2 Meat/Cheese/Fish/Egg servings
1 Fat serving

Mid-Afternoon Snack
1 Fruit serving

Dinner
3 Vegetable servings
1 Cereal/Starchy Vegetable/Grain serving
1 Legume serving
1 Fruit serving

2000 Calorie Lacto-Vegetarian Diet For Vata Types

Category 1: Fruits	3 servings/day
Category 2: Vegetables	6 servings/day
Category 3: Cereals, Starchy Vegetables, Grains	10 servings/day
Category 4: Legumes	4 servings/day
Category 5: Fats	4 servings/day
Category 6: Dairy	1 serving/day
Category 7: Meats, Cheese, Fish, and Eggs	–

Carbohydrate calories:	70%
Fat calories:	16%
Protein calories:	14%
Total Protein content:	61 g
Dietary fiber content:	33-68 g

Recommended Meal Design

Breakfast
2 Fruit servings
2 Cereal/Starchy Vegetable/Grain servings
1 Fat serving
1 Dairy serving

Lunch
3 Vegetable servings
5 Cereal/Starchy Vegetable/Grain servings
2 Legume servings
2 Fat servings

Mid-Afternoon Snack
1 Fruit serving

Dinner
3 Vegetable servings
3 Cereal/Starchy Vegetable/Grain servings
2 Legume servings
1 Fat serving

2000 Calorie Omnivore Diet For Vata Types

Category 1: Fruits	3 servings/day
Category 2: Vegetables	5 servings/day
Category 3: Cereals, Starchy Vegetables, Grains	6 servings/day
Category 4: Legumes	2 servings/day
Category 5: Fats	5 servings/day
Category 6: Dairy	1 serving/day
Category 7: Meats, Cheese, Fish, and Eggs	2 servings/day

Carbohydrate calories:	64%
Fat calories:	17%
Protein calories:	19%
Total Protein content:	79 g
Dietary fiber content:	22-82 g

Recommended Meal Design

Breakfast
1 Fruit serving
2 Cereal/Starchy Vegetable/Grain servings
1 Fat serving
1 Dairy serving

Lunch
2 Vegetable servings
2 Cereal/Starchy Vegetable/Grain servings
2 Fat servings
2 Meat/Cheese/Fish/Egg servings

Mid-Afternoon Snack
1 Fruit serving

Dinner
3 Vegetable servings
2 Cereal/Starchy Vegetable/Grain servings
2 Legume servings
2 Fat servings
1 Fruit serving

2500 Calorie Lacto-Vegetarian Diet For Kapha Types

Category 1: Fruits	5 servings/day
Category 2: Vegetables	8 servings/day
Category 3: Cereals, Starchy Vegetables, Grains	12 servings/day
Category 4: Legumes	4 servings/day
Category 5: Fats	5 servings/day
Category 6: Dairy	2 servings/day
Category 7: Meats, Cheese, Fish, and Eggs	–

Carbohydrate calories:	69%
Fat calories:	15%
Protein calories:	16%
Total Protein content:	91 g
Dietary fiber content:	35-102 g

Recommended Meal Design

Breakfast
2 Fruit servings
2 Cereal/Starchy Vegetable/Grain servings
1 Fat serving
1 Dairy serving

Lunch
4 Vegetable servings
6 Cereal/Starchy Vegetable/Grain servings
2 Legume servings
2 Fat servings
1 Dairy serving

Mid-Afternoon Snack
1 Fruit serving

Dinner
4 Vegetable servings
4 Cereal/Starchy Vegetable/Grain servings
2 Legume servings
2 Fat servings
2 Fruit servings

2500 Calorie Omnivore Diet For Kapha Types

Category 1: Fruits	3 servings/day
Category 2: Vegetables	7 servings/day
Category 3: Cereals, Starchy Vegetables, Grains	10 servings/day
Category 4: Legumes	2 servings/day
Category 5: Fats	7 servings/day
Category 6: Dairy	2 servings/day
Category 7: Meats, Cheese, Fish, and Eggs	3 servings/day

Carbohydrate calories:	63%
Fat calories:	18%
Protein calories:	19%
Total Protein content:	96 g
Dietary fiber content:	42-108 g

Recommended Meal Design

Breakfast
1 Fruit serving
2 Cereal/Starchy Vegetable/Grain servings
1 Fat serving
1 Dairy serving

Lunch
4 Vegetable servings
4 Cereal/Starchy Vegetable/Grain servings
3 Meat/Cheese/Fish/Egg servings
3 Fat servings
1 Dairy serving

Mid-Afternoon Snack
1 Fruit serving

Dinner
3 Vegetable servings
4 Cereal/Starchy Vegetable/Grain servings
2 Legume servings
3 Fat servings
1 Fruit serving

Herbal Supplements For Vata-Type Individuals

In addition to assisting with a generalized detoxification process throughout the body, the Sattva Vata Herbal Formulation is geared toward specifically up-regulating the cleansing processes in the large intestine, bladder and nervous tissues. These are all areas where Vata dosha tends to accumulate.

This formulation will support cleansing of the body's tissues and help up-regulate fat catabolism for people of all Ayurvedic Constitutional Types. For your convenience, here again is the **Sattva Basic Formulation**:

Guggulu (standardized to 2.5% guggulsterones) . . . . . . 125 mg. (1 part)
Citraka . . . . 500 mg. (4 parts)
Punarnava (standardized to 25% alkaloids) . . . . 125 mg. (1 part)
Garcinia (standardized to 10% hydroxycitric acid) . . . . 125 mg. (1 part)
Triphala powder . . . . 500 mg. (4 parts)
Ginger . . . . 250 mg. (2 parts)
Cayenne Pepper . . . . 250 mg. (2 parts)
Black Pepper . . . . 250 mg. (2 parts)

Vata-type individuals should add the following herbal components to the Basic Formulation:

Agnimantha	500 mg. (4 parts)
Vidanga	125 mg. (1 part)
Turmeric	125 mg. (1 part)
Garlic	250 mg. (2 parts)
Cinnamon	125 mg. (1 part)
Ginger	250 mg. (2 parts)

Mix all ingredients very well in a bowl and use the mixture to fill "00" veggie caps. Vata individuals should start by taking one "00" veggie cap twice a day before breakfast and dinner for the first week. If well-tolerated, you can increase to three times a day before breakfast, lunch and dinner.

It is safe to continue taking this herbal formulation for up to one year. However, every six to eight weeks it is recommended to stop the herbs for approximately one week. Then resume as before.

Here is some information about these additional herbs:

Agnimantha consists of the roots of a large shrub, *Premna integrefolia* Linn., which is found throughout India, Sri Lanka, and parts of southeast Asia. Decoction of the root was traditionally used for joint pains, poor digestion, constipation, neurological disease and inflammation. As its name indicates (*agni*, fire; *manthah*, rubbing), the stems were believed to be used to make sacrificial fires by rubbing them together. Today the herb is valued for its stomachic and carminative actions.

Vidanga is a medicinal herb that consists of the berries of a common shrub, *Embelia ribes* Burm. F., which grows throughout India and southern Asia. It is renowned as an anthelminthic (helps to expel worms!) in larger doses and as a skin purifier. It is part of many Ayurvedic formulations for ridding the body of toxins and improving digestion. It also is effective for many diseases that are caused by a combination of *Vata* and *Kapha* doshas.

Turmeric (*haridra*, in Sanskrit) consists of the bright yellow rhizomes of *Curcuma longa* Linn., found throughout India and in many parts of the world. In classical Ayurvedic medicine, turmeric is still used as a blood purifier, anti-parasitic, and as an anti-inflammatory in rheumatic diseases, as well as externally to treat certain forms of skin infections, eczema and insect bites. Recently, the component responsible for the rhizome's yellow coloration, curcumin, was isolated and is receiving a lot of attention as an effective anti-inflammatory in joint disease. It is given with coriander in this formulation also to increase the assimilation of the other herbs.

Garlic (*rasona*, *lasuna* in Sanskrit). The cloves of this perennial herb *Allium sativum*, Linn., has been used for centuries in the treatment of *vatavyadi*, or generalized *Vata* diseases. It is particularly useful in alleviating nervous disorders, lung congestion, abdominal bloating, hypercholesterolemia, and diminished digestive function. Externally it is often used to treat bacterial skin infections and ear infections.

Cinnamon (*twak*, in Sanskrit). Cinnamon consists of the inner bark of *Cinnamomum zeylanicum*, Breyn., found throughout India. The powdered bark is antispasmodic, antiseptic, mildly stimulating, carminative, and helpful in general digestive functions. In ancient times it was also used to improve the voice, alleviate cough, and treat headache.

Ginger (*ardraka*, in Sanskrit). Ginger is common to many parts of the world as the pungent-tasting rhizomes of the perennial herb *Zingiber officinale* Rosc.. Ginger root is highly valued in dyspepsia, gastritis, intestinal gas, indigestion, cough, motion sickness, and asthma. It is, however, used much more widely as a condiment than as a medicine. Even as a condiment it helps all varieties of non-specific digestive afflictions. It helps to assimilate other herbs and is excellent for *Vata-Kapha* disorders.

Exercise

As previously explained in the section on the general principles of the Sattva Program, an exercise program, like any other health-promoting activity or substance, is only effective when it suits the specific needs of the individual. Exercise that is done properly always creates vitality and energy; it does not destroy it. Regular exercise is not only important for the Sattva Program and weight loss, but is an essential component for maintaining optimal function of the human organism. It is an imperative initial step to be implemented in any health promotion strategy.

Vata individuals benefit most from exercises that balance, and do not tend to aggravate, the air element. Exercise must not cause exhaustion, negative attitudes, or mental agitation. This will include exercises that do not involve being suspended in the air for long periods of time or moving with excessive speed. For example, forms of exercise that would not be appropriate on a daily basis for Vata individuals are: trampoline, jumping rope, stationary bicycle or sprinting. Vata-friendly exercise regimens can include these exercises occasionally but not everyday. Rather, exercises that emphasize slow, gentle, coordinated movements should be performed.

It is common for Vata individuals to become very enthusiastic and over-zealous about their exercise regimen in the beginning, but too soon become distracted, lose interest and quit. They often expect too much, too soon, and become disappointed in themselves, their doctors, and their weight loss program when results are not immediate. Vata people, therefore, must invest some quiet time to reflect realistically about their condition and understand, *before* beginning an exercise program, the regularity and commitment which is required for optimum results. Vata people usually have ups and downs during their weight loss program, which is a reflection of their fluctuating mental energies. Regular physical exercise of an appropriate nature can help Vata individuals ground themselves and achieve a satisfied, peaceful state of mind. Vata individuals should take on only one or two forms of exercise and become very consistent with it. A simple and straightforward weight loss regimen will bring comfort and stability to the Vata mind and allow them to accomplish their goal.

Examples of healthy exercise for Vata individuals include:

Aerobics, low-impact	Horseback Riding
Archery	Ice skating (indoors)
Badminton	Judo
Baseball	Sailing
Bicycle (leisurely)	Step-training
Bowling	Swimming
Dancing	Tai Chi
Golf	Table tennis
Gymnastics	Walking
Hiking	Yoga

If you happen to be a bi-doshic (two doshic) type, for the purposes of exercise, refer to your overall physique to determine your type. If you normally have a light, thin frame, musculature which is not very thick, very little padding around the joints and over the hands and feet, and skin which is dry, consider yourself a Vata type for matters of exercise.

Vata individuals will benefit most from the forms of exercise listed above. In addition, as we have said elsewhere throughout this book, remember that *walking is the best form of exercise for all types*. Vata individuals benefit more from a gentle style of walking which is sustained for thirty to forty minutes, once a day. Like Pitta individuals, Vata types should also definitely drink water during every period of exercise that exceeds thirty minutes. The key to an exercise program for Vata types is that they approach themselves with calm determination and self love; they need to stop *thinking* about exercise and immediately begin to do it.

Pranayama For Vata Individuals

Pranayama connotes control of the breath. If performed consistently on a daily basis and with proper technique, pranayama can bring perfect balance to the nervous system, which results in a calm and perceptive mind. In what is considered the most authoritative of ancient texts on yoga practices, the *Hathayoga Pradipika*, this point is made somewhat more forcefully:

CHAPTER 12. RECOMMENDATIONS FOR SPECIFIC CONSTITUTIONAL TYPES

Performed well, pranayama destroys all disease.

Hathayoga Pradipika II,16

There is no question that the practice of breath control cultivates a calm, poised quality of mind. My own studies have shown that Vata individuals in particular who practice pranayama achieve a slower, fuller, steadier pulse. In other writings of ancient India we are told that breath control leads to the body becoming stronger and more flexible, a glowing complexion, and protection from anxiety and depression.

Prāṇa is a word with multiple meanings. This one word denotes "breath" and "air"; it also is the word for "life force". *Yāma* also has at least two interesting meanings. Commonly it is translated as "control or regulation", however, it also means "to expand and deepen". Thus, *prāṇāyāma* has a rich multi-layered significance. It describes a practice in which one learns to progressively expand and deepen the breathing. The pause between each breath is observed and controlled. Furthermore, the word hints that regular practice will help remove the impurities and obstructions covering the Life Force within, and allow it to shine forth in our thoughts, words and actions.

The Vata Pranayama Technique: Mridu Pranayama

This technique is a modification of the Deep Breathing Technique described on page 211, which is suggested for everyone of all Constitutional Types as a four to six week preliminary breathing exercise.

The word *mridu* means "gentle, showing compassion, soft". We will describe the technique in two parts: inhalation and exhalation. The inhalation technique is similar to the one utilized in the Deep Breathing Technique, with one variation: the inspiration is divided into two parts; the inspiration is interrupted at the half-way point by a four second pause.

Inhalation

1. Sit in a balanced, upright posture in a chair with a straight back. Feet should be flat on the floor about shoulder width apart; remove the shoes and socks. Place hands on the lap, palms up. Mouth should be closed. All breathing is through the nostrils.

2. Exhale whatever air is in the lungs.

3. Take a normal, slow, gentle inhalation filling the lungs *only half way*. This is a subjective measure that you will know precisely as you practice this technique for a few days. When you have reached what feels to be the half-way point in the inspiration, hold the breath there for four seconds.

(Count to yourself 1...2...3...4)

4. Then continue the inhalation until the lungs are full. At this point, again hold the breath there for four seconds, before exhaling as described below.

(Count to yourself 1...2...3...4)

Observe the following during inhalation:

a) the initial movement is that of the abdomen expanding slightly.
b) the chest expands next starting in its lower and middle zones.
c) do not constrict the throat in any way or make any sound during inhalation.
d) the sternum (breast bone) moves out away from the spine during the second part of the inhalation
e) do not strain to fill the lungs; the inhalation will stop naturally at the precise lung volume that is required. Observe this as it happens.
f) at the end of inhalation, a brief interval of no air movement occurs. Observe this for a moment and then begin the count of four.

Exhalation

4. Exhale slowly and gently while counting to *eight*.

This requires precise attention to the rate of exhalation. With a little practice it is easily mastered.

a) do not force the exhalation or use extra effort or undue haste.

b) relax the abdominal muscles as you exhale.

c) do not allow the head and chest to slouch forward during exhalation.

d) at the end of exhalation, a brief period of no air movement occurs. Observe this without in any way interfering or prolonging it. Let it be as long as it naturally needs to be before beginning the next inhalation.

5. This completes one cycle. At the end of exhalation, begin the next inspiration.

It is recommended to complete 8 cycles per session. Perform this exercise twice a day, morning and evening. It requires approximately two minutes to complete each session. After one month, you can increase the practice to 16 cycles per session.

This practice is especially recommended for those who experience anxiety, tremors, fears, restlessness, fatigue and lack of will power.

One brief note regarding retention of the breath. Although as described here it is a very safe and healthy practice, I ask that you do not extend the periods of retention for more than four seconds. Longer periods of retention are indeed utilized in Ayurveda, but require the individualized attention of an experienced prānāyāma master.

Remember too that your prānāyāma practice is a spiritual practice. Through inhalation one absorbs the universal Life Force (*prānā* = Life Force); during retention one creates a merging and union between the Individual Self and the Universal Self; and during exhalation one releases the hold on the separate ego structure and surrenders the Individual Self to the Universal Self.

Massage Oils For Vata Types

Vata individuals have a tendency to accumulate both nervous tension and muscular tension, the hallmarks of Vata excess, which can create muscular pain and fatigue. Chronic Vata excess often leads to a spread of painful sensations throughout the body, including the back of the neck, shoulders and lower back. These Vata-related tensions can also interfere with the efficient, innate elimination of metabolic wastes from the tissues. If not addressed, this can lead to a chronic syndrome of stress, which is usually poorly characterized and quite baffling to those seeking a western name for these symptoms.

One of the most effective ways to prevent or treat Vata imbalances (excesses) is with a regular regimen of self massage with an appropriate Vata-pacifying herbalized massage oil. Of all the Ayurvedic constitutional types, individuals with pure or partial Vata natures benefit the most from oil massage.

Vata massage oils should always be applied to the body after they have been warmed to at least the temperature of the blood or slightly warmer (99-105 degrees Fahrenheit). Besides being physically warmed before use, Vata oils should also be inherently warming oils. These oils should also be calming, have a pleasant, slightly sweet aroma, be somewhat viscous or thick, promote muscular relaxation, and have a sedative effect upon the nervous system.

Fortunately, Nature has provided us with several oils that have these characteristics. In fact, most oils—more than 70%—found in Nature are Vata-pacifying. What's more, almost any oil can be given Vata-reducing qualities by combining it with appropriate herbal materials. The oils listed below can be used individually or combined in any way. If you do combine two or more oils, it is best to use only one of the traditional oils in your formula. These are only the most common and available oils used; there are many others.

Vata Massage Oils

TRADITIONAL OILS	MODERN OILS
Narayana taila	Sesame
Mahnarayana taila	Castor bean
Dhanvantara taila	Almond
Ksheerbala taila	Jojoba
Nirgundi taila	Wheat germ
Bala taila	Apricot kernel

Individuals of Vata constitutions benefit from a gentle, rhythmic, soothing massage technique. When using the self massage technique known as *abhyanga*, the oil should be at body temperature or slightly warmer. The strokes should be long and slow—at a rate that is *less than* your pulse rate. The average pulse rate is approximately 72 beats per minute, which means the strokes should be slower than one stroke per second. A good place to start is to make each stroke (one cycle of "up and down") about two seconds long. Remember this is only a guideline to get you started. The best rate is the one that you intuitively adopt from your understanding of the term "slow speed".

Vata individuals also benefit from a massage technique that includes attention to the ears, fingers and toes. Be sure to devote time to these areas. Also, the head massage should be performed without exception once or twice per week.

Aromatherapy for Vata Types

As we have discussed earlier, the use of aromatic essential oils found in various plants is a time-honored aspect of Ayurveda. In Ayurveda we regard a plant's oil to contain its rasa, or essence, and that it is the vehicle which delivers the plant's life energy to human beings.

The physiological effect of aromas is understood to be mediated by the limbic lobe of the brain, which coordinates emotions associated with past experiences, instincts and mood. The limbic lobe also affects the respiratory rate, heart rate, memory, blood pressure and possibly hormonal secretions. We now know that even in concentrations that are too small to be consciously perceived, certain aromas can alter the electrical and neurochemical activity of the brain as well as produce mental and emotional changes in some individuals. This points to an effect of aromas that is subtler than the physical realm. According to Ayurveda, specific essential oils will benefit the various constitutional types.

Here are the essential oils that are used in Ayurveda to pacify Vata dosha:

Essential Oils Recommended for Pacifying Vata Dosha

Lavender	Ylang ylang
Geranium	Tulsi
Juniper	Myrrh
Patchouli	Vetivert
Mandarin	Bergamot
Vanilla	Spruce
Chamomile	Melissa
Lemon	Sandalwood
Neroli	Orange

To begin, try one or more of these Vata-pacifying combinations:

1. Lavender, Geranium, Vanilla

2. Mandarin, Lemon, Ylang ylang

3. Melissa, Bergamot, Vetivert

4. Juniper, Lavender, Patchouli

Continue to experiment with different combinations and quantities of these essential oils. You will undoubtedly discover your own unique blends.

Fasting Techniques For Vata Individuals

As I have described in previous discussions throughout this book, fasting is an overlooked, yet extremely effective and inexpensive way to increase the efficacy of therapy for a vast range of conditions, including obesity, arthritis, inflammatory diseases, hypertension, allergies, depression, and many other chronic degenerative conditions. It can and should be utilized, in addition, by healthy people who are seeking to optimize their overall physical, emotional and spiritual state of health.

However, there are certain *absolute* contraindications to fasting. Individuals who suffer from any of these conditions should not fast under any circumstances. These conditions include:

Diabetes	Epilepsy
Pregnancy	Renal Disease
Tuberculosis	Seizure Disorder
Anorexia/Bulimia	Lactation
Cancer	Severe Asthma
HIV Disease	Ulcerative Colitis
Anemia	Hemophilia

In addition, there are also *relative* contraindications to fasting. Individuals who have any of these conditions may fast under the guidance of a physician, nutritionist, nurse, or other licensed health-care provider. These conditions include:

Headache
Parasitic infections
Vertigo
Chronic Hepatitis

Included under this category of *relative* contraindications to fasting are individuals with pure or strongly Vata constitutions. Vata individuals can do a monthly fast using one of the following techniques, but should obtain consent from their physician first.

The reason for this seemingly extreme caution is based on past experience. Vata individuals, more than Pitta or Kapha types, will experience dizziness, insomnia, fatigue, hypotension, muscle aches, and even visual disturbances and cardiac arrhythmia's during even short fasts. Not all Vata-types will experience any of these negative effects, perhaps 15-20%. Some of these effects may be explained by the fact that during the first three days of fasting, significant water loss may occur. This can be significant even after only twenty-four hours. Vata people are less tolerant of this fluid shift and are therefore more prone to the symptoms listed above.

Properly supervised, however, Vata people can fast once a month with fruit juices, vegetable juices, and herbal teas.

Vegetable Juice Fasts

The following vegetable juice formulation works very well for Vata individuals. It is also excellent for Pitta (without the ginger) and Kapha types.

```
Carrot . . . . . . . . . . . . . . . . . . . . . . 33%
Celery      ⎫
Parsley     ⎪
Watercress  ⎬  . . . . . . . . . . . . 66%
Beet root   ⎪
Beet greens ⎪
Ginger Root ⎭
```

An alternative to the above juice is the elimination of the watercress and beet greens and the addition of zucchini.

Fruit Juice Fasts

Although fruit juices contain larger quantities of natural sugars and are therefore not generally as effective as vegetable juices for weight management, Vata types seem to do very well with them.

Vata Fruit Juice Fast #1

```
Grapefruit juice . . . . . . . . 4 oz.
Lemon juice . . . . . . . . . . 2 oz.
Strawberry . . . . . . . . . . . 1/2 cup, sliced
Water . . . . . . . . . . . . . . 2 oz.
```

Combine all ingredients and blend for 30-45-seconds.

Vata Fruit Juice Fast #2

```
Papaya juice . . . . . . . . . . 2 oz.
Pineapple juice . . . . . . . . 2 oz.
Lime juice . . . . . . . . . . . 2 oz.
Water . . . . . . . . . . . . . . 2 oz.
```

Combine all ingredients and blend for 30-45-seconds.

Vata Fruit Juice Fast #3

```
Honeydew melon . . . . . . . cup, cubed
Strawberry . . . . . . . . . . . 1/2 cup
Lime juice . . . . . . . . . . . 2 oz.
Water . . . . . . . . . . . . . . 3 oz.
```

Juice the honeydew and the strawberries. Add other ingredients and blend for 30-45 seconds.

Teas *(also see "Making Teas" on page 220)*

Herbal teas consisting of ingredients that have warming, calming, alkalinizing and hydrating qualities will be effective in detoxifying and balancing Vata individuals. There are many Ayurvedic herbal tea formulae that are known to promote gentle detoxification and are specifically good for weight loss programs.

One formula is the Vata Tea available through The National Institute of Ayurvedic Medicine which contains: Vidari (*Pueraria tuberosa*), Tamalpatra (*Curculigo orchiodes*) Bilva (*Aegle marmelos*), Cardamom, Cinnamon, Ginger, Pippali (*Piper longum*), and others.

Other excellent fasting teas for Vata types are

1) Two parts Ashwagandha (*Withania somnifera*), two parts cumin seed (*Cuminum cyminum*), one part freshly grated ginger root, one-half part cinnamon powder.

2) Two parts saunf (*Foeniculum vulgare*), one part coriander seed (*Coriandrum sativum*), one part sariva (*Hemidesmus indicus*), one part amalaki (*Emblica officinalis*).

3) Two parts fresh grated ginger root, one part cardamom and cinnamon, one-half part clove and nutmeg. Boil briefly in one cup of soy milk, strain and serve.

Vata Behavioral Therapies

Just as for Pitta and Kapha type individuals, there are various habits and behaviors that will lead to an excessive accumulation and excitation of Vata dosha especially in Vata types and are best avoided. Similarly other behaviors will tend to balance and nurture the unpredictable and changeable Vata nature.

Behaviors to be Avoided by Vata Types

- Excessive running, jumping, pedaling and other forms of fast-paced exercise created by the desire to lose weight
- Not obtaining sufficient sleep
- Staying up late at night
- Performing work after dinner that causes mental or physical strain
- Watching too much television or videos
- Spending excessive time on the telephone or in front of a computer
- Excessive travel, especially by airplane
- Excessive consumption of raw vegetables and fruits or green leafy vegetables
- Insufficient periods of quiet, contemplation and meditation
- Too much contact with friends and acquaintances
- Excessively emotional events one after another

- Lack of emotional support from family members
- Lack of physical contact
- Lack of a regular routine

Behaviors to be Encouraged by Vata Types

- Regular gentle and warm touch using warm oils such as sesame, almond or jojoba
- Tranquil colors used in clothing and the environment: deep blue, orange, red, green, purple, magenta and yellow
- Rhythmic, soft, and slow music including classical music, Indian ragas, and chants
- Warm, nourishing foods abounding in the sweet, sour and salty tastes
- Calming aromas such as lavender, neroli, bergamot, geranium and orange
- Gentle exercise: walking, yoga, tai chi, etc. (See Vata Exercise section)
- Moderate use of saunas, steam baths and hot tubs (if available)
- Defusing unwarranted fears and anxieties
- Cultivate quiet, peace, and self-love
- Regular meditation, both morning and evening

Chapter 13.

Seasonal Routines: Ritucharya

*I*n addition to making dietary and lifestyle recommendations according to your Ayurvedic Constitutional Type, *The Sattva Program* also considers another factor for encouraging weight loss and maintaining balance: *ritucharya*. Ritucharya means "the teaching of the seasons", and it encompasses all of the slight modifications one should make in their usual regimen with each season. A benefit of the ritucharya recommendations is that it brings some variety to your Constitution-based regimen and keeps you involved and alert to the energetic changes occurring around you as the year proceeds.

It is important to remember that your Constitution-based regimen is the main regimen to follow in *The Sattva Program*. Ritucharya simply provides some minor, yet important, variations you can make every few months.

Before looking at what Ayurveda advises for these seasonal variations it is important to understand something about the seasons themselves and their different energetic qualities.

The table below shows the classical Ayurvedic (Hindu) seasons and their Western equivalents. It also tells us which dosha dominates each season.

The Hindu and Western Seasons			
Hindu Season	Western Season	Corresponding Months	Dominant Dosha
Sisira	Late winter	January, February	Vata
Varsa	Rainy season	March, April	Kapha
Vasanta	Spring	April, May	Kapha
Grisma	Summer	June, July, August	Pitta
Sarad	Autumn	Sept., Oct., Nov.	Vata
Hemanta	Early winter	December	Vata

As you can see, the ancient Indians observed that the year could be divided up into six seasons. These seasons are very similar to the Western season to which we are accustomed with the addition of a "rainy season" and the division of winter into early and late. There is one important point to know about the rainy season. In India, as in other parts of the world, there is a *monsoon season*. This is literally a rainy season when it rains almost every single day, sometimes in huge amounts, for four to six weeks! In much of India, this season occurs during July and August. Although here in the West we do not have too many regions where the rainy season is quite so intense, we do generally have an increased amount of rainfall during March and April in most areas. Remember that the exact timings of the seasons may vary according to where you live. What truly determines the rhythm of the seasons in each part of the world is its proximity to the equator and its location in either the Northern or Southern hemisphere.

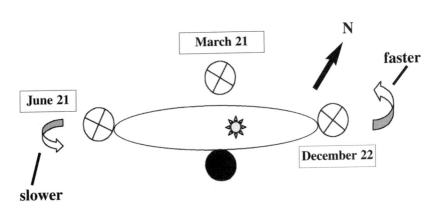

The above diagram illustrates how gravity holds the earth in a slightly elliptical orbit around the sun. Gravitational force depends on the mass of each body and the distance between them. As the earth moves closest to the sun—around December 22—gravitational force from the sun increases and the earth actually orbits faster (represented by the larger arrow). When the earth is farthest from the sun—around June 21—this force diminishes and the earth's orbit slows down.

The earth is closest to the sun in late December and early January and is also moving at its greatest velocity. This is in keeping with the fact that this is Vata season, which features quickness and movement. In the Northern Hemisphere, December, January and February correspond to the Winter season, which is shorter in duration than summer due to the earth's greater velocity. Similarly, the earth is farthest away from the sun in late June and early July and is moving relatively more slowly. This means that, in the Northern Hemisphere, summer season is longer.

What is interesting to observe is that it is not the absolute distance from the sun that determines the hot or cold seasons. Rather it is the *tilt* of the earth towards or away from the sun that determines this. Perhaps you can recall learning in grade school that the earth is tilted *23.5 degrees* from the perpendicular of its orbital plane. This is shown in the diagram below:

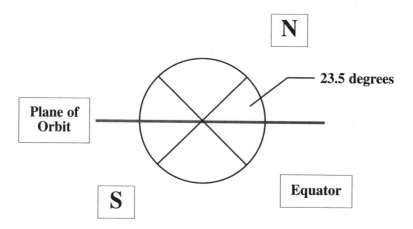

The earth's tilt causes the Northern Hemisphere to be closer to the sun than the Southern Hemisphere for half of the year, and the Southern hemisphere to be closer to the sun than the Northern Hemisphere for the other half of the year. The hemisphere that is tilted *toward* the sun receives more of the sun's rays and receives them more directly than the hemisphere tilted *away* from the sun. The hemisphere tilted toward the sun will be warmer and have the longest days. Thus when it is Pitta season (summer) in the Northern Hemisphere, this hemisphere is tilted toward the sun; at this time the Southern Hemisphere is tilted away from the sun and is experiencing Vata season (winter). If the earth's axis were not tilted, not only would each day and night everywhere on earth always be 12 hours long, there would be no seasons! By the way this does indeed occur twice every year on about March 21 and September 22 when both hemispheres are the same distance from the sun. When this occurs it is known as an *equinox;* the one which occurs in March is known as the *vernal equinox* and marks the start of Spring and the one in September heralds the beginning of Autumn and is called the *autumnal equinox.* On the equinoxes the sun is directly over the equator making day and night of equal lengths.

Now that we have some insight into the physical basis of the seasons, lets examine what Ayurveda says we should do differently during each of these periods.

Conduct in the Autumn Season

Fall is a time to assist the body and mind in eliminating excess Pitta dosha that may have accumulated over the hot summer months. The following modifications in your regimen are recommended.

- Small amounts of rice, barley, and wheat can be added to the diet. Otherwise, continue to follow your Constitution-based diet.
- Filtered water, clean and pure, should be taken both warm and cool at times.
- Avoid excessive sunbathing at this time of year.
- Avoid daytime sleep.
- Do not expose yourself to early frost or winds, especially coming from the north or east.
- Take time to be in Nature, especially in forests, near lakes, and in the rays of the moon.
- Place autumnal flowers in the home.
- Panchakarma therapies are recommended for purification; this should include massage with sandalwood oil, virechana (laxative) therapy, and alterative (blood-purifying) therapies.

Conduct in the Winter Season (both Early and Late)

Winter is dominated by Vata dosha. The atmosphere is cool and dry, the earth tilts away from the sun whose rays are weak, and cold wind and snow characterize the weather. Therefore, no matter what your Constitutional Type, everyone should make a few changes to protect against Vata dosha and its cold, windy, rough, agitating qualities.

- Include in the diet some foods with the sweet, sour and salty tastes (see Vata Pacifying Diet). Remember that if you are not a Vata Type, your Constitution-based diet is still the diet to follow with only a few Vata-reducing items added occasionally.
- Almost all food should now be warm or hot.
- Limit your intake of raw foods to 20% of your total diet.
- Do not consume cold water or beverages during Winter.
- Sipping hot water throughout the day is *highly* recommended.
- Increase the frequency of your oil massage to at least 3-4 times a week, if not everyday. Be sure the massage oil is nice and warm.
- Use sufficient warm and thick blankets to cover your body when you sleep.
- Winter is a time for enjoying frequent sexual activity, if appropriate.
- Exercise indoors whenever possible.

Conduct in the Spring Season

Spring is a time for renewal and new growth. Winds recede, the earth begins to lean toward the sun, and the atmosphere begins once again to warm. With Spring comes an increase in Kapha dosha which, when present in balanced proportion, supports the growth and rejuvenation of all living beings. However, when it accumulates excessively as it tends to do in the Spring it disturbs digestive functions, creates heaviness, obstructs the channels of the body, and causes weight gain. This is easily avoided if you do a few simple things to "defuse" the rise in Kapha to excessive proportions. Many of these recommendations are probably familiar to many of you.

- This is one of the most important times of the year to consider attending a residential Panchakarma detoxification retreat or at least have these therapies on an outpatient basis with an Ayurvedic physician. Even a short period (3-4 days) of therapies can be profoundly detoxifying.

- Avoid or greatly reduce heavy, oily, dense foods.
- Avoid or greatly reduce sweet foods and beverages, which will all aggravate Kapha.
- Add vegetable soups to your diet; use vegetables from the Kapha-reducing diet.
- Increase the amount of exercise that you do, especially in the beginning of the Spring season.
- Increase the intensity of your self-oil massage; use faster and more vigorous strokes.
- Include *Garshana* massage in your daily routine (see page 93).
- Avoid all daytime sleep.
- Come out of Winter hibernation, be more active, sing, dance, move, and even travel if your schedule permits.
- Whatever you do, whatever your constitution, it is wise to take as many measures as possible to not aggravate Kapha dosha during the Spring.

Conduct in the Summer Season

During the Summer, the hot sun tends to evaporate the moisture from the earth as well as from all organic life forms. Therefore, Ayurveda prescribes somewhat unctuous and moist foods and cool, hydrating beverages. As you can see from the list below, over-exposure to the sun and insufficient water intake are the two main conditions to avoid. Also, we are reminded that Summer is the season of *Vata Sanchaya*, accumulation of Vata dosha, which should be addressed as well.

- Avoid over-exposure to the sun, especially between the hours of 12 noon to 4 pm.
- Consciously make an effort to drink sufficient water.
- Skim milk (1%) and lassi can be included in the diet in moderation.
- Bath or shower in cool water once or twice a day, if possible.
- Only mild forms of exercise should be undertaken during the summer.
- Self oil massage should be performed less frequently with cooling, light oils such as coconut, sandalwood, sunflower, guduchyadi, or manjisthadi taila.

- Avoid excessively spicy foods.
- During the daytime try to be in a cool environment as much as possible.
- At night, if possible, sleep in an open area of the home that is naturally cool.
- A short daytime nap is permitted.

Conduct in the Rainy Season

Although the Rainy Season in most parts of the world does not rival the monsoons which arrive every year in India, Africa, and other areas, it is still wise to make the following variations in your regimen at this time. The main observation is that the digestive power—*agni*—tends to become weakened at this time and requires support. It can also be a time when Vata becomes aggravated.

- Eat primarily pungent, bitter, and astringent foods that are well cooked.
- Use generous amounts of spices to season your food.
- It is wise to be particularly careful not to overeat at any meal during this season.
- Try boiling your hot water; boiling is said to change the energetic quality and make it lighter and more kinetic.
- Exercise moderately.
- Perform regular self oil massage.
- Ginger root, garlic, and asafoetida are useful additions to the diet to maintain agni.

How the Seasons Affect the Doshas

As you now know, each of the three doshas tends to dominate in specific seasons throughout the year. Vata is most excessive in Autumn and Early Winter; Pitta is most excessive in the Summer, and Kapha in the Spring and Rainy Season. However, that is not the end of the story.

As you will recall, in Chapter 5 we described the Six Stages of Disease. We explained that all diseases, including obesity and overweight, proceed along distinct steps. The earlier we recognize that an imbalance has started and take measures to intervene and reestablish homeostasis, the easier and more completely we can expect to cure the condition.

The first three stages of any disease are easiest to treat:

Stage 1.   Accumulation
Stage 2.   Aggravation
Stage 3a.   Spread
Stage 3b.   Remission

Notice that after a disease process passes Stage 2 (Aggravation), it may proceed down one of two paths. It may further intensify and reach Stage 3a. where it will begin to spread throughout the physiology, or it may recede due to appropriate treatment or due to natural spontaneous remission. Remember that the human mind-body is capable of correcting a great number of imbalances and moving, even if unassisted, towards balance and healing. One of the reasons for this natural healing ability is that the doshas will naturally tend to recede during certain seasons, as long as the accumulation and aggravation has not been extreme. Also, be aware that the actual accumulation of excess doshas begins in a very subtle way earlier than you might realize. For example, there is accumulation of Pitta dosha during the rainy season (April/May); at this time the earth is just beginning to tilt toward the sun and to heat up. Then there is aggravation of Pitta during the summer season (June-August). In Autumn, there can be a natural remission of any aggravated Pitta dosha as long as the aggravation hasn't been too severe. If the degree of aggravation is too much, without supportive therapies the disease process will not recede and will begin instead to spread.

Here is a chart to remind you what effect the seasons are having on the doshas:

Effects of the Seasons on the Doshas

	Late Winter	Spring	Rainy Season	Summer	Autumn	Early Winter
Vata	Remission	Accumulation	Aggravation	Aggravation		
Pitta			Accumulation		Aggravation	Remission
Kapha	Accumulation	Aggravation	Aggravation	Remission		

CHAPTER 14.

THE BENEFITS OF A HEALTHY WHOLE FOODS VEGETARIAN DIET

As we enter the twenty-first century, food is finally beginning to be acknowledged in Western medical circles as an important facet of health and healing. Ayurvedic physicians have always known the importance of an appropriate diet. As more and more Westerners become conscious of what foods they choose to eat and begin to ask themselves about the nature of different food articles, they will require accurate and reliable information.

Certainly, if you have read this far into this book you realize that using foods to reduce weight or heal any condition is not haphazard. Foods have qualities and activities in the physiology just as herbs or medicines do—only usually less potent and radical. Used correctly, food is the solid foundation for all other treatments. It may take time to see the effects of dietary therapy, but when the effects occur they are widespread and affect all the tissues, organs, and systems of the body. This fact is emphasized in the *Charaka Samhita* where the author proclaims:

The entire body is born out of the food juice and all the diseases too are produced from unwholesome diet.

The modern American who is transitioning to a healthier way of eating soon encounters an avalanche of conflicting data regarding the necessity or harmfulness of eating meats and other flesh foods. Distilled down to their essence, the case for meat consumption is based on certain perceived dietary requirements while the case against meat consumption cite both the toxicity and ethical distaste for killing another sentient being.

Perhaps the best way to approach the issue is to ask the simple question: What is the purpose of eating? To most of us the answer will seem obvious: Eating provides energy for our daily physical and mental activities. Our activities, in turn, are determined by when, how, and where our individual karma moves us, in order that we may serve our life purpose. Our movements, in turn, consume energy—which is provided by our foods. Thus food enables us to fulfill our karmic roles and to evolve into more complete beings.

Scientifically speaking, all food articles contain potential biochemical energy, which are transformed in our bodies into forms that can be utilized by our cells. Modern science would point to glucose, fatty acids, amino acids, as well as literally hundreds of specific substances needed to create and maintain our vital organs and tissues. Ayurvedic medicine understands that all materials in creation derive from the same five elements. In both cases, we must be sure to consume a wide variety of foods to ensure that we obtain the right proportion of nutrients and elements for our unique constitution.

The Tamasic Quality of Flesh Foods

Within seconds of the slaughter of an animal, its flesh begins to deteriorate and putrefy. This decay proceeds as a rapid process even in an intact animal. However, once the flesh is butchered and separated from the animal this decay is additionally fostered by the growth of microorganisms (bacteria, fungi, and viruses) on its surface. By the time most flesh foods reach the supermarket, it has been dead for days and well into the decay process. To address this problem and mask its manifestations, chemical preservatives are added (to control the bacterial growth) and dyes are applied (to restore the red color which within hours naturally oxidizes to a less appetizing light brown).

Flesh food is dead food. Its *prana* ("vital energy") leaves it at the instant of death, and the inert material left behind (muscle, fat, and blood) is devoid of life-supporting energy. All dead food becomes *tamasic*: heavy, dull, stagnant, obstructing and destructive. Conversely, fresh vegetables and fruits retain their *prana* longer and can efficiently preserve and transfer their living energies to the human organism for longer periods of time. The seeds from all foods are a testament to this living energy; given water and a little warmth they will germinate and grow. Organic vegetables and fruits without chemical preservatives will keep their vital taste, smell, and appearance for several days; meat, poultry, and fish will continue to rapidly decay and become putrid in a matter of hours. In addition, meats remain in the gastrointestinal tract for a longer time than any other type of food, approximately *twenty-four hours.* This allows the already decaying, toxin-laden meat to further ferment and release unhealthy substances into the body.

When I was a student in Ayurvedic medical school we were asked to learn about the physiological effects of different foods in a brilliant way. This did not involve studying from textbooks or reviewing laboratory experiments. Instead we were asked to exclusively eat one single food over the course of one week and to make notes on how we felt. Each student would choose a food article (rice, cucumber, potato, orange, almond, etc.); some even chose the same food. After one week we would report on what we had observed. We understood that, normally, one should not live on any single food for an extended period of time; certainly this would result in a profound nutritional deficiency. The purpose of this exercise was to experience the physical, psychological, and subtle energetic effects of each food in our own bodies. Some foods have surprisingly potent effects on the elimination functions, heart rate, sleep patterns, breathing, emotions, mood and energetic status. Those of us who chose to perform this exercise with meat (chicken, lamb, or beef) found that its effects were profound. We felt heavy, lazy, unmotivated, physically strong, somewhat angry and impatient. We slept deeper, were constipated, congested, had an increase in mucous production, our breathe was more shallow, we were difficult to awaken in the morning, less romantic, resistant to exercise, and we consumed less water and other fluids on a daily basis.

Medical science has long recognized that meat consumption increases specific toxins in humans. Patients suffering from chronic renal failure as well as other kidney diseases are always told to drastically reduce, if not completely eliminate, meat from the diet. This is important because the kidneys have lost their capacity to filter out a toxin known as *uric acid.* Uric acid is contained in meat in large quantities. We know that if the uric acid level from flesh foods increases too much, lethargy, coma, and even death can occur. The same substance, uric acid, is responsible for causing gout and several other metabolic conditions.

In addition to uric acid, meat also poisons us with other toxic chemicals. Bile acids have been extensively studied for their cancer-causing effects in the colon. They were identified as likely carcinogenic substances because of their striking structural similarity to polycyclic aromatic hydrocarbons—known carcinogens. We now know that the concentration of bile acids is increased in the large intestines of people who eat beef in their diet. This higher quantity of bile acids causes the intestinal bacteria of meat-eaters to produce larger amounts of *7-alpha-dehydrolase*, which converts the bile acids into even more carcinogenic forms. Vegetarians from Africa and India have been found to have less of these bile acids and conversion enzymes in their intestines than in similar groups of carnivorous North Americans and Western Europeans.

Cooking meats presents still other problems and can generate a vast array of documented carcinogens. If during charcoal grilling, fat drippings are vaporized by the hot coals, benzo[a]pyrene forms. This potent carcinogen is then absorbed by the cooking meat. Cooking meat is also known to produce other carcinogens known as *heterocyclic-amines,* which cause mutations in human cells and in bacteria. They form easily when cooking meats of all types, especially when using high temperatures. Generally, cooking at lower temperatures results in the formation of less harmful substances. An exhaustive discussion of this subject is beyond our scope here, and is meant only to make you aware of the naturally occurring carcinogens in flesh foods. According to recent studies, our exposure to "natural" food-based carcinogens exceeds that of artificial ones by a factor of 10,000.

Women who suffer from uterine fibroids may want to re-assess the quantity of beef and other red meat that they consume. Uterine fibroids, or myomas, are benign tumors which can lead to infertility, recurrent miscarriages, uterine pressure and pain, uterine bleeding, urinary frequency as well as anemia. Approximately 20% of American women are diagnosed with this condition; the condition is more prevalent among African American women and less prevalent among women of Asian descent.

A recent Italian study examined the diets of over 1500 women without fibroid tumors and compared them to another group of 800 women with the condition. The study revealed that women who reported more frequent consumption of beef and other red meats and less frequent consumption of fruits, vegetables, and fish had a higher incidence of fibroid tumors. Conversely, women consuming less red meat and more plant-based and marine foods had a lower incidence of these tumors. The women who consumed the most meat had a seventy percent higher risk for fibroid tumors than the women who consumed the most vegetables. Because high estrogen levels are known to promote the growth of fibroids, it is likely that the estrogens contained in meats may play a role in the increased incidence in meat consumers. (*Obstetrics and Gynecology*, September, 1999).

Consider the emotional responses in an animal that occur during the process of transporting it to the slaughter house. From its familiar surroundings on the farm where it has spent its entire life, it is suddenly dragged into a dark, crowded truck or train where it will remain for hours and hours. It will be frightened further by the sudden turns and stops, strange sounds, bumps on the roads, and relentless vibrations. At the slaughter house, electric prods are used to herd the terrified animals through a confusing series of rooms, stalls, and baths. The smell of blood and sounds of the other terrified animals is everywhere.

Physiologically, animals experience fear and panic in response to extremely threatening situations much like humans do. Fear begins in the brain and through a complex series of neurohormonal events, reaches every fiber and cell of the body. Once fear is felt, the hypothalamus in the brain releases chemicals which in turn cause a flood of catecholamines (adrenaline and nor-epinephrine) and hormones to pour into the body of the animal. These create many effects that are summarized as follows:

First of all, the heart rate and blood pressure of the animal increases acutely; nostrils flare and the eyes dilate and tear reflexively. The adrenal glands pour out cortisol, which quickly causes the breakdown of proteins and a consequent increase of the waste product urea. Cortisol also causes the release of the stimulant angiotensinogen. Acidic gastric juices are released in large amounts in the stomach. Mast cells release histamine into the tissues and lactate levels soar in the muscles. Stool and urine are often spontaneously released in response to the terror.

Every fiber of the animal's body is filled with these chemicals and waste products, which are retained in the flesh after the butchering process. Regular consumption of these meats will increase the level of these substances in the human physiology, where they create similar effects. Thus the body of a meat consumer is often chronically fatigued and painful and the mind anxious, tense and confused. Unfortunately, advances in transportation, refrigeration, and chemical preservation have made meat more available than ever before. Before the era of refrigeration and transportation, flesh was primarily obtained from very local sources, where animals were sacrificed right on the farm. Today, in the affluent nations of the West, meat consumption has increased dramatically from a century ago. It is interesting that during this same period of time we have witnessed an equally dramatic increase in certain forms of cancer, irritable bowel, ulcers, and other gastrointestinal syndromes, anxiety, depression and heart disease.

A Vital Choice

Nature has evolved various species of animals that are carnivorous—they prey on other animals (which are almost exclusively herbivores) for their nourishment. Scientists understand that carnivores play an important role in the food chain of the world, because the herbivores that are killed are primarily the weak, sick, very old or very young. Thus these predators ensure the survival of only the fittest and strongest members of each species. Whereas carnivorous animals have no choice in their diet, mankind can rationally decide what he will and will not eat. Humans can and do survive extremely well without killing animals and eating their flesh. The fact that many millions of people do not consume meat is a testament to this fact. If experience and now science tell us that we not only can survive without eating meat, but that we can live healthier and longer lives, why then should any of us be meat-eaters? In Ayurveda, we acknowledge the divinity of all creatures and see no need or purpose in killing our fellow animals for our food.

In the case of plant foods, the fruit, vegetable, bean, or grain represents the final end-product of a natural process of growth that is designed for consumption by animals. In many cases, the plant itself is not harmed. In every case plants are recognized as appropriate foods for mankind at two times: either at the end of their natural reproductive cycle or at the end of their life-cycle. To harvest wheat at the end of the summer or to pick an apple from a tree in the autumn is among the most natural of human actions, for these foods are taken when fully formed, ripened, and at the end of their life-cycle. The plants produce fruits and vegetables which have interesting shapes, attractive colors, and delightful aromas, which beckon and attract us. Plants, too, benefit from the consumption of their ripened parts, which initiates another reproductive cycle and helps continue their species. The apple seeds eaten by an animal is activated but not completely digested in the digestive system and passes out with the feces. The feces, rich in nitrogen and other elements, becomes an early source of nutrition for the growth of these seeds. Thus we see a perfect harmony and mutually beneficial biological relationship between plants and the animals which consume them.

Specific Dietary Concerns

Despite the irrefutable health benefits of a vegetarian, whole-foods-based diet it is important to monitor your dietary pattern for a sufficient amount of several specific nutrients. When initially changing over from an omnivore (meat and vegetable eating) diet to one that is plant based, food intake can become haphazard, may lack variety at first, or be short on certain nutrients.

Protein

Over the past three decades, with the popularization of vegetarianism in the West, there has been an emphasis on the requirement for inclusion in the diet of so-called "complete protein". This means consuming a large enough variety of plant foods to ensure sufficient intake of all the necessary amino acids. This idea immediately made planning a vegetarian-based diet rather complicated and inconvenient and certainly turned off many people who were interested but intimidated. As a medical concept, the notion of "complete protein" is valid. However, in everyday common practice, planning out how to include individual amino acids and proteins is unnecessary. The body has the ability to constantly maintain an adequate supply of both essential and non-essential amino acids to accommodate the normal production and utilization of proteins even when a specific meal contains incomplete or no protein.

Iron

Iron-deficiency is not as common in the United States and Europe as it once was but it still does occur, especially in women and children. Legumes, most vegetables, and whole grains contain significant amounts of iron. In addition, seaweeds including dulse, wakame, and kelp are excellent sources of both iron and iodine. For vegetarians, foods that contain vitamin C are important because they will help to increase iron absorption. These vitamin C abundant foods include citrus fruits, tomatoes, cabbage, bell peppers, broccoli, sprouts, parsley, rose hip tea, and nearly all other vegetables and fruits. Be aware that excessive amounts of oxalates in the diet (i.e. spinach) can sometimes decrease iron absorption.

Vitamin D

Because Ayurveda recommends including some dairy products in the diet, vitamin D deficiency is rarely a problem. However, for people who avoid *all* dairy and animal products this can be problematic. All individuals should ensure that they get proper sunshine, which converts inactive to active vitamin D in the skin. Adequate sunshine exposure means approximately 20-25% of the skin exposed for thirty minutes daily at sea level. In the cold weather, most people expose only their face and hands; for your information this is equivalent to only 5% of the skin surface. If you work inside during the daylight, make sure you spend time outside on the weekends to compensate. If you live in a chronically cloudy area, the sunlight still reaches you but you require about double exposure. Of course, avoid excessive sunbathing and midday exposure whenever possible.

Vitamin B12

Vitamin B12 is necessary for red blood cell formation, normal growth and repair of tissues, fertility, pregnancy, immune competence and nerve function. Deficiency can result in weakness, fatigue, diarrhea, depression, numbness, palpitations, anorexia, shortness of breath, personality changes, and, if extreme, pernicious anemia—a condition of decreased red blood cell production.

Vitamin B12 can be depleted from the body by a number of factors that we should all guard against:

- Antibiotics
- Birth control pills
- Alcohol, tobacco, caffeine
- Excessive stress
- Chronic liver disease
- Stomach surgery
- Bacterial overgrowth in the colon

Plant sources of vitamin B12 include Brewer's yeast, fermented foods (like miso, tofu, tempeh, pickles, sauerkraut, sourdough breads, and nut yogurts), and algaes (like spirulina, chlorella, and blue-green algae). Eggs and cheeses also have small amounts of B12. The recommended daily requirement for vitamin B12 in both men and women of all ages is 2 mcg per day.

Zinc

This trace mineral is another important nutrient that unfortunately is found most abundantly in animal foods, although it does exist in plants as well. Deficiency can lead to cognitive (thought process) problems, prostate enlargement, fatigue, and abnormal blood formation. Exceptional plant sources of zinc are nuts—especially Brazil nuts—whole grains, tofu, wheat germ, and many legumes.

The most complete nutrient base is achieved when a plant-based, whole foods diet is allowed to include small amounts of dairy and eggs. The Sattvic Diets allow for flesh foods in small amounts if you are accustomed to eating these articles. The recommended daily requirement for zinc in both men and women of all ages is 12 mg per day for women and 15 mg per day for men.

Chapter 15.

Sattvic Recipes

A properly planned *Sattvic* meal will include food articles from many different categories all served at the same time. It is usually composed of the following elements:

1) a main dish, or *entrée*; this will consist of vegetables with legumes or grains

2) a second vegetable side dish; this will generally be a steamed or stir-fried simple preparation

3) a *dal* dish, a puree of lentils which ensures protein is included in the meal and adds moisture as well.

4) a raw vegetable salad

5) a yogurt salad, or *raita*, to provide a cooling, soothing sensation to the mouth and provide protein.

6) rice or another grain

7) chutneys, pickles, or relish, to provide sweetness, tartness, and pungent tastes.

The rationale behind this multi-faceted meal composition is to provide the body with the perfect balance of protein, carbohydrate, fats, minerals, vitamins, and trace elements so that they can merge, interact, and be assimilated by the tissues in the most nourishing way. If meat were to be part of the meal, it would serve as the main dish. Remember to keep the serving of meats, poultries or fish to a minimum.

As a child I was not brought up as a strict vegetarian, although I ate very little meat, usually at school. I truly did not miss it at all because the vegetarian meals we had at home were always delicious and very satisfying. I remember always feeling very happy and light after one of my mother's home-cooked meals and give much of the credit for my current excellent health (and normal weight) to the vegetarian-based meals of my early years.

Today, I am a practicing vegetarian and have learned to appreciate and prepare food according to the Brahmin tradition. The recipes that follow in this chapter are certainly not all strictly Indian affairs. They all do, however, adhere to the principles of sattvic cooking which not only makes them healthy, light and refreshing but gives them all a hint of fun and more than a little flavor and texture.

These recipes are included here because they are some of my favorites. This section is not intended to be an entire cookbook, but rather a way to get you to explore ways to use the Sattvic Food lists found in Chapter 12. It is my fervent hope that the recipes found here will stimulate you to add to the scope of your diet and teach you how Sattvic eating can be as sumptuous and satisfying as any style of cuisine you have ever known.

For each recipe in this section we have indicated its effect on the three doshas: ↑ indicates increase, ↓ indicates decrease, and **0** indicates a neutral effect.

Spices

Almost everyone knows that Indian food is famous for its spicy flavors and fragrant aromas. These tastes and smells are of course the creation of mixtures of spices and culinary herbs that are combined in specific proportions and added to the cooking process at various stages. Spices and herbs are the very foundation of Ayurveda and have many intriguing medical benefits. They are composed of organic materials that are often best used after some degree of processing before being added to foods (crushing, grinding, roasting, etc.). Volumes of knowledge about the medicinal value of herbs and spices are taught in Ayurvedic schools. The table below will at least give you some idea of the properties of some of the more commonly used spices in the *Sattva Program*.

TABLE 17.
SPICES AND CONDIMENTS

English Name	Indian Name	Whole/ Powder	Heating/ Cooling	Digestant/ Stimulant	Doshic Effect	
Aniseed	Variyala	W	H	D	-V, K	+P
Asafoetida	Hing/Hingra	P	H	D, S	-V, K	+P
Black Pepper	Maricha	W, P	H	D	-V, K	+P
Caraway	Jira	W	H	D, S	-V, K	+P
Cardamom	Elachi/Ela	W, P	H	D	-V, K	+P
Chili	Mirichi	W, P	H	D, S	-V, K	+P
Cinnamon	Twak/Dalchini	W, P	H	D	-V, K	+P
Clove	Lavanga	W	H	D, S	-V	+P
Coriander	Dhania	W, P	H	D, S	-P, K	
Cumin	Jeera	W, P	H	D, S	-VPK	
Dill seed	Sava	W	H	D	-V, K	+P
Fennel seed	Saunf	W	C	D	-V, K	+P
Fenugreek	Methi	W	H	D	-V, K	+P
Garlic	Rasona/Lasan	W ,P	H	D	-V, K	+P
Lovage	Ajowan	W	H	S	-V, K	+P
Mace	Javantari	W, P	H	D, S	-K	+P
Mustard seed	Rai	W	H	D	-V, K	+P
Nutmeg	Jaiphal	P	H	D	-VPK	
Onion seed	Kala jeera	W	C	D	-P	
Poppy seed	Afim	W			-V	+K
Saffron	Kesar/Kumkuma	W	H	D	-VPK	
Sesame seed	Til	W	H	D	-V, P	+K
Star anise	Badiyan	W, P	C	D, S	-VPK	
Turmeric	Haldi/Haridra	P	H		-VK	

Garam Masala

Garam masala is a wonderful aromatic blend of several dry-roasted and ground warming spices. Throughout India, most households have their favorite blends—some with only three or four ingredients and some with a dozen or more. Although the principal effect of *garam masala* is to generate internal digestive fire, in Ayurveda we have slightly different recipes for Vata, Pitta and Kapha constitutions.

Garam masala is easy and fun to make and imparts an exuberant touch to many recipes. Even if you are only dabbling in Ayurvedic cooking, experimenting with this spice blend is well worth the effort.

The procedure is the same for each recipe. All you will need is a heavy-bottomed pan or cookie sheet, an electric coffee grinder or spice grinder, and a fine meshed sieve. Before grinding to a powder, whole spice seeds are dry-roasted to release their flavors and lengthen shelf life.

To dry-roast spices on the stove, keep the heat low and stir every 4-5 minutes for about 15 minutes. Or you can place the spices in a pre-heated oven (200 degrees Fahrenheit) for 25-30 minutes. Also note that you will have to crush the cinnamon sticks into small pieces with a rolling pin or mallet before grinding and you will have to remove the cardamom seeds from their green pods as well. Grind small amounts of the roasted spices at a time until they are powdered; pass them through the sieve and mix well with the already powdered ingredients. Store away from heat and light in glass jars labeled with the date. Shelf life is about 6-9 months. Remember, the recipes given here are a guideline only—feel free to experiment.

Vata Garam Masala

2 dried whole chili pods
1/4 cup whole cloves
three 3-inch cinnamon sticks
20 cardamom pods
3/4 cup coriander seeds
1/2 cup cumin seeds
1/2 cup black mustard seeds
1/4 cup ginger powder
1/4 cup fennel seeds
1/4 cup black peppercorns
1/4 cup garlic powder
2 tablespoons ground nutmeg

Pitta Garam Masala

1 cup coriander seeds
3/4 cup cumin seeds
3/4 cup sesame seeds
1/2 cup fennel seeds
1/4 cup star anise
1/4 cup poppy seeds
1/4 cup grated coconut
1/4 cup ground nutmeg
1/4 cup turmeric
1 teaspoon saffron
10 cardamom pods

Kapha Garam Masala

3-4 dried whole chili pods
1 1/2 cups coriander seeds
1 cup mustard seeds
3/4 cup cumin seeds
3/4 cup black peppercorns
3/4 cup garlic powder
five 3-inch cinnamon sticks
1/2 cup ginger powder
1/2 cup turmeric
1/3 cup caraway seeds
1/3 cup whole cloves
1/4 cup fenugreek seeds
35 cardamom pods
8 bay leaves

Vegetables

Long before the advent of agriculture and the appearance of the earliest farms about 10,000 years ago, humans lived in wandering groups and obtained their food by hunting, fishing, and gathering plants from nature. No one is certain why at some point in the evolution of human civilization some of these nomadic tribes started to settle in one place; nor is it clear exactly how they learned to plant crops from seeds.

Vegetables have become a supremely important feature of the Ayurvedic diet, especially for those who wish to lose weight. Almost all of the vegetables used in Sattvic diets will be familiar to you and therefore need no introduction. Vegetables are always best when cooked soon after harvesting. This is now more possible in much of the United States than it ever was before due to the increasing number of farmer's markets that are springing up throughout the nation. Even in the midst of urban New York City, Chicago, Los Angeles, Detroit, Dallas, and almost every city I have recently visited, I have seen markets teeming with fresh produce of all varieties.

VEGETABLE CURRY I　　　　　　　　　*Serves 4*

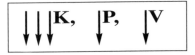

STEP 1	STEP 2
2 tablespoons ghee	1 cup chopped cauliflower
1 tablespoon minced fresh ginger	3/4 cup peeled and cubed
1/2 teaspoon black pepper	eggplant
1 teaspoon cumin seeds	3/4 cup finely cut string beans
1/2 teaspoon coriander seeds	3/4 cup peas
3/4 teaspoon brown mustard seeds	1 medium zucchini, cubed
1 large or 2 medium tomatoes, chopped	1 cup winter squash, cubed
	1 teaspoon turmeric
	1/2 cup water
	2 tablespoons fresh, chopped
	cilantro

STEP 1. Heat the ghee in a non-stick pot or wok. Add the ginger, cumin, black pepper and mustard seeds and sauté over low heat until the mustard seeds "jump", about 2 minutes. Add the tomato and cook for 3-4 minutes, stirring often.

STEP 2. Add the vegetables, turmeric and water. Bring to a boil. Cover, reduce heat and simmer 25-30 minutes until vegetables are tender. Add the cilantro during the last minute.

PER SERVING:	200 CALORIES
NUTRITIONAL INFORMATION	
Carbohydrate. . . . . 20 g	
Protein .. . . 8 g	
Fat . . . . 4 g	
Cholesterol. . . . . 0 mg	
Sat. Fat. . . . . 2 g	
Mono. Fat. 1.5g	

VARANASI VEGETABLE STIR-FRY   *Serves 4*

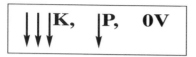

STEP 1	STEP 2
6 tablespoons vegetable broth (or water)	1/2 cup button mushrooms
1 carrot	1/2 cup bamboo shoots
1 small red bell pepper	1/2 cup snow peas
1 cup broccoli rosettes	1 bunch cilantro
3/4 cup baby corn ears	4 oz. diced tofu
3/4 cup Chinese cabbage (Napa)	black pepper
1/4 inch fresh ginger	salt
2 cloves garlic	
1/2 teaspoon mustard seeds	
1 tablespoon sesame oil	
1 dried chili pepper, crumbled	

STEP 1. Wash and trim all the vegetables. Cut the carrot, pepper, bamboo shoots, and cabbage into strips. Peel the broccoli stems, divide into smallest possible rosettes, and cut into small pieces. Halve the corn ears lengthwise, quarter the button mushrooms, and string the snow peas. Then peel the garlic and ginger and chop. Wash the cilantro and coarsely chop.

Heat the wok for five minutes and then add the sesame oil, garlic, ginger, mustard seeds, and chili pepper, stirring constantly. Then add the carrot, broccoli and corn and stir-fry over high heat for 2-3 minutes.

STEP 2. Reduce the heat to medium, add the button mushrooms, bell pepper, snow peas and bamboo shoots and cook an additional 2-3 minutes, stirring constantly, until all the vegetable are tender-crisp. Add the cilantro and tofu in the last 1-2 minutes. Season with pepper and a pinch of salt.

PER SERVING:	200 CALORIES
NUTRITIONAL INFORMATION	
Carbohydrate................20 g	
Protein ....8 g	
Fat ....4 g	
Cholesterol. ....0 mg	
Sat. Fat..................2 g	
Mono. Fat. 1.5g	

Eggplant in Mustard Yogurt Sauce   *Serves 4*

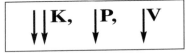

STEP 1	STEP 2
2 medium eggplants	1 tablespoon ghee
1/2 teaspoon salt	1 tablespoon mustard oil
1 teaspoon mustard seeds	1 teaspoon fresh grated ginger
1 teaspoon cumin seeds	3 dried red chili's, crumbled
1 tablespoon ghee	1/2 teaspoon turmeric
	1 teaspoon paprika
	1/4 teaspoon cayenne pepper
	2/3 cup plain low fat yogurt
	2 tablespoons cilantro leaves

STEP 1. Peel the eggplant and cut into 1/4" thick strips. Sprinkle with salt and let stand for 10 minutes. Meanwhile, dry roast the mustard seeds and cumin seeds in a pan or wok until they begin to "jump". Remove and set aside in a dish. Using paper towels, press the liquid out of the eggplant and pat dry. Heat the ghee in the wok or pan and cook the eggplant strips on both sides until golden brown. Drain on paper towels; discard any leftover oil.

STEP 2. Heat the mustard oil in the wok (pan) with the ginger and chili's. Stir in the remaining spices, stirring constantly. Add the yogurt and 4 ounces of water. Bring to a boil and simmer for 5 minutes. Grind the roasted mustard and cumin seeds finely and stir in. Add the eggplant strips and allow to braise, covered, for 5 minutes. Sprinkle with cilantro before serving.

PER SERVING:	220 CALORIES
NUTRITIONAL INFORMATION	
Carbohydrate. . . . . 20 g	
Protein . . . . 4 g	
Fat . . . . 10 g	
Cholesterol. . . . . 20 mg	
Sat. Fat . . . . 2 g	
Mono. Fat. 6.5g	

SEASONED SPINACH WITH SLICED POTATOES   *Serves 8*

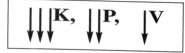

STEP 1	STEP 2
4 medium unpeeled potatoes boiled until almost tender	1 pound fresh spinach washed and coarsely chopped
1/2 teaspoon turmeric	1/3 pound each of: collard greens mustard greens, kale
1/2 teaspoon garam masala	
1/2 teaspoon ground cumin seeds	8 lime wedges
1/4 teaspoon paprika	pinch of salt
1 1/2 teaspoons ground coriander	
1 1/2 tablespoons lemon juice	
3 tablespoons water	
3 tablespoons ghee	

STEP 1. Peel the boiled potatoes and julienne into slices 1/3" wide and thick and 1 1/2" long. In a small pot or cup mix the *garam masala*, turmeric, cumin, paprika, coriander, lemon juice and water. Then heat the ghee in a non-stick wok or pan over high heat. Add the potatoes, turning until golden brown. Remove and set aside.

STEP 2. Reduce the heat to low and add the spice blend; cook until the liquid has evaporated. Stir in the greens, add the salt, cover, and cook for approximately 10 minutes. You can add a sprinkle of water during the cooking if the leaves appear dry. Add the potatoes, folding them into the greens. Cover, and cook an additional 5 minutes. Accompany each serving with a lime wedge.

PER SERVING:	134 CALORIES
NUTRITIONAL INFORMATION	
Carbohydrate.	20 g
Protein	4.5 g
Fat	5.1 g
Cholesterol..	12 mg
Sat. Fat	2 g
Mono. Fat.	2.5g

SATTVIC PASTA PRIMAVERA   *Serves 3*

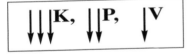

STEP 1	STEP 2
6 oz. uncooked linguini (or other pasta)	1 tablespoon grated Parmesan cheese
1 teaspoon extra virgin olive oil	fresh basil leaves, in strips
2 medium zucchini, sliced thin	
1 medium yellow squash, sliced thin	
1/2 cup mushrooms, sliced thin	
2 cloves garlic, minced	
8-10 cherry tomatoes, halved	

STEP 1. Cook the linguini or pasta in a pot according to box directions. Meanwhile, heat the olive oil in a wok or large pan. Add the zucchini, squash, mushrooms, and garlic and sauté for 5 minutes. Drain the pasta and return to its pot. Add the vegetables, mix gently, and place onto individual plates.

STEP 2. Top with grated Parmesan cheese and strips of fresh basil. Serve while hot.

PER SERVING:	126 CALORIES
NUTRITIONAL INFORMATION	
Carbohydrate. . . . . 22 g	
Protein . . . . 4 g	
Fat . . . . 2.5 g	
Cholesterol.. . . . . 0.5 mg	
Sat. Fat . . . . 0.5 g	
Mono. Fat. 1.5g	

CAULIFLOWER WITH BRAISED TOMATO   *Serves 4*

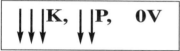

STEP 1	STEP 2
2 teaspoons ghee	3 pounds cauliflower florets
1-inch piece of fresh ginger root, thinly sliced	(2x 1x 1/2")
	1 tablespoon ground coriander
1 chopped red chili pepper	1/2 teaspoon turmeric
1/2 teaspoon black mustard seeds	pinch of salt
1 teaspoon cumin seeds	3 medium tomatoes (~3 pounds), peeled and cut into eighths
	1 teaspoon garam masala
	3 tablespoons of chopped fresh coriander

STEP 1. Heat the ghee in a large nonstick wok or sauté pan over moderately high heat. When hot, add the ginger, chili, mustard and cumin seeds. Heat until the mustard seeds pop.

STEP 2. Add the cauliflower, coriander, turmeric and salt. Stir-fry until the florets are slightly browned. Then add the tomatoes, cover and reduce to low heat. Cook 15-20 minutes, shaking the pan occasionally, until the cauliflower stalks are tender. Then uncover and stir-fry again over high heat to evaporate all the liquid. Just prior to serving add the garam masala and fresh coriander.

PER SERVING:	134 CALORIES
NUTRITIONAL INFORMATION	
Carbohydrate. . . . . 25 g	
Protein . . . . 8.5 g	
Fat . . . . 3.5 g	
Cholesterol. . . . . 6 mg	
Sat. Fat . . . . 1.5 g	
Mono. Fat. 1.4g	

CAULIFLOWER, EGGPLANT, AND POTATO KORMA   *Serves 6*

A *korma* is an old style of braising vegetables in a sauce made out of nuts. The vegetables are permitted to retain their shape and flavor during the cooking process. *Kormas* are definitely considered to be one of the most elegant dishes of Indian cooking and will usually be the main dish of the meal. The korma described here is one of my favorites and uses a coriander-fennel-cayenne sauce to create a delicious flavor.

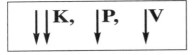

STEP 1	STEP 2
4 tablespoons canola oil	1 1/2 pounds cauliflower, stems
1 cup minced onions	removed, cut into 1 1/2 inch florets
2 teaspoons minced garlic	1 small eggplant (8 oz.), unpeeled,
2 tablespoons grated ginger	cut into 1 1/2 inch cubes
1/4 cup fresh minced coriander	2 medium potatoes (1/2 pound),
1 tablespoon ground coriander	peeled, cut into 1 1/2 inch cubes
1/4 cup ground almonds	1 1/2 cups water
1/2 teaspoon ground fennel	2 teaspoons of garam masala
1/2 teaspoon cayenne pepper	1 teaspoon toasted sesame seeds
1/4 teaspoon turmeric	salt to taste
1/2 cup canned tomato puree	
1/2 teaspoon oregano	

STEP 1. First, measure out all the spices and keep them nearby. Heat the oil in a wok or large pan over medium-high heat. Add the onion and stir until browned, about 8-10 minutes. Add the garlic and ginger and cook for 2 minutes, stirring. Add the minced coriander and almond and cook for another 2 minutes.

Now stir in the fennel, ground coriander, cayenne and turmeric. Then add the tomato puree and oregano, reduce the heat to low and cook for 2-3 minutes, stirring constantly. Do not allow to burn.

STEP 2. Add the water, cauliflower, eggplant and potatoes, increase the heat to high and bring to a boil. Lower the heat to low and simmer, covered, for 25 minutes. The cauliflower should be thoroughly cooked but not limp. Turn off the heat and stir in the garam masala. Cover and let stand for 30 minutes (important) allowing the flavors to combine. Sprinkle with sesame seeds and serve.

PER SERVING:	325 CALORIES
NUTRITIONAL INFORMATION	
Carbohydrate. . . . . 45 g	
Protein . . . . 9 g	
Fat . . . . 13 g	
Cholesterol. . . . . 0 mg	
Sat. Fat . . . . 1.5 g	
Mono. Fat. 5.2g	

BLACK BEANS AND EGGPLANT DAL
Serves 6

This hearty vegetable and bean combination which uses mustard oil and hot chilies is a specialty dish of the Himalaya foothill region. It is excellent for the Kapha and Vata doshas but can be enjoyed by those of Pitta constitution as well. It actually is a very mild preparation but can be made spicier by increasing the amounts of cayenne pepper and chilies.

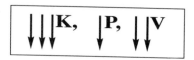

STEP 1	STEP 2
1 cup whole black gram beans	1/2 pound eggplant, unpeeled, cut into 3/4 inch cubes
3 tablespoons minced fresh ginger	1/2 pound ripe tomatoes, chopped
1 1/2 cups chopped onion	3 tablespoons mustard oil
1 chopped sweet green pepper	1 teaspoon dry mustard powder
2-4 hot chilies, minced	1 tablespoon garam masala
1/2 teaspoon cayenne pepper	1 cup chopped onions
1 1/2 teaspoons ground coriander	7 tablespoons fresh coriander, chopped
2 teaspoons marjoram	salt to taste
1/2 cup plain yogurt	
3 cups water	

STEP 1. *To soak the beans overnight:* Clean the beans well and place in a bowl. Cover beans with water by about 2 inches and let soak at least eight hours. Drain and rinse. Put the soaked beans into a large pot along with the ginger, onion, green pepper, chilies, cayenne, marjoram, coriander, yogurt, and 1 1/2 cups of the water and bring to a boil. Reduce heat to low and simmer, covered, for one hour. Add the remaining water and continue simmering for 30 minutes, or until the beans are soft.

STEP 2. Mix in the eggplant and tomatoes and cook for another 30 minutes or until the vegetables are very tender and the pot looks like a thick soupy stew. Let it continue to simmer over low heat.

Meanwhile measure out the cumin seeds, mustard powder, chopped onion and coriander and keep them nearby. Heat the mustard oil in a small pan until it smokes, then carefully add the cumin seeds and chopped onions, stirring constantly, for about 10 minutes or until they become caramel brown. Add the mustard powder and half the chopped coriander. While still sizzling, pour over the *dal.* Mix well and garnish with the remaining chopped coriander.

PER SERVING:	325 CALORIES
NUTRITIONAL INFORMATION	
Carbohydrate. . . . . .54 g	
Protein . . . . .19 g	
Fat .6.5 g	
Cholesterol. . . . . .1.3 mg	
Sat. Fat. . . . . .1.0 g	
Mono. Fat. 4.0g	

Owing to the black beans and yogurt in this dish, one serving contains approximately 235 mg of calcium, which is about 20% of the recommended daily requirement for both men and pre-menopausal women (1200 mg/day).

VEGETABLE STOCK   *1 quart*

The use of vegetable stock in place of water is an excellent way to provide extra nutrition to any soup. Equally important, stocks give interesting flavors and delicacy to any dish. Remember to use good quality vegetables to make your stock. If you use leftover peels and stems that were headed for the garbage, your stock will taste like...you get the idea. If you use truly palatable vegetables and vegetable parts, your stock will have a delicious flavor.

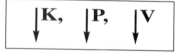

INGREDIENTS

4 1/2 cups of water	1 bell pepper (red or green)
2 carrots, sliced	1/2 cup chopped cilantro (leaves and stems)
2 stalks celery with leaves sliced	1/4 cup parsley, minced
1/2 cup peas	1 small onion, chopped

PREPARATION. Bring all the ingredients to a boil in a large pot. Cover, reduce to low heat, and simmer until the vegetables are tender, approximately 25 minutes. Strain out the vegetables and store the stock in glass jars in the refrigerator.

As a slight variation, puree a portion of the vegetables and add it back to the stock.

GRAINS

Grains are really an essential part of every meal, according to the Sattvic tradition. Grains are not only considered to be a food article, but in many cultures are symbolic of health, happiness and prosperity. Consider our own tradition of showering every newlywed couple with rice as they emerge from the marriage ceremony. Indians consume a wide variety of grains and prepare them in ingenious and delicious ways. No meal is ever considered complete from a nutritional or subjective viewpoint without grain being used in one of its innumerable forms.

CRANBERRY QUINOA   *Serves 4-6*

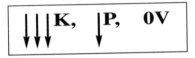

STEP 1	STEP 2
2 tablespoons olive oil	1 cup quinoa
asafoetida, pinch	2 cups water (or vegetable stock)
black pepper, pinch	salt, pinch
3/4 cup chopped fennel or celery	1/2 cup dried cranberries
	1/2 teaspoon ground cinnamon
	1/4 teaspoon cardamom seeds, crushed

STEP 1. Heat the olive oil in a saucepan. Add the asafoetida and after one minute add the fennel or celery. Sauté for 5 minutes over low heat.

STEP 2. Add the quinoa and sauté for two minutes. Add the water or vegetable stock, salt, dried cranberries, cinnamon and cardamom. Bring to a boil, cover, and simmer over low heat until the quinoa absorbs all the water and is tender, about 30 minutes.

PER SERVING:	325 CALORIES
NUTRITIONAL INFORMATION	
Carbohydrate.	20 g
Protein.	8 g
Fat.	4 g
Cholesterol.	0 mg
Sat. Fat	2 g
Mono. Fat.	1.5g

MILLET WITH HERBED TOMATOES   *Serves 4*

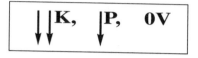

STEP 1	STEP 2
1 cup (500 g) dry millet	3 meaty vine-ripened tomatoes
pinch of salt	4 shallots
3 cups water	2 cloves garlic
	4 stalks of celery
	1 bunch parsley
	1 bunch basil
	1 tablespoon extra virgin olive oil
	1 tablespoon balsamic vinegar

STEP 1. Bring the millet, water and salt to a boil in a pot. Then cover and cook over low heat for 25 minutes.

STEP 2. Meanwhile, scald the tomatoes by placing them in a pot of boiling water for 30 seconds. Peel, remove the bases, and chop coarsely. Peel the garlic and shallots and mince finely. Clean and chop the celery. Wash the parsley and basil, discard the stems, and finely chop the leaves.

Heat the wok for 5 minutes and then add the oil, tomatoes, shallots and celery. Stir-fry for 5-7 minutes before adding the herbs and vinegar. Serve over the millet.

PER SERVING:	400 CALORIES
NUTRITIONAL INFORMATION	
Carbohydrate. . . . . .90 g	
Protein . . . . .22 g	
Fat . . . . .12 g	
Cholesterol.. . . . . .5 mg	
Sat. Fat . . . . .12 g	
Mono. Fat. 10g	

BARLEY WITH BAKED VEGETABLES　　　*Serves 6-8*

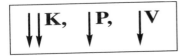

STEP 1	STEP 2
2 cups vegetable stock (or water)	turnips
3/4 cup hull-less barley	2 parsnips
1/4 tsp. salt	2 carrots
	1 tablespoon olive oil
	pinch of salt
	pinch of garam masala
	minced fresh parsley

STEP 1. Bring the vegetable stock (or water) to a boil. Add the barley, cover, and simmer over low heat until the liquid is absorbed and the barley is soft, approximately 40 minutes.

STEP 2. Preheat the oven to 400° F. Coat a baking dish with olive oil. Trim the turnips and carrots; trim and peel the parsnips. Lightly coat the vegetables with oil, place them in the baking dish, and sprinkle with salt. Cover and bake for about 35 minutes, or until tender.

Remove the vegetables from the oven, allow to cool a bit, and dice. Combine with the barley, add garam masala, and garnish with parsley.

PER SERVING:	155 CALORIES
NUTRITIONAL INFORMATION	
Carbohydrate. . . . . 30 g	
Protein . . . . 3.5 g	
Fat . . . . 2.4 g	
Cholesterol. . . . . 0 mg	
Sat. Fat . . . . 0.5 g	
Mono. Fat. 1.7g	

TRIDOSHIC PILAF WITH CHICKPEAS   *Serves 4*

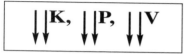

STEP 1	STEP 2
1 tsp. ghee	2/3 cup white basmati rice
1 medium onion, diced	1 tsp. garam masala*
2 cloves garlic, crushed	chickpeas, 10 oz. can
4 oz. button mushrooms, quartered	1 bay leaf
	1 1/2 cups vegetable stock
	1 tbs. toasted almonds, slivered

* add garam masala according to your Ayurvedic Constitutional Type

STEP 1. Heat the ghee in a medium-sized pan over medium heat. Add the onion, cover, and cook for three minutes, stirring once or twice. Add garlic and mushrooms and cook, uncovered, five minutes, stirring occasionally.

STEP 2. Add the garam masala and the rice and stir to combine. Add the chickpeas, bay leaf, and vegetable stock. Bring to a boil then reduce heat to very low. Cover and simmer for a minimum of twelve minutes, without lifting lid. Continue cooking if necessary until rice is tender and all the liquid has been absorbed.

Sprinkle with toasted almonds and serve.

PER SERVING:	252 CALORIES
NUTRITIONAL INFORMATION	
Carbohydrate. . . . . 45 g	
Protein . . . . 7 g	
Fat . . . . 5 g	
Cholesterol.. . . . . 3 mg	
Sat. Fat . . . . 1.0 g	
Mono. Fat. 3.7g	

VEGETARIAN LASAGNA   *Serves 6*

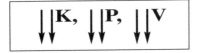

STEP 1	STEP 2
10 oz. spinach, washed	Cheese Sauce
12 lasagna sheets	
1 tablespoon grated Parmesan cheese	2 teaspoons ghee
	1 tablespoon besan flour
	1 cup skim milk
Vegetable Sauce	1/4 cup grated Parmesan cheese
	pinch of ground nutmeg
1 teaspoon virgin olive oil	1/4 teaspoon black pepper
2 medium onions, chopped	
2 teaspoons minced garlic	
6 oz. mushrooms, chopped	
1 small green pepper, chopped	
14 oz. can tomatoes, crushed	
1/2 cup tomato paste	
15 oz. can white beans, drained	

STEP 1. Lightly steam the spinach until slightly wilted; drain and set aside. *To make the Vegetable Sauce:* Heat the oil in a pan and add the onion and garlic and cook until soft, about five minutes. Add the green pepper and mushrooms and cook for three minutes, stirring occasionally. Add the tomatoes, tomato paste, and beans and bring to a boil. Simmer for 20 minutes, partially covered.

STEP 2. *To make the Cheese Sauce:* Melt the ghee in a pan and stir in the flour over one minute. Remove from heat and add the milk, stirring until smooth. Return to medium heat and stir until the sauce boils and thickens. Remove from heat and stir in the cheese, nutmeg and pepper.

STEP 3. *To Assemble:* Pour half the vegetable sauce over the base of an oven-proof dish, about 6 X 11 inches. Cover with a layer of lasagna sheets, then half the spinach. Then spread a layer of cheese sauce over the spinach. Then add the remaining vegetable sauce, followed by a layer of the remaining spinach. Cover with another layer of lasagna sheets and finish with the remaining cheese sauce. Sprinkle with Parmesan cheese.

Cover with aluminum foil and bake at 350° for about 40 minutes. Remove foil and bake an additional 30 minutes or until the top begins to brown.

PER SERVING:	330 CALORIES
NUTRITIONAL INFORMATION	
Carbohydrate.	52 g
Protein	10 g
Fat	9 g
Cholesterol..	3 mg
Sat. Fat	2.0 g
Mono. Fat.	6.7g

SALADS

Salads, as we commonly know them, or vegetable salads, as they are called in India, consist of chopped, sliced or minced vegetables. There are of course many varieties, but they all add a crunchy and cooling sensation to the palate. These salads are simple to prepare and some can be a meal in themselves. If part of a multi-item meal, they are usually eaten at the beginning of the meal as the first "course". In addition to being a wonderful counterpoint to the warmer, drier foods of a meal, salads actually provide fiber and essential vitamins and minerals which may be absent in the other foods. The fruit salads are great as complete meals on very warm evenings when a lighter meal feels right.

Main Course Greek Salad   *Serves 6-8*

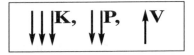

STEP 1	STEP 2
8 cups bite-size pieces of romaine lettuce	3/4 cup cucumber slices
1 cup tomato wedges	10 green bell pepper rings
1/2 cup sliced scallions	1/3 cup black olives
1/2 cup sliced radishes	1 cup crumbled feta cheese
1 tablespoon extra virgin olive oil	
1 teaspoon fresh lemon juice	
1/4 teaspoon dried oregano	

STEP 1. Combine the lettuce, tomatoes, scallions, and radishes in a large bowl and toss. In a small bowl combine the vinegar, olive oil, lemon juice, and oregano; stir and pour over the salad. Toss to mix.

STEP 2. Arrange salad on the serving plate. Top each with 1-2 green bell pepper rings, 6-8 cucumber slices, and 4-5 olives. Sprinkle about 2 tablespoons of feta cheese over each serving.

PER SERVING:	200 CALORIES
NUTRITIONAL INFORMATION	
Carbohydrate.	20 g
Protein	8 g
Fat	4 g
Cholesterol..	0 mg
Sat. Fat	2.0 g
Mono Fat.	1.5g

MAIN COURSE ANTIPASTO SALAD   *Serves 6-8*

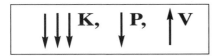

STEP 1	STEP 2
3 cups iceberg lettuce	3 tablespoons red wine vinegar
1 cup cooked chickpeas	tablespoon extra virgin olive oil
(or canned and drained)	1 clove minced garlic
1 cup sliced celery, 1" pieces	1/4 tsp. dried oregano
1 cup tomato wedges	
1/2 cup sliced red bell peppers	
1/2 cup marinated artichoke hearts	
10 green olives	
1/3 cup sliced red onions	
1/4 cup roasted red peppers	

STEP 1. In a large bowl toss the lettuce, chickpeas, celery, tomatoes, bell peppers, artichoke hearts, olives, onions and roasted peppers.

STEP 2. In a small bowl combine the vinegar, olive oil, garlic and oregano. Pour over the salad and toss to mix.

PER SERVING:	200 CALORIES
NUTRITIONAL INFORMATION	
Carbohydrate. . . . . 20 g	
Protein . . . . 8 g	
Fat . . . . 4 g	
Cholesterol.. . . . . 0 mg	
Sat. Fat . . . . 2.0 g	
Mono. Fat. 1.5g	

KAPHA-REDUCING FRUIT SALAD   *Serves 4*

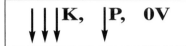

STEP 1

1 cup Apple
1 cup Pear
1 cup Strawberry
1 cup Blueberry
1 cup Grapefruit
1 cup Kiwi

STEP 1. Wash and cut the fruits and whole berries and mix together in a large bowl.

PER SERVING:	200 CALORIES
NUTRITIONAL INFORMATION	
Carbohydrate.	16 g
Protein	2 g
Fat	0 g
Cholesterol..	0 mg
Sat. Fat	0 g
Mono. Fat.	0g

PITTA-REDUCING FRUIT SALAD   *Serves 4*

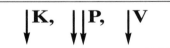

STEP 1

1 cup Apple
1 cup Red grapes
1 cup Honeydew
1 cup Cantaloupe
1 cup Sweet plums (not sour)
1 cup Pomegranate

STEP 1. Wash and cut the fruits and whole berries and mix together in a large bowl.

PER SERVING:	200 CALORIES
NUTRITIONAL INFORMATION	
Carbohydrate. . . . . 16 g	
Protein . . . . 2 g	
Fat . . . . 0 g	
Cholesterol.. . . . . 0 mg	
Sat. Fat . . . . 0 g	
Mono. Fat. 0g	

Vata-Reducing Fruit Salad   *Serves 4*

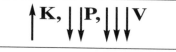

↑K, ↓↓P, ↓↓↓V

STEP 1

1 cup Peach
1 cup Cherries
1 cup Honeydew
1 cup Cantaloupe
1 cup Ripe mango
1 cup Banana

STEP 1. Wash and cut the fruits and whole berries and mix together in a large bowl.

PER SERVING:	200 CALORIES
NUTRITIONAL INFORMATION	
Carbohydrate. . . . . 16 g	
Protein . . . . 2 g	
Fat . . . . 0 g	
Cholesterol.. . . . . 0 mg	
Sat. Fat . . . . 0 g	
Mono. Fat. 0g	

LEGUMES (DAL)

This large family of plants has approximately 13,000 species, which all produce a distinct type of "bean" or pod. Legumes provide three to four times more protein than grains. More importantly, the amino acid patterns of legumes and grains complement each other so as to provide every *essential* amino acid required by human beings. Legumes are basically divided into three types: lentils, beans and peas. Beyond that, they are categorized as *split* (skin removed) or *unsplit* (skin still attached). The split varieties cook in less time, are easier to digest, and are therefore the main type of legume used in the *Sattva Program*. By the way, all legumes are known as *dals* even though *dal* also refers to a particular kind of liquid preparation.

TRADITIONAL DAL

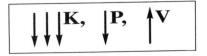

> 1 1/2 cups of:
>   yellow lentils, or
>   red lentils, or
>   yellow split peas, or
>   yellow mung dal
> 1/4 teaspoon turmeric
> 2 bay leaves
> 1 teaspoon salt
> 1/4 teaspoon asafoetida
> 1 teaspoon garam masala

Pick through the lentils, split peas, or dal removing stones and debris and then wash in several changes of cold water. Place the washed legumes in a deep pot along with the turmeric, bay leaves, salt, and asafoetida. Add 4 1/2 cups of cold water and bring to a boil, stirring occasionally. Cook partially covered for the following times:

Yellow lentils or split peas: 45 minutes
Red lentils or mung dal: 25 minutes

Then cover and continue cooking for an additional 25 minutes (15 minutes for red lentils and mung dal) or until soft.

Remove from heat and measure the volume of dal; there should be 4 1/2 cups. If less, add water to bring to that volume. If you prefer a smoother consistency, whisk the dal for 2 or 3 minutes. Mix in *garam masala* and serve. Cooked dal can be kept for three days if well-covered and refrigerated.

PER SERVING:	210 CALORIES
NUTRITIONAL INFORMATION	
Carbohydrate. . . . . 37 g	
Protein . . . . 15 g	
Fat . . . . 0 g	
Cholesterol.. . . . . 0 mg	
Sat. Fat . . . . 0 g	
Mono. Fat. 0g	

URAD DAL (WHITE GRAM BEANS)   *Serves 6*

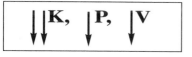

STEP 1	STEP 2
1 cup split urad dal	2 tablespoons ghee
4 green cardamom pods	1 cup chopped onion
2 bay leaves	1 teaspoon minced garlic
1/8 teaspoon turmeric	1 teaspoon grated ginger
1/8 teaspoon asafoetida	6 whole cloves
1/2 half cup skim milk	1 teaspoon garam masala
1 1/2 cups water	1/2 teaspoon black pepper
1 teaspoon salt	

STEP 1. Pick through the dal removing stones and debris and then wash in several changes of cold water. Place them in a bowl and cover with water by about two inches. Soak for three hours. Drain and put into a deep pot with the cardamom pods, bay leaves, turmeric, asafoeti-

da, milk, water and salt. Cook over low heat, partially covered, for one hour, stirring occasionally to avoid sticking. Add an additional 1/2 cup of water and cook for 20 more minutes over low heat.

STEP 2. While the beans finish cooking, in a pan heat the ghee, onion, ginger, garlic, and cloves over medium heat until the onions turn golden brown (about 10 minutes). Turn off the heat, add the *garam masala* and black pepper, and pour the contents over the dal. Stir gently to mix the ingredients and serve.

PER SERVING: 166 CALORIES
NUTRITIONAL INFORMATION
Carbohydrate. . . . . 23 g
Protein . . . . 8.5 g
Fat . . . . 4.5 g
Cholesterol. . . . . 11 mg
Sat. Fat . . . . 1.5 g
Mono. Fat. . . . . 1.5 g

YELLOW LENTILS WITH SPICED MANGO   *Serves 6*

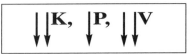

STEP 1	STEP 2
1 1/2 cups yellow lentils	1 tablespoon ghee
1/4 teaspoon turmeric	1 tablespoon safflower oil
1 medium mango, peeled	1 teaspoon cumin seeds
and sliced	1/2 teaspoon cayenne pepper
2 bay leaves	1 teaspoon garam masala
1 teaspoon salt	1/3 cup chopped fresh coriander
1/4 teaspoon asafoetida	
4 1/2 cups water	

STEP 1. Pick through the dal removing stones and debris and then wash in several changes of cold water. Place them in a bowl and cover with water by about two inches. Soak for three hours. Drain and put into a deep pot with the bay leaves, turmeric, asafoetida, water and salt.

Cook over low heat, partially covered, for 45 minutes, stirring occasionally to avoid sticking. Then cover, reduce to low heat, and cook for an additional 25 minutes.

STEP 2. While the beans finish cooking, in a pan heat the ghee over medium heat. When it is hot add the cumin seeds, which will brown in about 15 seconds. Then add the mango slices and cook, turning often, for 6-8 minutes, until soft. Reduce the heat, sprinkle the mangoes with the cayenne pepper, garam masala, and half the coriander and cook for 2-3 additional minutes. Turn off the heat, and pour the contents over the dal. Stir gently to mix the ingredients. Garnish with remaining coriander and serve.

PER SERVING:	213 CALORIES
NUTRITIONAL INFORMATION	
Carbohydrate. . . . . .36 g	
Protein . . . . .7.0 g	
Fat . . . . .4.5 g	
Cholesterol.. . . . . .7 mg	
Sat. Fat . . . . .0.5 g	
Mono. Fat. . . . . .2.5 g	

THREE BEAN COUNTRY DAL

Serves 6

↓↓K, ↑P, ↓↓V

STEP 1	STEP 2
3/4 cup split yellow mung beans	2 tablespoons ghee
1/2 cup split white gram beans	2 tablespoons sunflower oil
1/4 cup red lentils	1 teaspoon cumin seeds
1/2 teaspoon turmeric	1 teaspoon mustard seeds
1/4 teaspoon asafoetida	1/2 teaspoon paprika
1 teaspoon salt	2 medium onions, chopped
4 1/2 cups water	3 medium tomatoes, 3/4 inch wedges
	1/3 cup fresh coriander, chopped

STEP 1. Pick through the dal removing stones and debris and then wash in several changes of cold water. Place them in a bowl and cover with water by about two inches. Soak for three hours. Drain and put into a deep pot with the bay leaves, turmeric, asafoetida, water and salt. Cook over low heat, partially covered, for 45 minutes, stirring occasionally to avoid sticking. Then cover, reduce to low heat, and cook for an additional 25 minutes.

STEP 2. While the beans finish cooking, heat the ghee in a pan over medium heat. When it is hot add the onions, garlic, and ginger and cook for about 15 minutes, stirring constantly. Then increase the heat to high and add the tomatoes, stirring, until they appear slightly browned (about five minutes). Pour entire contents over the dal, mix and continue simmering.

In the same pan, which you have wiped clean, add the sunflower oil over medium heat and then the cumin seeds, which will brown in about 15 seconds. Then add the cayenne, paprika, and half the coriander and cook for 2-3 additional minutes. Turn off the heat and pour the contents over the dal. Stir gently to mix the ingredients. Garnish with remaining coriander and serve.

PER SERVING:	265 CALORIES
NUTRITIONAL INFORMATION	
Carbohydrate.	46 g
Protein	9.0 g
Fat	5.0 g
Cholesterol..	4 mg
Sat. Fat	0.5 g
Mono. Fat.	2.0 g

SOUPS

Whereas soups are often used in the West as a first course or appetizer, in the *Sattva Program* they can actually be the entire meal along with a salad, especially those that have one or more legumes as ingredients. Soups, in smaller quantities, are also used as an integral part of a multi-component meal. These soups below are all fragrant and aromatic but not too spicy.

CURRIED TOMATO LENTIL SOUP   *Serves 8*

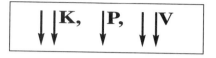

STEP 1	STEP 2
1 pound ripe Italian plum tomatoes	2 teaspoons ground coriander
3 cups cooked lentils	1/4 teaspoon cayenne pepper
1 cup water	1 tablespoon onion, minced
1 teaspoon cumin powder	1 tablespoon garlic, minced
1 tablespoon ghee	1 teaspoon salt
1 teaspoon mustard seeds	1 tablespoon lemon juice
6 curry leaves	1 tablespoon canola oil

STEP 1. Blanch the tomatoes in hot water, peel, and cut in half. Scoop out the pulp and puree in a blender. Put the cooked lentils in a deep pot, add the water and whisk for 1-2 minutes. Add the pureed tomatoes, cumin, coriander, cayenne, onion, garlic and salt and bring to a boil. Lower the heat and simmer, partially covered, for 10 minutes. Next add the lemon juice and cook for another 2 minutes. Turn off the heat and cover for a few minutes.

STEP 2. Heat the canola oil until hot and add the mustard seeds, which may spatter (be careful). When the spattering stops, add the curry leaves and turn off the heat. Stir briefly and pour contents into the soup, mixing well. Add more water if necessary to achieve a thin consistency. Serve hot.

PER SERVING:	177 CALORIES
NUTRITIONAL INFORMATION	
Carbohydrate.	25 g
Protein	10 g
Fat	5.0 g
Cholesterol.	5.0 mg
Sat. Fat	1.5 g
Mono. Fat.	2.0 g

Mung Bean Soup with Lemon Juice   *Serves 4*

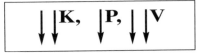

STEP 1	STEP 2
1 1/2 cups yellow split mung beans	3/4 teaspoon dill
2 hot green chilies, diced	1/2 teaspoon ground cumin
8 dry curry leaves	1/2 teaspoon black pepper
2 1/2 cups water	1 teaspoon salt
1 cucumber, peeled and sliced thin	1 tablespoon ghee
Juice of 1/2 lemon (or more)	1/2 teaspoon mustard seeds
	1/4 teaspoon asafoetida
	2 tablespoons chopped fresh coriander

STEP 1. Add the cooked mung beans, water, green chilies, cumin, pepper and curry leaves in a pot and bring to a boil. Then add the cucumber, cover and simmer over medium-low heat for 5 minutes. Turn off the heat, add the lemon juice and salt, and allow to stand covered during Step 2.

STEP 2. Heat the ghee. When hot, add the mustard seeds; cover with a lid if spattering occurs. After 1 minute add the asafoetida and mix. Add contents to the soup. Garnish with coriander and add the salt to taste.

PER SERVING:	215 CALORIES
NUTRITIONAL INFORMATION	
Carbohydrate. . . . . 33 g	
Protein . . . . 14.5 g	
Fat . . . . 2.0 g	
Cholesterol.. . . . . 4.0 mg	
Sat. Fat . . . . 0.5 g	
Mono. Fat. . . . . 1.5 g	

ZUCCHINI YOGURT SOUP   *Serves 6*

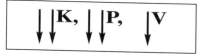

STEP 1	STEP 2
1 pound zucchini	2 teaspoons sesame oil
1/2 pound yellow squash	2 teaspoons mustard seeds
2 cups water	1 teaspoon coriander seeds
2 cups plain yogurt	1 teaspoon salt
6 hot green chilies	2 tablespoons chopped fresh coriander
2 inches fresh ginger root	

STEP 1. Wash and cut the zucchini and squash into 1/8-inch slices. Put into a 4 quart pan with 2 cups of water and bring to a boil. Lower the heat and cook, covered, for 8-10 minutes. Meanwhile, in a blender put the yogurt, chilies, ginger and salt and puree until smooth. Add this to the vegetables, cook for 5 additional minutes then turn off the heat.

STEP 2. Heat the sesame oil and, when hot, add the mustard and coriander seeds. Protect yourself from spattering with a pot lid. When the spattering stops, add the contents to the soup. Garnish with coriander and serve *cooled*.

PER SERVING:	215 CALORIES
NUTRITIONAL INFORMATION	
Carbohydrate.	33 g
Protein	14.5 g
Fat	2.0 g
Cholesterol.	4.0 mg
Sat. Fat	0.5 g
Mono. Fat.	1.5 g

CHUTNEYS

Chutney is probably derived from the Sanskrit root word *chak*, which means "to be satisfied or satiated". Chutneys are certainly prepared just for that purpose. They provide many different taste sensations—sometimes all at once—sweet, sour, bitter, pungent, salty and astringent. They are an accompaniment to a meal, which ensures that all six of the primary tastes are present which creates satisfaction in the subtle mind. Chutneys are made from fruits and spices and can be thick and chewy or smooth and velvety. They are a low-calorie, low fat way to add zest to any lunch or dinner.

TRIDOSHIC MANGO SAFFRON CHUTNEY   *Makes 12 ounces*

↓K, ↓P, ↓V

STEP 1	STEP 2
2 large mangoes (~1 1/2 pounds)	1 1/2 teaspoons cayenne pepper
1 tablespoon salt	1 teaspoon cardamom powder
1/2 cup brown sugar	1 teaspoon cumin powder
1/2 teaspoon saffron threads	2 tablespoon seedless raisins

STEP 1. Peel and coarsely grate the mangoes; you should have about 2 1/2 cups of mango shreds. Mix the shreds with the salt in a bowl and let sit for 30 minutes.

STEP 2. Combine the shreds and all the other ingredients in a pan. Bring to a boil, stirring constantly. Then reduce to low heat and cook for about 20 minutes, or until a thick syrup forms. Pour into glass jars; refrigerate after use.

PER SERVING:	52 CALORIES
NUTRITIONAL INFORMATION	
Carbohydrate.	10 g
Protein	0 g
Fat	0 g
Cholesterol.	0 mg
Sat. Fat	0 g
Mono. Fat.	0 g

CORIANDER CHUTNEY

Makes 12 ounces

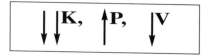

PREPARATION

1 ripe medium pineapple
2 teaspoons cumin powder
1 teaspoon fennel powder
1/4 teaspoon cinnamon powder
1/2 teaspoon cayenne pepper

3/4 teaspoon black pepper
fresh juice of 1 lemon
3/4 cup brown sugar
salt to taste (1-2 teaspoons)

Place all the ingredients in a blender (or food processor) and blend until finely pureed.

Pour into a glass jar or a bowl, cover and chill. Keeps for 4-5 days.

PER SERVING:	28 CALORIES
NUTRITIONAL INFORMATION	
Carbohydrate. . . . . 7 g	
Protein . . . . 0 g	
Fat . . . . 0 g	
Cholesterol.. . . . . 0 mg	
Sat. Fat . . . . 0 g	
Mono. Fat. . . . . 0 g	

SWEET PINEAPPLE CHUTNEY   *Makes 12 ounces*

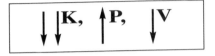

PREPARATION

2 cups packed fresh coriander leaves
  coarsely chopped
1/3 cup water
2 hot green chilies, chopped
1/4 inch piece of fresh ginger

1 teaspoon brown sugar
1 tablespoon fresh lemon juice
1/4 cup fresh mint leaves
salt to taste

Peel and core the pineapple and blend in a blender (or chop with a knife) until coarsely pureed. Put the pureed pineapple and all the other ingredients in a pan and cook over medium heat, bring to a boil. Reduce to low heat and simmer for about 30 minutes, or until a jam-like consistency is achieved. Pour into glass jar. Flavor improves over next two days. Refrigerate after use.

PER SERVING:	56 CALORIES
NUTRITIONAL INFORMATION	
Carbohydrate.	14 g
Protein	0 g
Fat	0 g
Cholesterol.	0 mg
Sat. Fat	0 g
Mono. Fat.	0 g

DESSERTS

Desserts every evening are probably not such a great idea for those trying to control their weight, however, for those times when it seems in order here are a few of my favorite recipes, which are low in fat and calories. Desserts are actually many times a way to balance the Vata and Pitta dosha, but the ones I've included here can also have a Kapha-decreasing effect—if taken in the proper measure.

BAKED APPLE CRUMBLE   *Serves 6*

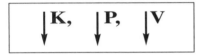

STEP 1	STEP 2
3 large Granny Smith apples, peeled, cored, and sliced	3/4 cup rolled oats
3/4 teaspoon allspice	1 1/2 ounces unprocessed oat bran
	1/3 cup brown sugar
	1 teaspoon cinnamon
	1 1/2 tablespoons ghee

STEP 1. Combine the sliced apples and allspice in a 9-inch pie dish. In a food processor or blender combine the remainder of the ingredients until crumbly.

STEP 2. Sprinkle the crumble over the apples and bake at 375° F for 30 minutes.

PER SERVING:	217 CALORIES
NUTRITIONAL INFORMATION	
Carbohydrate.	40 g
Protein	3 g
Fat	5 g
Cholesterol..	8 mg
Sat. Fat	1.5 g
Mono. Fat.	2.0 g

AROMATIC FRUIT SALAD   *Serves 4*

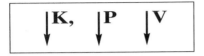

STEP 1	STEP 2
1 small ripe banana, 1/4 inch slices	1/8 teaspoon cayenne pepper
1 ripe papaya, 1 inch wedges	1/8 teaspoon mango powder
1 ripe pear, 1/2 inch slices	1/8 teaspoon asafoetida
1 orange, separated into segments	1/8 teaspoon black salt or coarse salt
1 sweet apple	1/2 teaspoon garam masala
4 lettuce leaves	1 ounce fresh lemon juice
	1 teaspoon brown sugar

STEP 1. Combine all the fruits in a bowl except for the bananas and sprinkle on all the spices, sugar, and lemon juice. Cover and refrigerate for at least an hour

STEP 2. Just prior to serving, mix in the banana slices and serve on lettuce leaves.

PER SERVING:	132 CALORIES
NUTRITIONAL INFORMATION	
Carbohydrate. . . . . 31 g	
Protein . . . . 1.3 g	
Fat . . . . 0.5 g	
Cholesterol. . . . . 0 mg	
Sat. Fat . . . . 0.1 g	
Mono. Fat. . . . . 0.1 g	

WATERMELON SHERBET   *Serves 8*

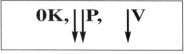

INGREDIENTS

2 quarts (64 ounces) of ripe, de-seeded, cubed watermelon
1/2 cup brown sugar
3/4 cup water
8 mint leaves

PREPARATION. Put the watermelon cubes and sugar into a large plastic bag and shake to coat the cubes. Seal the bag and freeze for 6-8 hours. Put the cubes into a blender or food processor 2-3 cups at a time. Add about 1-2 ounces of water for every 2 cups of cubes. The resulting sherbet should be pinkish and fluffy. Place in a bowl and refrigerate. Serve in parfait or wine glasses with a mint leaf.

You can also use cantaloupe, honeydew, oranges, strawberries, mangoes, papayas, or a combination of fruits.

PER SERVING:	78 CALORIES
NUTRITIONAL INFORMATION	
Carbohydrate. . . . . 19 g	
Protein . . . . .5 g	
Fat . . . . 0 g	
Cholesterol.. . . . . 0 mg	
Sat. Fat . . . . 0.1 g	
Mono. Fat. . . . . 0.1 g	

SATTVA RICE PUDDING   *Serves 12*

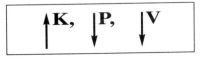

STEP 1	STEP 2
2 quarts 2% fat milk	1 tablespoon flaked coconut
1/2 cup long grain basmati rice	2 tablespoons raisins
1/8 teaspoon cardamom powder	1/2 cup brown sugar
1/8 teaspoon nutmeg	

STEP 1. Combine 1 quart of the milk and the rice in a pan and bring to a boil. Then lower the heat and cook for about 25 minutes, stirring constantly to prevent burning. After cooking, the mixture will have a somewhat creamy texture. Now add the remaining milk, cardamom and nutmeg and continue cooking for 60-75 minutes until the milk thickens to a pudding consistency. Stir often to prevent sticking and burning.

STEP 2. During the final 10 minutes add the coconut flakes and sugar. Allow to cool, then refrigerate and serve with a few raisins on top.

PER SERVING:	140 CALORIES
NUTRITIONAL INFORMATION	
Carbohydrate.............. 21.5 g	
Protein .... 6.0 g	
Fat .... 3.0 g	
Cholesterol.. .... 12.2 mg	
Sat. Fat .... 2.1 g	
Mono. Fat. .... 1.0 g	

CHAPTER 16.

PANCHAKARMA THERAPY

As the life of an individual unfolds, the body encounters many stresses and undergoes innumerable changes as it continuously adapts to its environment. Throughout the days and nights, throughout the changing seasons, and during the different stages in one's life the products of normal metabolism are produced in the tissues and are carried away for elimination via one of three major routes:

- feces
- urine
- perspiration

In addition to physical forms of by-products which arise, excess doshas also are being continuously formed and removed from the body by its natural eliminatory processes. Although the pathways for the removal of these excess doshas are multiple, the gastrointestinal tract is the main route for their elimination. Furthermore, specific parts of the gastrointestinal tract are the main site of elimination for a specific dosha: the stomach for Kapha, the jejunun and ileum for Pitta, and the colon for Vata.

Normally, the body has the innate ability to efficiently process and remove these waste materials, including the vitiated doshas. However due to one's repeated dietary indiscretions, poor exercise patterns, lifestyle and genetic predisposition, the digestive enzymes, metabolic co-factors, hormones and agnis which regulate the body's internal homeostasis become disorganized. This can lead to the accumulation and spread of toxins throughout the physiology—resulting in disease. A modern example of this situation occurs when you eat a (non-organic) apple treated with a pesticide. The chemical is absorbed into the bloodstream and eventually arrives at the liver where it normally undergoes two biochemical processes known as *functionalization* and *conjugation.* These processes convert the pesticide into a water-soluble form, which can be eliminated in the urine or feces. A simple example of how these processes operate is the conversion of the toxin benzene into its non-toxic metabolite as illustrated below:

Benzene

(unsoluble) **FUNCTIONALIZATION**   **CONJUGATION**   (soluble)

Furthermore, for these important processes to proceed effectively many specific complex enzymes are required in proper proportion to be released at the correct moment. If the liver is properly nourished and is in a clean state, the pesticide will be eliminated from the body before its can exert its neuro- or immunotoxic effect. Consider that like any machine, the human body requires regular cleaning to ensure long and proper functioning. The organs and tissues that act as filters (liver, spleen, kidneys, lymphatics, mucous membranes, etc.) must be purified and have any accumulated toxins removed to prevent the channels that carry life's quintessential substances from becoming impeded. The ancient Ayurvedic physicians knew that without such maintenance, bothersome mental and physical conditions were more likely to arise, which could then give rise to more advanced disease states and eventually premature mortality.

Although most reasonable individuals recognize the value in maintaining a clean internal physiology, modern medicine has yet to accept this idea as a central tenet of health-care and has therefore provided no practical guidance for detoxification therapies. The result is that few of us give the same care and attention to our internal organs and tissues that we confer on our vacuum cleaners, cars or washing machines. However, recently more and more men and women are becoming aware of the dangers of living in environmentally toxic, over-populated and over-stressed conditions. On a planetary scale there is an increasing awareness of the need to purify our minds and bodies, to remove toxins and to maintain a balanced lifestyle. Only in this way can we expect to remain vital, strong and immune to disease.

Panchakarma Chikitsa, the detoxification therapies of Ayurveda, may well be the most effective method of cleansing and rejuvenating the various cells, tissues and organs of the human physiology.

Panchakarma therapy (chikitsa) is regarded as the means by which the body can once again reestablish its innate intelligence and regain the ability to naturally assimilate nutrients and eliminate wastes. The health of each and every individual depends on these processes. Panchakarma therapies are designed to effect the radical purification of the bodily tissues through the elimination of vitiated doshas, which are the causative agents of disease. Unlike many health-promoting recommendations of Ayurveda, these are not self-administered therapies. These procedures must be administered by specially trained therapists in a definite sequence for a specified period of time. In addition, although Panchakarma is for the most part a delightful and comfortable therapy, there can be periods of discomfort associated with the profound release of toxins that does occur. It is therefore essential that the therapy be supervised by a knowledgeable expert who can recognize the signs of properly and improperly administered Panchakarma. Fortunately these signs were meticulously recorded by the ancient practitioners and can be learned by the dedicated student.

The ancient physicians were very clear and direct in their assessment of the importance of Panchakarma Chikitsa in one's overall health care. It is considered important for everyone to regularly undergo these treatments regardless of one's state of health, with the exception of certain patients with absolute and relative contraindications to the treatments (which we will cover later on). If one is generally in good health, Panchakarma can prevent the accumulation of toxins, enhance your vital energies, and prevent the occurrence of subsequent disease. If suffering from diseases of either acute or chronic natures, it can assist the body in the removal of obstinate, stubborn waste products that have become toxic.

Thus the importance of Panchakarma is apparent even for people living under the best of circumstances. However, it becomes an even higher priority for individuals living in more stressful, polluted, and unnatural environments. Over-worked and under-rested members of our society often eat unsatisfactory meals in a rushed manner, get insufficient exercise, sit at sedentary jobs under artificial light, breath stale oxygen-depleted air, and then watch hours of mind-numbing television, take synthetic medicines, and live surrounded by noise, electromagnetic fields, and harmful radiation far removed from nature.

Normally, human beings adapt well to changes in their environment and over time develop physiological modifications to prevent disease. However, as we move into the twenty-first century, it is clear that our exposure to harmful conditions and substances, especially bioactive chemicals, is increasing at a rate that surpasses the adaptive capacity of the human physiology. Because the vast majority of toxic substances are lipophilic ("lipid loving"), they accumulate primarily in fat tissues. When toxic accumulation reaches a critical state, symptoms manifest that we recognize as a clinical imbalance or disease. Examples of this would be intestinal malabsorption, joint pains, sinus congestion, bronchitis, dermatitis, nausea, fatigue, menstrual pain and others.

However, some individuals do not reach the point of toxicity where any of these recognizable symptomatologies occur. Instead, many of us incur subclinical levels of toxic accumulations in our fat tissues and the result is a derangement of the metabolism of this tissue. Ultimately, this toxic-induced physiological derangement results in a higher fat:muscle ratio, which leads to obesity.

To further exacerbate our situation, we learn to suppress many of our natural bodily functions in order to assimilate politely into an unnatural society: coughing, sneezing, expelling intestinal gas, belching, yawning, eating, drinking, sleeping, sweating, urinating and defecating. As members of society we give our tacit agreement to suppress these natural urges in public and therefore we eat according to the office schedule, drink insufficient water, yawn self-consciously, sneeze while squeezing our noses, and rush to visit the toilet only between meetings.

The unavoidable consequence of this lifestyle is the formation and bioaccumulation of toxic substances and residues in the physiology. They can take a myriad of forms including: senescent (dead) cells, mucous secretions, bacterial overgrowths, excessive fats and fatty acids, and many forms of toxins which are so unique that they defy classification in modern terms. You can be reasonably certain you suffer from toxicity if you are experiencing headaches, joint pains, recurrent respiratory infections, constipation, hemorrhoids, sinus congestion, psoriasis, acne, non-structural low back pain, mood changes, depression, food allergies, ulcers, or generalized aches and pains. Panchakarma detoxification is perhaps the "missing link" to restoring optimum function of our cells and tissues. Whether undertaken to prevent disease or treat conditions like obesity, most individuals who avail themselves of authentic panchakarma chikitsa will feel physically and mentally revitalized with a commensurate amelioration in symptoms of toxicity.

Overview of Panchakarma Chikitsa:

What Does Panchakarma Involve?

Like all medical procedures, Panchakarma Therapy always must begin with an initial consultation by a qualified health professional who can determine the individual's prakriti (constitutional type), the nature of the health problem (if any), and the appropriate degree of intensity of the prescribed therapies. There are certain special circumstances in which panchakarma should be administered only with strict medical supervision: recovering drug addiction, alcoholism, hypertension, diabetes and eating disorders are the most common. Panchakarma may also not be appropriate for individuals who are significantly under-weight or physically weak or for persons with inadequately treated (or undiagnosed) hypothyroidism or hypoglycemia. The same is true of persons with cancerous diseases, immune-deficiency states, or those recovering from recent surgery. All potential patients, but especially those identified above, should always consult a qualified health professional before initiating any form of detoxification program.

When Panchakarma is indicated, seven to twenty-eight day programs are recommended, according to the individual's specific needs. Occasionally, this can be extended for up to 90 days. Each daily session requires from one-and-a-half to two hours.

Panchakarma can be easily understood as being comprised of three components:

– Preliminary therapies
– Primary therapies
– Follow-up therapies

1. PRELIMINARY THERAPIES

The preliminary procedures are often under-appreciated in the grand scheme of proper administration of Panchakarma. In practice, you will find that without well-planned preliminary therapies, the primary procedures will not be effective. These preliminary therapies are three in number and we will examine them individually; they include:

– Oleation Therapy
– Fomentation Therapy
– Digestive Therapy

The importance of these three preliminary measures can be explained in the following way. Due to dietary, behavioral, and various other factors, one or more doshas has become aggravated and "overflowed" beyond its natural site where it has become lodged in some peripheral tissue. In every case, an excess of Vata dosha is present, providing the moving force for this spread of the aggravated dosha (which may also be Vata itself). It is the quality of pressure inherent in Vata dosha that pushes the vitiated dosha towards the periphery and into the tissues. After some critical time, the dosha becomes firmly adherent and stagnant in its new location. In addition, the channel (srota) through which the dosha has moved from its original (central) site to its new (peripheral) site also becomes vitiated and obstructed. This obstruction of the channel prevents the easy return of the vitiated dosha to its original (central) site in the alimentary canal.

The general purpose of the preliminary therapies is to begin to loosen, liquefy and move the disturbed doshas from their abnormal sites in peripheral tissues to the appropriate central site within the alimentary canal. Let's briefly describe what each of these three preliminary procedures involve.

A. Oleation Therapy

Oleation means to make oily or unctuous and that's exactly what these therapies do—both externally and internally.

Externally, oleation therapy involves receiving a series of warm oil massages usually once a day for one or two weeks. The oils that are used are special herbalized Ayurvedic oils that are selected according to the Ayurvedic Constitutional Type of the individual. Each individual massage usually lasts one to one and a half hours.

Internally, oleation therapy involves the ingestion of an oily substance, usually ghee (clarified butter), olive oil, or particular herbs which have a slightly oily composition (e.g. long pepper). The oily substance is usually taken early in the morning on an empty stomach for a period of 4-7 days.

The purpose of all this oil is to provide an appropriate solvent for various lipid soluble impurities that are lodged in the digestive system and body tissues.

B. Fomentation Therapy

Fomentation therapy is nothing more than inducing a person to sweat at a specific intensity and for a specific period of time. It is instrumental in helping to liquefy the sticky and adherent toxins that have become lodged in the tissues. Properly timed and combined with oleation and digestive therapies (to be described in the following section,) fomentation can soften and melt toxins sufficiently for the body to efficiently expel them with the help of the main detoxification therapies.

Fomentation therapies in Ayurveda are classified in several different ways. Here is the most practical way to classify them:

1. With or without the use of fire.
2. Applied to the entire body or to one individual area.
3. Wet or dry
4. Intensity: mild, moderate or strong.

With this general classification in mind, here is the list of specific procedures used in Ayurveda to promote sweating:

Thirteen Types of Fomentation Which Utilize Fire

1. Application of steam therapy to a clothed or unclothed patient.
2. The patient lies on a bed of leaves of *Ricinus communis* and *Calotropis gigantea*, corn, pulse, pippali, ginger, maricha and ghee. Paayasa (a milk reparation) or krushara is also added. The patient is covered with silk or wool blankets.
3. Medicated steam is directed through a hose or tube (nadi) to specific areas of the body.
4. Hot herbal decoction is showered over the body from a pitcher, pot, or pipe that has many small holes in it.
5. The patient enters a circular room built near a pond or small lake which has an oven burning special herbs to heat it; similar in some respects to an Indian "sweat lodge".
6. The patient lies on a stone slab on which has been burning special varieties of wood. The wood is removed and the patient is clothed in cotton, leather and silk.
7. Same as above except the patient lies directly on the earth instead of on a stone slab.
8. The patient lies in the bottom of a pit, which has a smokeless fire, well wrapped in protective clothing. The heat is produced by burning wood.
9. The patient lies on a woven bamboo bed suspended over a pit containing the burning dung of the following animals: cow, elephant, horse, ass or camel.
10. The patient lies on a woven bamboo bed, which is over a steaming decoction of herbs buried in the ground.
11. The patient lies on a bed inside a thick-walled, round cottage with no windows and which contains several ovens or furnaces.
12. The patient lies on a thin bed resting on the burnt ashes from animal dung.
13. The patient takes a hot bath in a tub filled with an herbal decoction of oil, meat juice, ghee, or milk for a specified period of time.

In addition to methods of inducing sweat which involve the use of fire in one form or another, Ayurveda also recognizes treatments that *do not* require the use of fire:

1. Exercise
2. Being inside a warm chamber
3. Wearing of heavy clothing
4. Hunger
5. Excessive drinking of alcohol
6. Fear
7. Application of thick poultice
8. Anger
9. Wrestling
10. Exposure to the sun

Choosing the Type of Fomentation

The physician must take into account the Ayurvedic Constitutional Type of the patient, the disease and bodily organs most affected, the season, the age of the patient, and the place where the treatment is being given. For example, an elderly patient who is obese and of a Vata constitution also suffering from an arthritic left shoulder, in a very cold season high in the mountains might warrant techniques which are mild in intensity, localized and Vata alleviating. Similarly, a Kapha individual, also obese with mild depression, bronchial congestion, and cravings for sweets would receive fomentation of a more intense, prolonged and penetrating nature.

Ayurvedic Herbs Used In Fomentation Therapy

There are many herbal substances mentioned in the ancient Ayurvedic medical texts (*samhitas*) for the purpose of producing and enhancing fomentation. For full details of these herbs please refer to the original books on the subject. The following is an abridged summary of some of the more common herbal medicines used in Fomentation (the *italicized* postscript indicates the Ayurvedic Constitutional Type which is benefited most). The majority of these herbs are available from any good mail order distributor of Ayurvedic herbs (see Appendix).

Calotropis gigantea	k	Crataeva religiosa	k	Trachyspermum mami	v
Boerhaavia diffusa	v,p,k	Tinospora cordifolia	v,p,k	Oroxylum indicum	v,p,k
Sesamum indicum	v,p,k	Moringa oleifera	v,k	Aegle marmelos	v,k
Dolichos biflorus	v,k	Adhota vasica	k	Foeniculum vulgare	v
Zizyphus jujuba	v,p	Bambusa arundinacae	v,p,k	Nelumbe nucifera	v,p,k
Ricinus communis	v	Ocimum sanctum	k	Glycyrrhiza glabra	v,p
Embelia ribes	v,k	Mesua ferrea	v.k	Valeriana walachi	v,k
Vitex negundo	v.p,k	Elettaria cardamomum	v,k	Nardostachys jatamansi	v,k
Coriandrum sativum	v,p,k	Santalum album	p	Cedrus deodara	v,k
Sida cordifolia	v,p	Azadirachta indica	p,k	Cinnamomum tamala	v,k
Tribulus terristris	v,k	Gmelina arborea	v,p,k	Solanum indicum	v,k

C. Digestive Therapy

Digestive Therapy is the process by which toxins in the various tissues and channels of the body are digested and liquefied through the use of herbs. The preliminary procedure primes the digestive organs to be able to process the large toxic load that will imminently follow. This is accomplished by increasing the Agni, or digestive fire, of the body. This includes not only the main digestive fire (Jathagni) located in the stomach and proximal small intestine, but also the seven agnis associated with each of the seven dhatus (Dhatagnis) and the five agnis which correspond to the five elements which compose the physiology (Bhutagnis).

Digestive Therapy involves the ingestion of Agni-promoting (fire-promoting) herbs. These herbs are generally pungent and bitter in taste (Rasa), heating in potency (Veerya), and pungent in post-digestive taste (Vipaka). Their physiological effects are to increase internal heat, stimulate the metabolism, enkindle the digestive enzymes, increase peristalsis, improve the circulation and promote mental focus. These are herbs which warm the gastrointestinal tract, are commonly diaphoretic, stimulate gastric and intestinal digestive juices, provide kinetic energy to the circulatory system and sharpen the five senses. Many of these herbs happen to have antiparasitic or antibacterial properties and some may have immune-enhancing effects. They all decrease Kapha and revive lethargic digestive systems. They are generally Vata-decreasing as well except for the herbs with a predominantly drying quality. They can be used, in smaller amounts, in persons with a Pitta prakriti or in those with a Pitta excess-related condition, especially if that condition involves ama.

Digestive Therapy is known in Sanskrit as *pacana*. The word *pacana* derives from the Sanskrit root *pac* which means "to cook, ripen, to cook to completion, mature". Hence, these are herbs that will help cook or digest any toxins, or ama, already in the body as well as any toxic substances that are subsequently released by the tissues.

How And When To Administer Digestive Therapy

The best time to initiate preliminary digestive therapy is approximately two weeks prior to Oleation; in other words before any other form of therapy. If this is not possible, digestive therapy can be started concurrently with Oleation.

The principles of administering the herbal medicines are actually very simple. Herbs are given in very small amounts during the two largest meals of the day (lunch and dinner). For some patients this will be reduced to only during one meal (generally lunch in this situation). For some patients, special herbs may be recommended thirty minutes before the meal or immediately following its completion. As with all preparatory or main detoxification therapies, the constitution of the patient, the primary doshic imbalance, the digestive power, the season, and the general state of health must be carefully considered. In addition, the physician must assess the patient's state of hydration, any signs or symptoms of inflammatory diseases especially involving the bowels (e.g. colitis, Crohn's Disease, etc.), any degree of Pitta aggravation, and any tendency toward dryness. It is important to remind patients that during this phase of preliminary therapy it is particularly important to stay well-hydrated with warm water being the best choice of fluid. With very few exceptions, almost all patients can receive some form of appropriately chosen digestive therapy.

Commonly used single and combination herbs for digestive therapy include:

Trachyspermum roxburghianum
Emblica officinalis
Zingiber officinale
Calotropis procera
Terminalia chebula
Syzygium cumini
Strychnos nux-vomica
Piper nigrum
Panchakatu (Five Pungents): Piper longum (seed)
                            Piper longum (root)
                            Piper chaba
                            Plumbago zeylandica
                            Sunthi (dry ginger)

Garcinia Indica
Trichosanthus dioca
Zanthoxylum alatum
Allium sativum
Andrographis paniculata
Premna obtusilfolia

Coriandrum sativum
Citrus limon
Ocimum sanctum
Carum carvi
Cuminum cyminum
Operculina turpethum
Ferula foetida
Elettaria cardamomum
Angelica glauca
Nigella sativa
Urginea indica
Cinnamomum zeylanicum
Cinnamomum tamala
Crocus sativus
Syzygium aromaticum
Solanum xanthocarpum
Alpinia galanga
Carum copticum
Trikatu (Three Pungents):
          Piper nigrum
          Piper longum
          Zingiber officinale

These herbs are generally prepared in powders, pastes or decoctions. These recipes are numerous and therefore beyond the scope of these notes. However, it would be appropriate to list certain guidelines for the administration of some of these materials to individuals according to prakriti.

	Digestive Therapy Herb	Dosage	When to Take In Relation To Meals
VATA	panchakatu	1/4 tsp.	During the meal
	trikatu	1/4 tsp.	During the meal
	C. tamala	1/2 tsp.	15 min. before the meal
	F. foetida	1/4 tsp.	During the meal
	A. sativum	1 clove	During the meal
PITTA	O. turpethum	1/2 tsp.	During the meal
	C. cyminum	1/2 tsp.	15 min. before the meal
	C. sativus	1/8 tsp.	15 min. before the meal
	A. paniculata	1-2 oz	15 min. before the meal
KAPHA	panchakatu	1/2 tsp.	During the meal
	trikatu	1/2 tsp.	During the meal
	Z. officinale	1/2 tsp.	During the meal
	S. xanthocarpum	1/2 tsp.	15 min. after the meal
	O. sanctum	1/2 tsp.	During the meal
	A. sativum	1-2 cloves	During the meal

*The following herbs are used for all three constitutional types in dosages of 1/4 – 1/2 tsp. taken during meals:

E. cardamomum   P. nigrum
C. sativum   E. officinalis
C. carvi

2. PRIMARY THERAPIES

We now come to an examination of the five-fold procedures that are the main therapies of Panchakarma Treatments. First, we must be clear on a few terms that are important for an overall view of these therapies.

According to Ayurveda, the treatment of almost all diseases depends on three approaches; these are:

a) Purification: the elimination of toxins and waste products from the body,

b) Homeostasis: the maintenance of equilibrium among the doshas through correct lifestyle regimens, herbal medicines, and meditative practices, and

c) Nutrition: the use of proper diet and herbal supplements.

Purification, or eliminative therapy, is considered by many of the ancient physicians to be the most important aspect of the treatment of disease. Much is said by Charaka, the most famous of the ancient Ayurvedic physicians, about the benefits of purification type of treatments. To summarize his comments, he said that these therapies remove the possibility of the disease ever recurring, as opposed to Homeostasis, or maintenance therapies, which alleviates the disease but the possibility of re-provocation still exists. Purification increases the digestive power, causes disease to disappear, brings clarity to the mind and senses, clears the complexion, increases vigor and off-spring, regulates plumpness and virility; it retards aging, and gives the individual a long life free from disease (CS Su. 16/17-19).

The main therapies are five in number and these have become known as *panchakarma* (pancha = five; karma = actions).

Charaka and Sushruta, another famous ancient physician, differ slightly in their opinions of which five procedures actually constitute panchakarma.

CHAPTER 16. PANCHAKARMA THERAPY

Charaka identifies the following five procedures:

1. Vamana	(Therapeutic Vomiting)
2. Virechana	(Purgation)
3. Nasya	(Nasal Medications)
4. Niruha Vasti	(Decoction Enema)
5. Anuvasana Vasti	(Oily Enema)

Sushruta combines the two types of Vasti as one procedure and adds a fifth process known as raktamokshana, or blood letting. This comes as no surprise, knowing Sushruta's surgical orientation.

Sushruta's final formulation of panchakarma looks as follows:

1. Vamana	(Therapeutic Vomiting)
2. Virechana	(Purgation)
3. Nasya	(Nasal Medications)
4. Vasti	(Decoction and Oily Enemas)
5. Raktamokshana	(Blood-letting)

Panchakarma is designed to remove the excessive doshas, which have been brought to the digestive system by the preliminary measures, from either the upper part of the body (i.e. the mouth, nose) or the lower part of the body (i.e. the anus).

Vamana Therapy is normally the first main therapy to follow preparatory therapies. It will therefore be the first to be described.

Vamana

The use of emetic herbs to induce a therapeutic vomiting of the stomach contents. It is preceded by the consumption of cool water or specific teas to fill the stomach. Excellent in treating all kapha-type conditions including asthma, bronchitis, allergies, depression and many digestive problems.

Snehana-Virechana

A two-part procedure that involves an initial consumption of an oily or unctuous substance followed by the administration of an herbal laxative. The oleation acts as a solvent and mobilizer for certain toxins in the body and also promotes strength, good complexion, efficient digestion, and proper function of the sense organs. The subsequent laxative therapies eliminates the toxins loosened by the oleation and causes a maximal dilation of the hepatic, biliary, and other channels which allows for the removal of lipid-soluble impurities.

Basti

Gentle, herbalized enemas which cleanse the rectum and lower colon and eliminate excess vata dosha from the physiology.

Nasya

The application of specially herbalized nasal drops that cleanse the sinuses and remove impurities from the throat, facial and supraclavicular areas.

Raktamokshana

The removal of a small quantity of blood from the patient using modern sterile techniques; traditionally this was accomplished with special *jaluka*, or leeches. This procedure is valuable if there is toxicity in the blood; it also stimulates production of fresh blood cells from the bone marrow.

Additional specialized therapies are administered when medically indicated. These are often luxurious and spa-like while deeply and completely purifying the targeted tissues. These procedures may include:

Shirodhara

A continuous stream of warm, herbalized oil flows from an overhead vessel through a small aperture onto the forehead. This treatment is said to purify the mind-body, and profoundly relax the nervous system. Individuals experience twilight states of consciousness between waking and dreaming. Very meditative and pleasurable.

Udvartna

A general term for therapies in which herbal pastes (or muds) are applied to all parts of the body. Patients are wrapped in warm blankets and the paste removed when dry. This treatment exfoliates the skin, penetrates to the muscles and fat tissues, and removes impurities. Useful in stimulating weight reduction.

Shirobasti

The placement of a leather crown around the head, which is filled with warm herbalized oil and remains on the head for up to thirty minutes. The weight of the column of oil causes penetration down the thousands of hair shafts to their junctions with the tiny nerves that innervate them. Creates a decrease in Vata dosha and a state of calm.

3. FOLLOW-UP THERAPIES

It is best to follow a regimen after the detoxification therapies to promote a continued removal of toxins from the body for several weeks even after the therapies have ended. The most important aspect of the follow-up therapy is a specific, light diet that is recommended for a period of time equal to the length of the treatment period.

Other recommendations include specific herbal supplements, exercise recommendations, spices, and simple hygienic procedures.

Appendix I

Technical Jargon

*O*ver the more than four years that it has taken to complete this book, I have constantly reviewed both the conventional allopathic as well as the complementary medical literature on the subject of overweight and obesity. Although this is a book that deals primarily with the Ayurvedic approach to weight loss and maintenance, I feel it is the responsibility of any physician author to be conversant with the allopathic medical concepts that relate to his subject.

This appendix contains short paragraphs that summarize the current conventional medical understanding of topics related to obesity. I realize that this material may seem unnecessarily technical and dry to many readers. However, in the spirit of being comprehensive, I have included it for those of you who may find it relevant and interesting.

Review Of Our Current Understanding Of Obesity and Its Treatment

Obesity is one of the most common disorders in clinical practice. Defined by the National Institutes of Health as a body weight 20% or more above "desirable" weight, over one third of adult Americans are now considered overweight. Positioned at the epicenter of chronic disease risk and psychosocial disability for millions of Americans, successful management of obesity is truly an opportunity to avert a national health disaster in the coming century. If all Americans were to achieve a normal body weight, it has been estimated that there would be a 3-year increase in life expectancy, 25% less coronary heart disease, and 35% less congestive heart failure and stroke.

Unfortunately, obesity is also one of the most difficult and frustrating disorders to manage successfully. Considerable effort is expended by primary care providers and patients with little benefit. Using standard treatments in university settings, only 20% of patients lose 20 pounds at two year follow-up while only 5% of patients lose 40 pounds. Regrettably, this includes results from even the most well-known and best-selling weight loss programs available today. Despite what the proponents of these programs may say, the cold hard fact is that they are all equally ineffective when followed out past two years. This lack of clinical success has created a never-ending demand for new weight loss treatments. Approximately 50% of women and 25% of men are involved with weight loss regimens at any one time. Americans spent over $50 billion last year on diet books, diet meals, weight-loss classes, diet drugs, exercise tapes, "fat farms" and other weight loss aids!

The challenge for health care providers is to identify those patients with obesity who are most likely to medically benefit from treatment and most likely to maintain weight loss, and to provide them with sound advice, skills for long-term lifestyle change and support. The purpose of this book is to present a time-tested method to promote weight loss in an intelligent, scientifically-supported, *sustainable* way while simultaneously greatly improving your general health.

Our Current Understanding of Obesity

Definitions

Obesity is an excess of *body fat*; overweight is an excess of *body weight*, including all components of body composition (muscle, bone, water and fat). In clinical practice, the two are used interchangeably to refer to excess body fat. The two most commonly used terms to quantify obesity are relative weight (RW) and body mass index (BMI). The RW is the actual weight divided by the "desirable weight" (derived from "acceptable weight" tables). The BMI, or Quetelet index, is the actual body weight divided by the height squared (kg per m2). This index more closely corresponds to measurements of body fat and better differentiates "overweight" due to an increase in muscle mass from true obesity.

A recent National Institutes of Health Consensus Conference defined obesity (somewhat arbitrarily) as a RW of greater than 120% (BMI > 27 kg/m2). "Morbid" obesity is commonly defined as a RW greater than 200% (BMI >40 kg/m2).

Health Consequences of Obesity

The relationship between body weight and mortality is curvilinear, similar to other cardiovascular risk factors. Most studies have demonstrated a J-shaped or U-shaped relationship, suggesting that the thinnest portion of the population also have an excess mortality. This is thought to be primarily due to the higher rate of cigarette smoking in the thinnest group.

The relationship of body weight to mortality is also affected by age. The body weights associated with the lowest mortality increase with age, and the newest weight tables take this into account. In addition, as age increases to over 65, the relationship of body weight and mortality takes on a more striking U-shape. This suggests that although obesity remains an important risk factor in the elderly, malnutrition is also extremely important.

The increase in total mortality related to obesity results predominantly from coronary heart disease (CHD). Evidence is mixed whether obesity is an independent risk factor for coronary heart disease. For example, the 1993 cholesterol treatment guidelines omit obesity as a risk factor for CHD, while the previous edition in 1988 included obesity. Nonetheless, obesity is clearly an important risk factor for the development of many other CHD risk factors. Obese individuals age 20-44, for example, have a 3.8 times greater risk of type II diabetes, 5.6 times greater risk of hypertension, and 2.1 times greater risk of hypercholesterolemia. As a result, type II diabetes and stroke also contribute to the increase in obesity-related mortality. The obese also have an increased risk of certain cancers including colon, rectum, and prostate in men and uterus, biliary tract, breast and ovary in women.

As a result of these conditions, relative weights of 130% are associated with an excess mortality of 35%. Relative weights of 150% have a greater than two-fold excess death rate. Patients with "morbid" obesity (relative weights greater than 200%), have a greater than 10-fold increase in death rates.

Obesity is also associated with a variety of other medical disorders including degenerative joint disease of both weight-bearing and non-weight bearing joints, diseases of the digestive tract (gallstones, reflux esophagitis), thromboembolic disorders, heart failure (both systolic and diastolic), respiratory impairment, and skin disorders. Obese patients also have a greater incidence of surgical and obstetric complications and are more prone to accidents. Although obesity is not associated with an increased risk of major psychiatric disorders, obese patients are at increased risk of psychological disorders and social discrimination.

Regional fat distribution

Recent investigations suggest that the location of the excess body fat (regional fat distribution) is a major determinant of the degree of excess morbidity and mortality due to obesity. At least three components of body fat are associated with obesity-related adverse health outcomes. These are:

(1) the total amount of body fat (expressed as a percentage of body weight),
(2) the amount of subcutaneous truncal or abdominal fat (upper body fat), and
(3) the amount of visceral fat located in the abdominal cavity.

These three are partly correlated with each other but exhibit a fairly high degree of independence. Each of these components of body fat is associated with varying degrees of metabolic abnormalities and independently predict adverse health outcomes. In each of 6 prospective epidemiologic studies, increased abdominal obesity was associated with increased cardiovascular and total mortality.

Body fat distribution can be assessed by a number of measurement techniques. Measurements of skin folds (subscapular and triceps) reflect subcutaneous fat. Measurement of circumferences (waist and hip) reflect both abdominal and visceral fat. CAT and MRI scans measure subcutaneous and visceral fat. Clinically, measurement of the waist and hip circumference is most useful. The waist is measured at the umbilicus and the hips at the greater trochanter.

A waist to hip ratio of 1.0 and 0.8 are considered normal in men and women, respectively. Ratios above these values reflect abdominal and/or visceral obesity and a greater risk of obesity-related disorders.

Appendix I. Technical Jargon

Etiology of Obesity

Numerous lines of evidence suggest strong genetic influences on the development of obesity. Most convincing are genetic studies of adoptees and twins. In a study of 800 Danish adoptees, there was no relationship between the body weight of adoptees and their adopting parents but a close correlation with the body weights of their *biological parents*. In a study of approximately 4000 twins, a much closer correlation between body weights was found in monozygotic than dizygotic twins. In this study, genetic factors accounted for approximately two thirds of the variation in weights. More recent studies of twins reared apart and the response of twins to overfeeding showed similar results. Studies of regional fat distribution in twins has also shown a significant, but not complete, genetic influence.

The exact mechanisms by which such genetic factors result in obesity are considerably less clear. Differences in both energy intake and energy expenditure have been investigated. Genetic influences on control of appetite and eating behavior have long been considered. Animal studies have demonstrated the influence of dozens of factors on eating behavior, and it is likely that similar factors are at work in humans. Observational studies of eating behavior have suggested that the obese both eat more food and do so more rapidly than the non-obese.

Differences in energy expenditure are also likely to be at least partially determined by genetic influences. Differences in the resting metabolic expenditure (RME), for example, could easily result in considerable differences in body weight since RME accounts for approximately 60-75% of total energy expenditure. The RME can vary by as much as 20% between individuals of the same age, sex, and body build; such differences could account for approximately 400 kcals of energy expenditure per day! Recent evidence suggests that the metabolic rate is similar in family members, and as expected, individuals with lower metabolic rates are more likely to gain weight. Differences in the thermic effect of food, the amount of energy expended following a meal, may also contribute to obesity. Although some investigators have shown a decreased thermic effect of food in the obese, others have not.

I am including this review of information on the genetic influences of obesity not to sound a pessimistic voice, but rather to address the subject in the full light of the truth. We need to hear the voice of reason when discussing this subject, which has become fraught with such intense emotional overlay that lay persons are tempted to believe what this month's weight loss guru has proclaimed. I wish to present the clear, objective truth of the situation. The fact is that genetic influences are at work in the treatment of obesity. It will not help to ignore this fact, though many physicians and lay persons conveniently do. Fortunately, the situation is not at all dismal because these genetic factors appear capable of being modified in most, if not all, people by environmental factors.

Environmental factors are also clearly important in the development of obesity. Decreased physical activity and food choices that result in increased energy intake also clearly contribute to the development of obesity. Medical illness and some medications can also result in obesity, but such instances account for less than 1% of cases. Hypothyroidism and Cushing's syndrome are the most common, but these are both rare. Diseases of the hypothalamus can also result in obesity but these are quite uncommon. Major depression, which usually results in weight loss, can occasionally present with weight gain. Consideration of these causes is particularly important when evaluating unexplained, recent weight gain.

Thus, the etiology of obesity is multi-factorial, and almost certainly under both genetic and environmental influences.

Who Should Lose Weight?

According to modern Western medicine, the answer to this question is rather straightforward. Weight loss is indicated to treat any patient who is obese (RW>120%, BMI>27 kg/m2). In fact, weight loss is the first-line treatment for heart disease, diabetes, hyperlipidemia, hypertension, arthritis, and many other degenerative disorders. In addition, many patients with relative weights of 100-120% (BMI 25-27 kg/m2) who have one of these conditions (particularly hypertension, diabetes, lipid disorders or significant psychosocial disability) will often dramatically benefit from weight reduction.

I find it very interesting to note that weight loss to prevent complications of obesity in patients without active medical complications or metabolic consequences of obesity is more controversial. In young and middle aged individuals, particularly those with a family history of obesity-related disorders, treatment is based on the degree of obesity (RW >120%) and body fat distribution. Such individuals with upper body obesity (waist-hip ratios >1.0 in men and >0.8 in women) are considered for treatment in medical circles; those individuals with lower body obesity, and no medical complications or metabolic consequences of obesity, are only reassured and followed for development of additional upper body obesity and its metabolic consequences.

This algorithm is the one currently (2001) recommended by physicians to select patients who require treatment. Of course it gives not the slightest consideration to how the patient feels and thinks. Modern Ayurvedic wisdom teaches that what your ideal weight should be is more a subjective decision than previously thought. Assuming that you are not obese (BMI>27kg/m2), the most important factor is whether you feel in command of your general health picture. If your weight gain was the result of a recent period of indiscretion that has temporarily interrupted an established healthy lifestyle, then the best thing to do for weight loss is to resume that lifestyle again. No specific measure may be required. However, if you perceive the sensation as something which somehow transpired while you were sleeping, like a fire in your house, you must take action now! On the other hand, if you are comfortable with your weight and are not obese, do not allow the opinions of others influence you. If you are not comfortable with your weight, this book will show you how to attain it without emotional pain or physical martyrdom, and how to maintain it for your lifetime.

A medical or personal indication for weight loss is necessary but not sufficient, however, to begin treatment. Only *motivated* people should begin a treatment regimen. Considerable effort should be made to assess your motivation for the modest dietary and exercise changes that will inevitably be necessary. Questions you ask yourself should focus on how the current attempt compares to previous attempts, a realistic assessment of your goals for the amount and rate of weight loss, the extent to which outside stresses, emotional disorders, or substance abuse might impair the attempt, and the degree to which others can provide support.

Your motivation can be simply assessed by completing specific preliminary assignments. For example, make a resolution to complete a 3-5 day diet record and to write down on paper an exercise plan that includes both the type of aerobic exercise that you plan to begin and how you plan to fit it into your schedule.

Diet Therapy

Standard dietary treatment of obesity should utilize the same nutritional principles as diet recommendations for healthy people. Total fat intake should be limited to 20% or less of total calories, protein 15%, and carbohydrate (primarily complex carbohydrates) 65% or greater. A total energy intake should be recommended to result in a daily energy deficit of 500-1000 calories. Since one pound of fat equals approximately 3500 calories, these deficits will result in a 1-2 pound weight loss per week.

No dietary manipulation of macronutrients or other nutritional components can change these basic thermodynamic concepts; yet sadly, virtually all popular diets are based on attempts to circumvent thermodynamics.

It is impossible for the clinician to keep up with each new popular diet. Categorizing diets, however, can allow generalizations that allow for a basic understanding of the most common diets. Major categories of diets include low carbohydrate diets, vegetarian diets, single-food diets, high carbohydrate diets, very-low-calorie diets, and prepackaged diet programs.

Low Carbohydrate Diets

Low carbohydrate diets are the most resilient popular diet concept. Examples include the Atkins diet, the Stillman diet, and the Scarsdale diet, to name a few. These diets are based on the correct observation that at equal calorie intakes, low carbohydrate diets result in more rapid weight loss than high carbohydrate diets. Unfortunately, the greater weight loss observed during low carbohydrate feeding is entirely due to changes in water balance. During carbohydrate restriction, ketonuria increases and results in greater sodium excretion and water loss. The resumption of even modest carbohydrate feeding reverses this process and results in sodium and water retention. No other differences in body composition or weight loss are observed. Low carbohydrate diets are by definition high in fat and/or protein and are thus unsuitable for long-term weight loss. These diets are also commonly deficient in calcium and/or dietary fiber. The high protein content of these diets can lead to kidney dysfunction and osteoporosis if continued for long periods of time.

Vegetarian Diets

Vegetarian diets are typically low fat, high carbohydrate, high fiber diets and thus consistent with dietary goals. Vegetarian diets, however, can be either nutritionally adequate or inadequate depending on food selection. Diets that restrict all animal products (vegan) require particular attention to protein intake and vitamin B-12. Diets that include dairy products (lacto-vegetarian) or dairy and eggs (lacto-ovo vegetarian) are easier to plan. Most large weight loss programs include a vegetarian option. The Sattva Program diets are closest to this category.

Single-Food Diets

Single-food diets are based on the concept that it's not only what you eat but when you eat it that is important. The Beverly Hills diet, for example, suggests that by ingesting foods one at a time, digestion is made more efficient, resulting in fewer calories getting "stuck" and less weight gain. The diet relies primarily on fresh fruit and is inadequate in protein, niacin, calcium and iron. As expected, it commonly results in diarrhea.

High Carbohydrate Diets

High carbohydrate diets are typically balanced, hypocaloric diets. Most are also high fiber diets. Although the intake of large quantities of dietary fiber offers no particular weight loss benefit, these diets are consistent with current dietary recommendations and can be encouraged. Most large commercial diet programs such as Weight Watchers, TOPS, etc. use high carbohydrate diets and can be recommended to patients.

Very-Low-Calorie Diets (VLCD's)

A major development in the dietary treatment of obesity is the use of safe and effective very-low-calorie diets (VLCD's). Also known as protein-sparing modified fasts and protein-formula-liquid diets, these diets restrict calorie intake to 400-800 kcals per day. Patients ingest only preformulated, usually liquid, food that provides adequate protein, vitamins and minerals. Additional intake is limited to 2-3 quarts of calorie-free beverages per day. The major advantage of these diets is the "complete removal of patients from the food environment" to facilitate compliance. In addition, the significant energy deficit results in rapid weight loss, usually 3-4 pounds per week, encouraging the patient to continue. Major ongoing concerns about these diets include their cost, side effects and complications and long term results.

A recent concern, for example, has been the observation that significant numbers of patients using VLCD's develop gallstones. Studies using serial ultrasound examinations of the gallbladder before, during and after VLCD's have shown that approximately 25% of patients develop gallstones or "sludge." Approximately 25% of these become symptomatic and require surgery, approximately 50% resolve spontaneously, and approximately 25% remain asymptomatic. VLCD-related gallstones can be prevented with ursodeoxycholic acid and possibly by aspirin. Some authorities recommend the use of ursodeoxycholic acid (or aspirin) in individuals at particularly high risk of gallstone disease (e.g. those with a prior history).

Patients on VLCD's have marked improvements in obesity-related metabolic parameters. Within weeks blood sugars, blood lipids, and blood pressure are significantly reduced. Most diabetic, hypertensive and hypercholesterolemic patients can have medications markedly reduced or discontinued.

As with standard diet therapy of obesity, VLCD's require compliance during the diet and long term nutritional and behavioral changes to maintain weight loss. Well planned programs that combine VLCD's with behavior modification, exercise, and social support report improved long term results. For example, Nunn et. al. reported an average weight loss of 55 pounds with 75% and 52% of the loss maintained at one and 2 1/2 year follow-up, respectively. Hartman et. al. reported maintenance of an average of 24 pounds after 2-3 year follow-up. The largest study reviews the 18 month follow-up for over 4000 patients treated with Optifast. 25% of patients dropped out of the program early. Of those remaining in the program, 68% lost considerable weight but did not reach their goal. Of this group only 5-10% maintained weight loss after 18 months. Of the 32% of patients who attained their goal weight, 30% of women and 50% of men maintained their weight loss at 18 months. Thus, of the entire initial cohort, approximately 15% of patients met their weight loss goal (typically >40 pounds of weight loss) and maintained it at 1 1/2 years. Although these results are significantly better than results from most standard programs (in which approximately only 5% of patients lose and maintain 40 pounds at one-year follow-up), the expense and risks of such programs continue to raise considerable controversy.

A recent trend in the use of liquid supplements has been the use of similarly formulated 800 kcal/day diets. Most authorities feel that at 800 kcals per day or more there is little risk of the medical complications seen at lower levels of energy, including gallstones. Thus, although such patients continue to require extensive counseling and support during and after such programs, considerably less medically monitoring (and expense) is necessary. A recent comparison of 400 kcal and 800 kcal liquid diets demonstrated that although the rate of weight loss was greater in the lower calorie group (as expected), the long-term results were equivalent.

Liquid Diets

A variety of other liquid diets are available commercially over the counter. Those that provide <800 kcals per day are potentially quite dangerous due to the lack of medical supervision and their use in individuals with mild obesity (who develop greater degrees of protein loss than those with more significant obesity). Ultra Slimfast is a variant on this concept available in most supermarkets. Patients are instructed to use two shakes per day (approximately 200 kcals each) and then eat a sensible dinner (400-600 kcals). Since this results in >=800 kcals per day, and contains adequate quantities of protein, vitamins and minerals, it is generally considered to be safe. Although no studies have been published on its efficacy, it is unlikely to work for most individuals since most problem eaters take in most of their calories at the evening meal. If such individuals were able to eat a "sensible dinner" (and no additional calories just before and afterwards) in the first place, they would lose weight successfully without the product. It too also suffers from the difficulty of weight maintenance after the patient makes the transition to regular food.

Pre-packaged Meals

Another important development in the treatment of obesity is the tremendous expansion of commercial weight loss programs that provide the client with prepackaged meals in combination with varying degrees of nutrition education, exercise, and behavior modification. As with VLCD's, these programs offer the advantage of "removing the patient from the food environment," by limiting the patient's choices in regards to shopping, meal planning, food preparation and at meal time. As with VLCD's, these programs may be helpful to some patients who need considerable structure to initiate weight loss. Unfortunately, these programs also have difficulty at maintaining weight loss when the patient again makes the transition to regular foods. Because these diets contain >800 kcals per day intensive medical monitoring is not necessary during dieting.

Effects of Weight Loss on Morbidity and Mortality

Surprisingly, few studies have examined the effects of weight loss on morbidity and mortality. Studies examining the effect of weight loss on cardiovascular risk factors generally show beneficial changes with weight loss as predicted. Descriptive studies on mortality, however, show inconsistent results. Some studies show reduction in mortality in the obese (Wannamethee, 1990; Lean,1990) and some show increased mortality (Garrison, 1985; Pamuk, 1993; Wilcosky, 1990). Such descriptive studies are unable to clarify whether changes in mortality is caused by the weight change, whether disease or other factors which contribute to disease such as cigarettes causes weight loss, or whether both are related to a third factor. No randomized trials of long-term effects of voluntary weight loss on mortality have been published.

Effects of Weight Fluctuations

Since so many Americans are dieting at any one time, and having so little long-term success, considerable interest has been focused on the potential adverse effects of weight cycling ("yo-yo dieting"). At least 9 potential adverse effects of weight cycling have been hypothesized, primarily from animal studies. These include making further weight loss more difficult, increasing total body fat and central obesity, increasing subsequent calorie intake, increasing food efficiency, decreasing energy expenditure, increasing levels of adipose-tissue lipolytic enzymes and liver lipogenic enzymes, increasing insulin resistance, increasing blood pressure, and increasing blood cholesterol and triglyceride levels. Most experts currently feel that these phenomena occur inconsistently, if at all.

More recently, seven descriptive studies have attempted to address this question by looking at the impact of weight fluctuations on CHD incidence, CHD mortality and total mortality. Five demonstrated an effect on at least one of these endpoints, while two others did not thus suggesting a link between weight variability and disease outcomes. It should be noted, however, that these studies were not designed to assess the contribution of dieting (and voluntary weight loss) to weight fluctuation. Other factors that influence weight were also not considered.

Thus, at the present time, it remains uncertain if dieting-induced voluntary weight fluctuations have a negative health impact in humans. This remains an important question, however, and reinforces the idea that casual attempts at quick weight loss should be avoided. At the present time, however, committed attempts at long-term weight loss should not be discouraged because of the potential of regaining weight.

Metabolic rate

As every dieter has observed, the rate of weight loss slows during the course of dieting. Because this can be quite discouraging to the unwary patient (or uninformed physician), it is important to inform the patient prior to initiating a weight loss diet that this is likely to occur. Weight loss is most rapid during the initial days of hypocaloric feeding due to changes in sodium and water balance. This is due to early loss of glycogen and protein (both contain water) and, depending on the degree of calorie deficit and type of diet, to sodium losses associated with ketonuria. Following this initial phase, weight loss will depend on the extent of energy deficit. With time, however, the rate of weight loss slows again as the body's metabolic rate decreases and the energy deficit becomes smaller. This change in metabolic rate can be 2-3 times greater than that predicted from changes in body weight. The lower the energy content of the diet, the lower the metabolic rate will be. Although it was initially suggested that exercise occurring during a period of hypocaloric feeding could prevent this decrease in metabolic rate, recent studies have suggested that it has no beneficial effect during hypocaloric feeding (but will increase the post-diet metabolic rate by preserving lean body mass).

Following the period of hypocaloric feeding (resumption of normal energy intakes), the metabolic rate will increase, but to a level below that observed before beginning the diet. In this instance, the extent of decrease is appropriate for the amount of weight lost. Nonetheless, an individual who has successfully lost weight will have a significantly reduced total energy expenditure as compared to before weight loss. This is not only due to reductions in metabolic rate, but also reduction from the thermic effect of food (the individual eats less), and in differences in physical activity (it takes less energy to perform the same amount of activity for a smaller person). Thus, in order to maintain weight loss, individuals need to consume less energy than before dieting (and increase energy expenditure by increasing the amount of physical activity).

Exercise

Aerobic exercise offers a number of significant advantages to patients attempting to achieve long-term weight loss. First and foremost, exercise increases energy expenditure, helping to create the energy deficit necessary for weight loss. Unfortunately, the amount of energy expended during most aerobic exercises (walking, jogging, swimming, etc.) for the typical periods of time performed (20-30 minutes 4-5 times per week) is modest, approximately 500-1000 kcals per week. Thus, exercise can be predicted to have little effect on short-term weight loss. Clinical trials reflect this modest effect: some studies demonstrate weight loss with exercise alone or extra weight loss when exercise plus diet is compared to diet alone, but some studies do not.

The importance of exercise for successful maintenance of weight loss is more clearly established. In addition to the cumulative effect of increased energy expenditure (500-1000 kcals/week x 52 weeks=7-15 pounds per year), exercise effects the composition of the body substance lost during weight loss. When exercise is directly compared to diet, or when exercise plus diet is compared to diet alone, exercise results in greater preservation of lean body mass. That is, for each pound of weight lost, less fat and more muscle is lost during weight loss programs without exercise. This is particularly important since the body's resting metabolic expenditure (a major portion of the total daily energy expenditure) is closely correlated with lean body mass.

The observation that much of the long-term impact of exercise is through preservation of lean body mass has resulted in an increased interest in the potential role of resistance training (weight lifting, circuit training, etc.). Preliminary results suggest that resistance training during dieting does result in maintenance of lean body mass compared to dieting alone. Thus, highly motivated patients can be instructed to add resistance training to their aerobic exercise program.

Regular aerobic exercise results in a number of other benefits to the obese patient including improved cardiovascular training effect (increased exercise tolerance), decreased appetite (per calorie expended), a general sense of well-being, decreased blood pressure (in hypertensives), improved glucose metabolism and insulin action (in diabetics), improved blood lipids (in lipid disorders) and, in the long-term, decreased cardiovascular and all-cause mortality.

Young patients with mild to moderate obesity can be started directly on a regular aerobic exercise program. Patients are commonly instructed to select two exercises and to perform either one of them 4-5 times per week for 20-25 minutes per day. Patients are taught to take their pulse and to generate a sustained tachycardia at 50-70% of their maximum predicted heart rate. Older patients and patients with severe obesity are instructed to begin walking programs without initial concern about meeting target heart rates. As weight loss proceeds, and patients become used to exercising regularly, patients can be advanced to formal aerobic programs.

Although many authorities recommend formal exercise stress testing prior to prescribing an exercise program for all patients, our practice has been to reserve testing for sedentary men over 40 and women over 50; for patients with known or suspected coronary artery disease; and for patients with two additional cardiovascular disease risk factors (in addition to obesity and sedentary lifestyle). Patients on VLCD's should be prescribed exercise programs in the same manner as patients on standard weight loss programs.

Behavior Modification and Social Support

Sustained weight loss requires long term changes in eating behavior. Patients must learn specific skills to facilitate decreased calorie intake and increased energy expenditure. Although formal behavior modification programs are available most patients can be taught basic behavioral strategies in the office.

The single most useful behavioral skill is planning and record keeping. Patients can be taught to plan both menus and exercise programs in advance. Patients are then instructed to record actual dietary and exercise behaviors. While the act of record keeping itself will aid in behavioral change, the availability of records will also help the health care provider assess progress and make specific suggestions for additional problem solving. Specific reward systems are also useful for many patients. Refundable financial contracts have been shown to be effective in a number of small studies.

Social support is an additional essential component for any successful weight loss program. Most successful programs use peer group support. Involvement of family members is also particularly important. A comprehensive review of published results of weight loss programs strongly suggests that close provider-patient contact is a better predictor of success than the particular weight loss intervention.

APPENDIX I. TECHNICAL JARGON

Medications for treatment of obesity

Medications for the treatment of obesity are widely available both over the counter and with prescription. Medications include amphetamines (with high abuse potential-DEA Schedule II); non-amphetamine schedule IV appetite suppressants fenfluramine (Pondimin), phentermine (Ionamin), diethylproprion (Tenuate, Tepanil), mazindol (Sanorex, Mazanor) and pemoline (Cylert); the over-the-counter medication, phenylpropanolamine; and the antidepressants fluoxitene (Prozac) and sertraline (Zoloft).

Considerable controversy exists as to the safety and efficacy of these agents and specific indications for their use. Numerous barriers to the use of medications for obesity have been recently described by advocates for their use. These include public perception of obesity as a disease of lack of willpower, expectation that medications should "cure" obesity, hindrance by state licensing agencies, limited research on long term efficacy, and the abuse potential of some of the medications. Numerous short term studies of appetite-suppressant drugs (ASD's) have been conducted. A recent meta-analysis of 36 studies using mazindol and fenfluramine showed that a median duration of 12 weeks use resulted in a mean weight loss 3 kg greater than placebo. However, in those studies with follow-up, discontinuation of the drugs most commonly resulted in rebound weight gain.

Even more ominous was the 1997 Mayo Clinic report on the association of the use of "fen-phen" with heart valve disease. Fen-phen refers to a weight loss product containing fenfluramine and phentermine, which became popular in the early 1990's. Both had been approved by the FDA as short-term appetite suppressants. However, when used in combination it was found that up to 30% of patients may develop a leaky condition of the aortic valve, one of the four major valves in the heart. The product has since been withdrawn from the market.

Surgery

Although generally considered to be the last resort for the treatment of obesity, over 100,000 obese patients have had surgical therapy. Few controlled trials exist, and the development of rational indications for surgery has been difficult.

Gastric operations are now the procedures of choice. Most popular are the vertical-banded (Mason) gastroplasty in which a smaller stomach pouch is created, and gastric bypass procedures. Although both procedures result in significant weight loss, randomized trials comparing the two procedures tend to favor gastric bypass procedures. This is particularly true in patients who consume large amount of sweets. Perioperative mortality averages <1%, but ranges between 0-4% in different centers. Complications are common and include wound dehiscence, peritonitis, nausea and vomiting, vitamin deficiencies, and hair loss. When all necessary reversals, revisions, and patients lost to follow-up are considered, failure rates approach 50%.

Jejunoileal bypass was the first major surgical procedure popularized for the treatment of obesity. Although weight loss was effectively produced and maintained (average 100 pounds in 5 years), diarrhea and fluid and electrolyte disorders occurred chronically in over half of patients. One-third of patients develop progressive liver disease. This procedure has been abandoned. Two newer bypass operations under investigation are a biliointestinal operation and a biliopancreatic operation. Jaw wiring is another commonly used, but not recommended, surgical treatment. Initial weight loss is similar to gastric procedures on average but data on weight maintenance is quite variable. Suction lipectomy, or liposuction, is a surgical procedure permitting the removal of fat from specific areas of the body. Usually performed by plastic surgeons, 5 pounds of fat can be removed with each procedure in an attempt to reshape thighs and waists resistant to more traditional weight loss and exercise treatments. No advantageous metabolic changes are induced by the procedure.

Summary

No magic bullet exists for the very difficult, but medically important, task of weight loss. Although many of the most common problems encountered in medical practice can be treated by weight loss alone, only motivated patients should be started on weight loss programs. Weight loss treatments vary considerably in terms of risk, cost, and efficacy. For most patients with mild or moderate obesity, a multifactorial approach including diet, exercise, behavior modification and social support can be prescribed. Close patient-provider contact and long-term follow-up with emphasis on exercise are key ingredients for success. Motivated patients with severe obesity should be considered for supervised VLCD's, again emphasizing long-term dietary change, exercise, behavior modification and social support.

Selected References

Andres R. Muller DC, Sorkin JD. Long term effects of change in body weight on all-cause mortality: A review. Ann Int Med 1993:119:737-743

Alford, B.B., Blankenship A.C., and Hagen R.D. "The effects of variations in carbohydrate, protein, and fat content of the diet upon weight loss, blood values, and nutrient intake of adult obese women." J Am Diet Assoc. 1990; 50:534-40.

Aswal, BS, Bhakuni, DS, Goel, AK, Kar, K, Mehrotra, BN, abd Mukerjee, KC, Screening of Indian plants for biological activity, Ind J Exp Biol., 22,312,1984.

Ballor, D. L., Katch V.L., Becque M.D., and Marks C.R. "Resistance weight training during caloric restriction enhances lean body weight maintenance."

Am J Clin Nutr 1988; 47:19-25.

Bhakuni, DS, Dhar, ML, Dhar, MN, Dhawan, BN, and Mehrotra, BN, Screening of Indian plants for biological activity, II, Ind J Exp Biol., 7,250,1969.

Blair SN, Shaten J, Brownell KD, et al. Body weight change, all-cause mortality and cause-specific mortality in the Multiple Risk Factor Intervention Trial. Ann of Int Med 1993; 119: 749-757

Bouchard, C. Is weight fluctuation a risk factor? N Engl J Med 1991; 324: 1887-9

Bouchard, C., Tremblay, A., Despres J. et al. The response of long-term overfeeding in identical twins. N Engl J Med 1990; 322: 1477-82

Bray, G.A. Pathophysiology of obesity Am J Clin Nutr 1992; 55: 488S-494S

Bray, GA. Barriers to the Treatment of Obesity. Ann Int Med 1991; 115:152-3

Brownell KD and Rodin J. The dieting maelstrom: Is it possible and advisable to lose weight? Am Psychologist 1994; 49:781-791

Charaka Samhita, Jamnagar, 1949

Consensus Development Conference Panel. Gastrointestinal surgery for severe obesity: Consensus Development Conference Statement. Ann Int Med 1991; 115:956-61

Danford, D. and Fletcher, S.W. Methods for voluntary weight loss and control: National Institutes of Health Technology Assessment Conference. Ann Int Med 1993; 119: 641-770

Foster GD at al. A controlled comparison of three very-low-calorie diets: Effects on weight, body composition, and symptoms. Am J Clin Nutr 1992; 55:811

Frank, A. Futility and avoidance: Medical professionals in the treatment of obesity. JAMA 1993; 269:2132-2133

Gupta, LP, Sen, SP, and Udapa, KN, Pharmacognostical and pharmacological studies on *Terminalia arjuna*, J Res Ind Med Yoga Homeop., 11,4, 1976.

Gupta SS, Seth, CB, Experimental studies on pituitary diabetes, Ind J Med Res., 50, 708, 1962.

Gupta, SS, et al., Effect of gurmar and shilajit on body weight of young rats, Ind J Physiol. Pharm., 9, 87, 1965.

Guru, LV, Mishra DN, Effect of alcoholic and aqueous extractives of Embelia ribes in patients infested by ascarides. J Res Ind Med, 1, 47, 1966.

Jeffery RW, Wing RR, French SA. Weight cycling and cardiovascular risk factors in obese men and women. Am J Clin Nutr 1992; 55: 641-644.

Kholkute, SD et al, Ind J Exp Biol, 16:1035, 1978

Lee IM, Paffenberger RS. Change in body weight and longevity. JAMA 1992;268:2045

Lee IM, Manson JE, Hennekens CH, Paffenber RS. Body weight and mortality: A 27-year follow-up of middle-aged men. JAMA 1993; 270:2823-2828

Levy AS, Heaton AW. Weight control practices of US adults trying to lose weight. Ann Int Med 1993; 119: 661-666.

Appendix I. Technical Jargon

Lissner L, Odell PM, D'Agostino RB, et al. Variability of body weight and health outcomes in the Framingham population NEJM 1991; 324:1839-1844.

Manson JE, Colditz GA, Stampfer MJ, Willett WC, et al. A prospective study of obesity and risk of coronary heart disease in women. NEJM 1990; 322:882-889

Menon, MK and Kar, A., Planta Medica, 19, 333, 1971.

Mukherji, M., and Vaidya, AB, Abstr., Indian Pharm. Soc. Annual Conf., Srinagar, 1986.

Pandey, VN and Chaturvedi, GN, J. Res. Ind. Med., 3:25, 1963.

Pandey, VN, Ph.D. Thesis, Clinical studies on certain lever diseases with special reference to

the indigenous drug kutaki (*Picrorhiza kurroa*) in the treatment of jaundice, Banaras Hindu University, Varanasi, 1966.

Rajaram, D., Preliminary clinical trial of P. Kurroa on bronchial asthma, Bombay Hosp. Journ., 18(2),14-66, 1976.

Rathinam, K, et al, J Res Ind Med, Yoga, Homeo. 11:4, 1976.

Singh, RH, Udupa, KN, Studies on the Indian indigenous drug punarnava. Experimental and pharmacological studies, *J. Res. Indian Med.,* 7, 28, 1972.

Singh, N., et. al., Planta Med.,45(2):102, 1982.

Singh, N., et. al., Ind J Pharm., 11(1):33, 1979.

Stahl KA, Imperiale TF. An overview of the efficacy and safety of fenfluramine and mazindol in the treatment of obesity. Arch Fam Med 1993; 2:1033-37

Stamler, J. Epidemic Obesity in the United States. Arch Int Med 1993;153:1040-43

Stunkard, A.J., Harris J.R., Pedersen N.L., and McClearn G.E. "The body mass index of twins who have been reared apart" NEJM 1990;322:1483-87.

Tewari, NS, and Jain, PC, A clinical evaluation of Arogyavardhini as a hypocholesterolemic agent , J. Res. Ayur. Siddha, 1(1), 121, 1980.

Wadden, TA, Foster GD, Letizia KA, and Mullen JL. "Long-term effects of dieting on resting metabolic rate in obese outpatients." JAMA 1990;264:707-11.

Wilber JF. Neuropeptides, appetite regulation and human obesity. JAMA 1991;266:257

Wilson GT. Relationship of dieting and voluntary weight loss to psychological functioning and binge eating. Ann Int Med 1993; 119: 727-730

Williamson, D.F. Madans J., Anda R.F. et al. Smoking Cessation and Severity of Weight Gain in a National Cohjort. N Engl J Med 1991;324:739-45

Yanowski SZ. Are anorectic agents the "magic bullet" for obesity? Arch Fam Med 1993; 2:1025-26

Ayurvedic Herbal Medicines Useful In Weight Management

Latin: *Embelia ribes* Burm. f.   **Family: Myrsinaceae**

Vernacular names: *Sanskrit,* Vidanga; *Hindi,* Baberang,Viranga; *English,* Vidanga; *Unani,* Baubring; *Bengali,* Biranga; *Marathi,* Vavadinga; *Tamil,* Vivlangam; *German,* Embeila Fruchte; *Tibetan,* Bidan; *Nepalese,* Bayubidang.

Description: A shrub with cone-shaped eminences on the stems; leaves are alternate and ovoid to eliptic in shape, 5-7 cm long and 0.5 cm wide with wide glandular depressions on the undersurface. the flowers are numerous, white or yellow (sometimes greenish-yellow). The fruits are small, black, globose berries with a rough surface.

Distribution and Habitat: Found throughout India especially in low hillside areas stretching from the Himalayan foothills down through central India, the eastern and southern plateau regions and down into tamil Nadu and Sri Lanka. Also found throughout Southeast Asia.

Part Used: berries, leaves, root, bark

Ayurvedic Energetics: *Rasa:* pungent *Veerya:* heating
                Vipaka: pungent
                Guna: light, dry, sharp
                Doshas: VK- ; P+

Pharmacological actions: anthelminthic (tapeworms), carminative, laxative, alterative

Clinical Research: Both the alcoholic and aqueous extracts were found to be very effective against Ascaris lumbricoides. In addition, there are reports of antifertility effects of the petroleum, methanol, and fall in serum bilirubin levels in patients with infective hepatitis. Other

aqueous extracts of *Embelia ribes*. Anti-implantation effects were reported in albino rats and rabbits that were given 10 mg/kg embelin, the biologically active benzoquinone component of the plant.

Latin: *Picrorhiza kurroa* **Royal ex Benth** **Family: Scrophulariaceae**

Vernacular names: *Sanskrit*, Katuki; *Hindi*, Katki, Kutaki; *Unani*, Kutki; *Bengali*, Kuru; *Tamil*, Kadukurokani; *Punjabi*, Kali Kutki; *Persian*, Kharbaq Siyah; *Chinese*, Hu Huang Lin; *Japanese*, Kooren

Description: A perennial, woody herb with rhizomes that are cylindrical, - 2 cm. diameter, and grayish brown. Leaves are 4-10 cm in length and rounded, serrated, and spatulate. Flowers are dark violet and in spikes, braceate and lanceolate; fruits 1-2 cm.

Distribution and Habitat: Found only at higher altitudes of 8,000 to 12,000 ft. throughout the northwestern regions of the Himalayas

Part Used: rhizome

Ayurvedic Energetics: **Rasa:** bitter   **Veerya:** cooling
Vipaka: pungent
Gunas: light, dry
Doshas*: PK- ; V+*

Pharmacological actions: laxative, cathartic, cholagogic, anti-inflammatory

Clinical Research: Protective and therapeutic actions against hepatocellular damage have been demonstrated by several investigators using various models of liver damage in animals. Different preparations of the plant including the crude aqueous extract have been shown to protect the liver from damage due to alcohol, carbon tetrachloride, paracetamol, and galactosamine. Bile flow has been shown to increase in dogs. Mukherji and Vaidya reported an inhibition of CCl4 -induced lipid peroxidation of liver microsomes by the active glycoside fraction. Anti-inflammatory action and diminished mast cell degranulation have also been reported. *P. Kurroa* has been shown to promote a more rapid

investigators have found benefits of the plant in the management of asthma and hypercholesterolemia.

Traditional Uses: The root powder given with asafoetida, triphala, salt, and pepper is an effective treatment for chronic constipation; given with hot water and jaggery its laxative effect is mild. It is combined in equal amounts with the powdered roots of calamus and chitraka and triphala and taken with cow's urine to treat painful dyspepsia. It is also given with patola (*Trichosanthus dioica*) for the same indication. It is used commonly to treat fever, anemia, jaundice, scorpion sting, and heart disease.

Indications: viral hepatitis, bronchial asthma, dyspepsia, constipation

Dosage and Formulations: root powder : 0.5-1.0 g. three times a day
                                 decoction : 2-3 oz. three times a day
                                 root extract : 5-7 ml. three times a day
                                 Arogyavardini 500 mg three times a day

Latin: *Gymnema sylvestre* R.Br.   Family: Asclepiadaceae
     (syn. *Asclepias geminata* Roxb.)

Vernacular names: *Sanskrit,* Meshasringa; *Hindi,* Gurmar; *English,* Gurmar; *Unani,*Gokhru; *Bengali,* ChhotaDudhilata,*Tamil,* Siru-kurinjan

Description: A climbing shrub with leaves opposite, usually ovoid or elliptic, 3 to 5 cm. in length, hairy; flowers are yellow, small in umbels; lamina is ovate or ovate-lanceolate with pubescent surfaces.

Distribution and Habitat: Found throughout the Western Ghats, Goa, Western and Southern Plateau regions and in Central India.

Part Used: root, leaves

Ayurvedic Energetics: *Rasa:* astringent, pungent *Veerya:* heating
                             Vipaka: pungent
                             Guna: light, dry
                             Doshas: KV- ; P+

Pharmacological actions: diuretic, astringent, hypoglycemic, refrigerant, stomachic

Clinical Research: The leaf powder caused a clinically insignificant decrease in serum glucose in normal rats but a significant reduction in serum glucose in experimentally induced hyperglycemic animals. Body weight and urine output both increased in rats treated with the herb. Both of these effects may be due to stimulation of pancreatic insulin secretion. There is however currently no good evidence to show that *G. sylvestre* powder or extract has any effect on the serum or urine glucose concentrations of humans suffering from diabetes mellitus. no water-soluble or alcohol-soluble constituents that have glucose-destroying action in vitro have been isolated.

Research conducted at the University of Madras showed that water-soluble extracts of *G. sylvestre* increased the number of pancreatic beta cells in laboratory animals, which are responsible for insulin production. The extracts were at concentrations of 33:1. The dosage used, 20 mg extract per kg body weight per day, was equivalent to 40 grams of dried herb per day for the average 65 kilogram adult.

Traditional Uses: Diabetes mellitus, snakebites (root powder), fever, and cough. In Ayurveda, *G. sylvestre* is also used to treat somatic burning sensations, biliousness, hemorrhoids, and urinary disorders. When chewed the leaves have the remarkable property of abolishing the ability to taste sweet and bitter substances. It also has a mild laxative effect, probably due to its anthraquinone content that irritates the bowel walls (similar to Cassia angustifolia, rhubarb, or the aloes.)

Indications: type 2 diabetes mellitus as an adjunct to other treatments, snakebite.

Formulations and Dosage: leaf powder 2-4 g. three times a day
leaf decoction 2-4 oz. three times a day

Latin: *Boerhavia diffusa* Linn.   **Family: Nyctaginaceae**

Vernacular names: *Sanskrit,* Punarnava; *Hindi,* Biskhafra; *Bengali,* Gadhapurna; *English,* Spreading hogweed; *Unani,* Bishkhapra

Description: A diffuse herb with a stout, woody root and erect branches. The taproot is long and tapering. The leaves are opposite, glabrous, and thick 1 to 2 in. long. The flowers are hermaphrodite, oblong, and pedicellate; the fruit is detachable and the radicle long.

Distribution and Habitat: All over India usually in sandy soil and near dumping areas.

Part Used: whole plant, root

Ayurvedic Energetics: *Rasa:* sweet, bitter, astringent *Veerya:* heating
                                            Vipaka: sweet
                                            Doshas: V,P,K -

Pharmacological actions: laxative, diuretic, expectorant, purgative

Clinical Research: Singh and Udupa reported that the alcoholic extract of roots and leaves showed significant anti-inflammatory activity against carageenin-induced hind paw edema in rats. Both the aqueous extract and its isolated alkaloid, punarvarine, inhibited the increased serum aminotransferase activity in arthritic animals, similar to hydrocortisone; liver ATP phoshohydrolase activity was also increased. Punarnava is also known to have potent diuretic properties.

Traditional Uses: Decoction of the root is used as a laxative, expectorant, and a diuretic. It is used to treat asthma, bronchitis, edema, anasarca, and internal inflammations.

Indications: fluid retention, nephritic syndrome, asthma, constipation, as an antidote to snake venom.

Formulation and Dosage: decoction: 30 ml three times a day
                                                milk decoction: 30 ml. three times a day
                                                as powder with guggul (one gram each)
                                                twice daily

Latin: *Terminalia arjuna* Wight &Arn.   **Family: Combretaceae**

Vernacular names: *Sanskrit*, Arjuna, Dhavala, Raktarjuna; *Hindi*, Arjuna, Anjana, Khawa, Kahu; *English*, Arjuna myrobalan *Unani*, Arjun; *Marathi*, Shardul; *Gujarati*, Sajadan, Sadado; *Tamil*, Vellamarda, Marutham

Description: A large deciduous tree growing to 20 to 30 meters in height and a trunk circumference of 3 to 4 meters with spreading branches and white bark. Leaves subopposite, ovate, coriaceous, sometimes clustered terminally on twigs; flowers small green or yellowish-white in short axillary spikes, bracteoles minute; bark slightly curved, outer surface white and smooth, inner surface soft and reddish-brown.; fruit ovoid, 5-7 winged, smooth, size variable.

Distribution and Habitat: Found throughout India along rivers, streams, and in the hotter, drier regions as well; especially abundant in Kerala, Maharashtra, Madhya Pradesh, and in the south of India.

Part Used: bark

Ayurvedic Energetics: *Rasa*: astringent *Veerya:* cooling *Vipaka:* pungent
Gunas: light, drying
Doshas: KP- ; V+

Pharmacological actions : cardiac tonic, astringent, hypocholesterolemic, hypotensive, diuretic

Clinical Research: Arjuna is commonly utilized as a cardiac tonic and there appears to be at least some scientific support for this use. Gupta, et. al. demonstrated that the water-soluble fraction of the alcoholic extract of the bark increased the force of contraction of perfused frog heart. Intravenous administration of the aqueous extract of the bark decreased blood pressure and heart rate in dogs. This extract also has been shown to inhibit the carotid occlusion hypertensive response. Hypotension and bradycardia were also observed and thought to be of central origin, possibly vagally mediated. Further, a diuretic effect has been reported which is attributed to the triperpene saponin content of the bark. Udupa reported a series of studies, some as long as twenty years in duration in assessing the value of long-term administration of arjuna in the prevention of myocardial infarction. It was found that rabbits fed arjuna were more resistant to myocardial ischemia and the development of cardiac arrhythmias. Another study showed a decrease in total cholesterol, triglycerides, and an increase in HDL cholesterol in young rabbits given T. arjuna in their diets. Finally, *arjuna* has been reported to increase prothrombin times from 10.01 to 20.0 seconds (which is an anticoagulant effect) and to have a thrombocytopenic effect (platelet reducing) in rabbits. A small study involving six patients with hypercholesterolemia who were treated with *Terminalia arjuna* 1.5 grams bid showed a statistically significant decrease in total cholesterol, triglycerides, LDL cholesterol, and serum cholesterol/HDL cholesterol ratio. No effect was seen on serum HDL cholesterol levels.

Traditional Uses: Ayurvedic physicians use arjuna bark in the treatment of cardiac decompensation due to derangements of all three doshas, *vata*, *pitta*, and/or *kapha*. It is given especially where there is a component of edema. It also is used commonly in stable angina and non-bacterial pericarditis and endocarditis. It tends to lower the blood pressure in hypertensive individuals but to have no effect on normotensive patients. It is also used in diarrhea, dysentery, and sprue as well as in acne and other skin disorders. Arjuna has an unusually high content of calcium salts and not surprisingly it has been prescribed both internally and externally to help bones heal following fracture.

Indications: congestive heart failure, chronic stable angina, hyperlipidemia. It is not recommended that *Terminalia arjuna* be taken in place of modern cardiac medications, but rather as a tonic and adjunct to allopathic treatments.

Formulation and Dosage: bark powder : 1-3 g twice daily
arjunarista : 2-4 oz. twice daily
bark decoction : 2-4 oz. twice daily

Latin: *Plumbago zeylanica* Linn.   Family: Plumbaginaceae

Vernacular names: *Sanskrit,* Chitraka; *Hindi,* Chitra, Chiti; *English,* White leadwort, Ceylon leadwort; *Bengali,* Chita; *Tamil,* Kodiveli; *Gujarati,* Chitaro; *Punjabi,* Chitrak; *French,* Dentelaire de Ceylon; *German,* Ceylonische Bleiwurz

Description: A perennial, branching undershrub with long tuberous roots, yellow when fresh, brown when dried; leaves 7 to 8 x 3 to 4 cm. simple, alternate, short-petioled, ovate-oblong, with entire margins; flowers white in terminal spikes, bisexual, tubular; corolla tube slender, 5-lobed; fruit is a membranous capsule within the persistent calyx.

Distribution and Habitat: Grows wild throughout tropics and sub-tropical regions throughout India and commonly cultivated in gardens.

Part Used: roots

Ayurvedic Energetics: *Rasa:* pungent *Veerya:* heating *Vipaka:* pungent
    Gunas: dry, light, sharp
    Doshas: KV- ; P+

Pharmacological actions: alterative, digestive stimulant; it has a specific action (*prabhava*) on the uterus and is abortifacient; in large doses it is an arconarcotic poison.

Clinical Research: Most of the research on *P. zeylanica* has centered around its antifertility activity and the reports to date have been contradictory. Gupta, et. al. reported anti-implantation activity in the 50% alcoholic extract of the root and fruits. Premakumari et.al.. observed similar effects in addition to abortifacient effects as well. However, Bhakuni, et. al.. and Aswal, et. al. could not confirm these findings in later studies. Other studies showed antibacterial effects but not antifungal effects. Plumbagin oil (isolated from the related *Plumbago indica*) was found to be active against common warts.

Traditional Uses: The root powder mixed with sesame oil is used in an external application for arthritic joints and enlarged lymph nodes. It is also useful to treat hemorrhoids mixed with buttermilk. It is commonly used for treating skin diseases, sometimes taken with cow's urine. Other traditional indications include flatulence, edema, cough, dyspepsia, and vata and kapha diseases. It is useful as a digestive stimulant when mixed with equal amounts of amalaki, pippali, ginger powder, and rock salt and given in 500 mg doses with meals. For mental agitation and anxiety two parts each of Chitraka and Brahmi whole plant (Bacopa monniera) and one part each of Jyotishmati seeds (Celastrus paniculatus) and Vacha root (Acorus calamus) are ground into a powder and given 0.5 gram bid. The root paste is applied as a local irritant to the os uteri to induce abortion.

Indications: intestinal gas, hemorrhoids, skin diseases

Formulation and Dosage: root powder : 0.25-0.5 gr. twice daily

Index

A

Abhyanga Self-Massage, 77, 95
Activity level, determination, 136-7
Agni, 41, 44-48, 58-59, 293, 354
Allopathic Medicines For Weight Loss, 185-8
    Orlistat, 186-7
    phen-fen, 186
    Sibutramine, 187
Ama, 46, 59, 355
amylopectin, 109, 111, 115, 117
amylose, 109, 111, 115, 117
Aromatherapy,
    for Kapha types, 224
    for Pitta types, 253
    for Vata types, 275
Atharvaveda, 9
ATP, 171
Attention Exercise, 91-93
Ayurvedic Caloric Need, determination, 137-8
Ayurvedic Herbal Medicines
    allopathic medicines derived from, 12
Ayurvedic Herbology
    Ayurvedic pharmacodynamics, 181-2
Ayurvedic Herbs
    for Kapha types, 207
    for Pitta types, 241
    for Vata types, 270
    for weight loss, 175
    Sattva Basic Formulation, 207, 241, 271
Ayurvedic Medicine, 10, 181, 185
    degrees, 10
    eight sub-specialties, 10
Ayurvedic questionnaire, 31-5

BIOGRAPHICAL SKETCH

SCOTT GERSON, M.D.

Scott Gerson, M.D. is one of the country's leading authorities on complementary medical treatments and their integration with conventional modern medicine. His specialty is in Ayurvedic Medicine; however, he is well versed in virtually all modalities of alternative medicine. He received his medical degree from the Mount Sinai School of Medicine in New York City, where he helped to establish that institution's first course for medical students on alternative medical treatments. Currently, he lectures on alternative medicine at both Mount Sinai and Columbia Presbyterian College For Physicians and Surgeons. He served as a staff physician at the New York University Medical Center, Bellevue Hospital, and New York Downtown Hospital where he completed his residency training in Internal Medicine.

Dr. Gerson received his formal training in Ayurvedic Medicine at the Ayurvedic College in Trivandrum, India and is currently in the Ph.D. program at the prestigious Benaras Hindu University in Varanasi, India. He was awarded his Fellowship in Ayurveda from the Institute of Indian Medicine, in Poona. His other main affiliations in India are with the Central Council for Research in Ayurveda and Siddha Medicine in New Delhi and the International Federation of Ayurveda (vice-president) in Poona. He is the author of *Ayurveda: The Ancient Indian Healing Art* (Element Books, 1993*), Medicinal Plants of Ayurveda* (completed 1998, unpublished), in addition to numerous articles and papers on Ayurveda and holistic medicine. He founded *Ayurvedic Medicine of New York* in 1982, where he consults with private patients. He is currently president of *The National Institute of Ayurvedic Medicine*, the most respected source of accurate information on Ayurveda in the U.S. He also serves as the executive director of *The Foundation for Holistic Medical Research*, a non-profit organization that objectively evaluates complementary medical therapies for safety and efficacy. He also serves as editor-in-chief for *Alternative Medicine Practice*, a peer-reviewed journal for physicians. Finally, he is the co-host of *Integrative Healing,* his very popular live call-in radio show which airs throughout the New York metropolitan area.

Dr. Gerson lives with his wife and two dogs in Brewster, New York where he often gathers locally growing medicinal plants for his patients throughout the year. He is a great believer in the healing power of humor, which he satisfies by maintaining his membership in the American Medical Association and by coaching Little League.

Herbs and other natural health products and information are often available at natural food stores or metaphysical bookstores. If you cannot find what you need locally, you can contact one of the following sources of supply.

Sources of Supply:

The following companies have an extensive selection of useful products and a long track-record of fulfillment. They have natural body care, aromatherapy, flower essences, crystals and tumbled stones, homeopathy, herbal products, vitamins and supplements, videos, books, audio tapes, candles, incense and bulk herbs, teas, massage tools and products and numerous alternative health items across a wide range of categories.

WHOLESALE:

Wholesale suppliers sell to stores and practitioners, not to individual consumers buying for their own personal use. Individual consumers should contact the RETAIL supplier listed below. Wholesale accounts should contact with business name, resale number or practitioner license in order to obtain a wholesale catalog and set up an account.

Lotus Light Enterprises, Inc.

PO Box 1008 WL
Silver Lake, WI 53170 USA
262 889 8501 (phone)
262 889 8591 (fax)
800 548 3824 (toll free order line)

RETAIL:

Retail suppliers provide products by mail order direct to consumers for their personal use. Stores or practitioners should contact the wholesale supplier listed above.

Internatural

PO Box 489 WL
Twin Lakes, WI 53181 USA
800 643 4221 (toll free order line)
262 889 8581 office phone
EMAIL: internatural@lotuspress.com
WEB SITE: www.internatural.com

Web site includes an extensive annotated catalog of more than 14,000 items that can be ordered "on line" for your convenience 24 hours a day, 7 days a week.